D0838545

Cancer, Culture, and Communication

Cancer, Culture, and Communication

Edited by

Rhonda J. Moore
National Institutes of Health
Bethesda, Maryland

and

David Spiegel
Stanford University School of Medicine
Stanford, California

Kluwer Academic/Plenum Publishers
New York   Boston   Dordrecht   London   Moscow

Library of Congress Cataloging-in-Publication Data

Cancer, culture, and communication / edited by Rhonda J. Moore, David Spiegel.
    p. cm.
Includes bibliographical references and index.
ISBN 0-306-47885-4
    1. Cancer—Social aspects. 2. Social medicine. 3. Culture. 4. Communication. I. Moore,
Rhonda J. II. Spiegel, David, 1945–

RC262.C285 2004
362.196'994—dc22

2003055933

ISBN 0-306-47885-4

© 2004 Kluwer Academic/Plenum Publishers
233 Spring Street, New York, New York 10013

http://www.wkap.nl/

10 9 8 7 6 5 4 3 2 1

A C.I.P. record for this book is available from the Library of Congress

Permissions for books published in Europe: permissions@wkap.nl
Permissions for books published in the United States of America: permissions@wkap.com

Printed in the United States of America

Contributors

Ludovico Balducci, MD is Chair of the interdisciplinary Oncology Program at the H. Lee Moffitt Cancer Center and Research Institute in Tampa, Florida. His research interests include cancer prevention, cancers in the life course, and the impact of culture and aging.

William Brietbart, MD is Chief of the Psychiatry Service at Memorial Sloan-Kettering Cancer Center. Dr. Brietbart's interests include pain in the terminally ill, quality of life, and spirituality and meaning after chronic illness.

Phyllis Butow, PhD is Associate Professor of Medical Psychology Unit at the University of Sydney, Australia. Dr. Butow's interests include psychological factors that affect people who have already developed cancer, quality of life, and cultural differences in clinician-patient communication in oncology.

Edzard Ernst, MD, PhD, FRCP (Edin.) is Professor of Complementary Medicine, the Institute of Health and Social Care Research, Peninsula Medical School, the Universities of Exeter and Plymouth. Dr. Ernst has written extensively on CAM, including the *Desktop Guide to Complementary and Alternative Medicine* (Mosby, 2001). His research interests also include evidence-based medicine, clinical trials, and toxicity in CAM therapies.

Edward J. Estlin, MD is Macmillan Consultant in Paediatric Oncology at Royal Manchester Children's Hospital in Manchester, England. His interests include clinical trials, pediatric oncology, QOL, and the development of novel therapies for children with drug-resistant tumors.

Christopher Gibson, PhD is on staff in the Department of Psychiatry at Memorial Sloan-Kettering Cancer Center, where he is coordinating several studies examining the efficacy of meaning-centered interventions for cancer patients. In addition, Dr. Gibson is an Assistant Professor of Psychology at John Jay College of Criminal Justice as well as a Senior Staff Psychologist at the Center for Cognitive Behavioral Psychotherapy. He has published in the areas of end-of-life issues, behavioral medicine, and anxiety disorders.

Carolyn Cook Gotay, PhD is Associate Professor of Cancer Research at the University of Hawaii. Her research interests include quality of life in culturally diverse patient populations.

Samuel Mun Yin Ho, PhD is Associate Professor in the Department of Psychology, the University of Hong Kong, and Honorary Associate Director, Centre on Behavioral Health, the University of Hong Kong.

Darlene Johnson (MBA) is Program Administrator for the Senior Adult and Radiation Oncology Programs at the H. Lee Moffitt Cancer and Research Institute in Tampa, Florida; she also holds a Research Associate Faculty Appointment at the University of South Florida. She is a Fellow of the American Academy of Medical Administrators and Editor-in-Chief of the *Journal of Oncology Management*. Her research interests include quality of life, patient satisfaction, outcomes in senior adult patients, and patients receiving radiation treatment for cancer.

Javier Kane, MD is Assistant Professor of Pediatrics at the University of Texas Health Science Center, Medical Staff Member, Cancer and Blood Disorders, Center Medical Director, Supportive and Palliative Care Program, Christus Santa Rosa Children's Hospital.

Patricia T. Kelly, PhD is Medical Geneticist at Saint Francis Memorial Hospital in San Francisco, California. Dr. Kelly's interests include clinical and medical genetics, bioethics, risk assessment, and the impact of these factors on clinician-patient communication in oncology.

Collen McClain is a doctoral candidate at Fordham University. Her dissertation project,which is funded by a National Service Award by the NIH, is investigating the importance of religioisity and spirituality on immune functioning in people with terminal cancer. During her time at Fordham working with the MSKCC research team, she has researched the importance of spirituality and religiosity on coping with illness and death.

Rhonda J. Moore, PhD is a cultural anthropologist and postdoctoral fellow in the Department of Epidemiology at The University of Texas M.D. Anderson Cancer Center in Houston, Texas. Dr. Moore's interests include cultural issues that impact oncology care, the impact of pain and suffering in advanced stage cancers, and social inequality in cancer care.

Joseph O'Donnell, MD is Professor of Medicine and Dean of the Medical School at Dartmouth School of Medicine. Dr. O'Donnell's interests include medical education, cancer pain, and quality of life.

Judith A. Paice, PhD, RN, FAAN is Research Professor of Medicine at Northwestern University. Dr. Paice's research interests include pharmacological management of pain, adverse effects of analgesic therapies, complementary techniques to relieve pain, and quality pain management and research.

Richard Penson, MD, MRCP is Assistant in Medicine and Director of Clinical Research in Medical Gynecologic Oncology at Massachusetts General Hospital and Instructor in Medicine, Harvard Medical School. His interests include gynecologic oncology, novel therapeutics, and psychosocial oncology.

Hayley Pessin, PhD is currently overseeing the study at the Memorial Sloan-Kettering Cancer Center assessing the influences on end-of-life attitudes among terminally ill cancer patients. Her research interests in the area of palliative care are focused on examining end-of-life despair, reasons for living and dying, the burden and benefit of research participation, the impact of cognitive impairment on desire for death, and developing psychotheraphy interventions that target the needs of terminally ill patients.

Nathalie Rapoport is a visiting scholar at the Psychosocial Treatment Laboratory, School of Medicine, Stanford University. After completing her medical studies and a master's degree in psychology in France, she graduated in medical psychology from Tel-Aviv University. She has more than ten years of clinical experience in France and Israel in the field of medical psychology and behavioral medicine. Her main interests are psychosocial interventions for the medically ill and doctor-patient interactions in chronic disease.

David Spiegel, MD is the Willson Professor and Associate Chair of Psychiatry and Behavioral Sciences and Director of the Center for Integrative Medicine at Stanford University School of Medicine. Dr. Spiegel is an internationally recognized expert on psychosocial issues in breast cancer patients. His other interests include trauma, hypnosis, dissociation, and complementary and alternative medicine in cancer patients.

Pierre Saltel, MD is Chief of the Psycho-Oncology Service, Comprehensive Cancer Center Leon-Berard, Lyon, France, and general secretary of the French Psycho-Oncology Society. His areas of interests include early detection of psychological distress in cancer patients, psycho-oncology networking, and the continuous training of professionals.

Ami Shah received her BA degree from Columbia University. After fourteen years teaching mathematics and computing at Saint Ann's Private School in Brooklyn, New York, she went on to pursue a career in medicine at the Mount Sinai School of Medicine in New York, where she is currently in her second year. As of this writing, she is considering the fields of psychiatry, pediatrics, and family medicine as possible future specialities.

Claire Stevinson, BSc, MSc is currently working toward a doctorate with the assistance of a Cancer Research UK scholarship. At the time she coauthored Chapter 10 with Edzard Ernst, she was a research fellow in the Department of Complimentary Medicine at the University of Exeter. Currently she is at the University of Bristol, Department of Exercise and Health Sciences, where she teaches and researches cancer rehablitation with a focus on physical activity.

John Weisburger, MD, PhD is Senior Member and Director Emeritus of the American Health Foundation in New York. Dr. Weisburger is an internationally known expert in the fields of cancer prevention and control, and dietary and nutritional factors related to cancer risk.

Foreword

As a young man from time to time I found myself sitting with my left leg upon a hassock, for no obvious reason. One day, however, it came to me that quite unconsciously I had been imitating the posture of my grandfather who in his later years had had a bad leg. Now that I am older, there is reason enough, for that leg was the site of a vein that some years back short-circuited a block in my coronary vessels. Actions like mine as well as habits or codes of behavior can be inherited without the intervention of DNA, so to speak, and so can attitudes – from Republicanism to abhorrence of spiders, or a distaste for fatty foods. In the very same way, I am convinced, many symptoms – digestive ones high on my list – are passed on from one generation to another not by the genetic code, but as appropriate- or at least customary-ways to respond to stress, embarrassment, or other situations, just like voting for the Democratic Party.

Heartburn, recently promoted to the status of a disease by gastroenterologists and pharmaceutical manufacturers as GERD (Gastroesophageal Reflux Disease), offers a pertinent example. That new designation has turned heartburn into a thing, reified as the philosophers say, changed from a symptom that once was a badge of industry to a disease that must be guarded against and tamed. An often harmless symptom that could be ignored has been made into an icon of disease that must be treated forever, no matter the evidence that about half the people who complain show no evidence of its organic/structural basis. More than likely it seems to me, if your father or mother had heartburn when aggravated (mine did not), you will learn that complaint as a family/familiar response, and the ability of your lower esophageal sphincter to guard against acid reflux may not really matter.

If the family matters, culture has an even broader influence in the genesis of symptoms and the response to disease or disability. Long ago, Walter Alvarez of the Mayo Clinic wisely observed that symptoms, like many other habits, were transmitted as a cultural/idiosyncratic reaction from one generation to the next That seems self-evident once you think about it; it may have been easier in the innocently more homogeneous early 20th century for physicians to understand and empathize with the emotional responses of people much like them. The change in American society over the past century, however, has turned the founding British culture into a cosmopolitan Americanism that is still refining itself. That is certainly true of the medical scene. In the 1920s at Yale Medical School, Dean Milton Winternitz, though an early pioneer in social medicine, sympathetic to the new science of psychoanalysis, and himself a Jew, continued the racial restrictions on admission: "Five Jews, 2 Italians, no Negroes." At Harvard Medical School even in the early 1940s, we students were all white men, largely because of the conviction that after medical school women would get married and so be lost to the active care of patients. The change in these two medical bastions by the 21st century reflects the diversity that now has so improved America. More than half the students at Yale and Harvard are women, there are many blacks, Asian-Americans abound, gays are welcomed as faculty and students, and one can go on and on. The elderly, the aged, alone face prejudice that remains unremitting because, it is argued, everyone ages.

To the happy intermingling of cultures under the American flag there has been added the contributions of science to medical practice. Science and technology have let physicians cure diseases that in the past killed so many, and have led doctors to believe that medicine has turned into a science, that rules are everything and that medical practice can be modular and "evidence-based" with guidelines. Every patient resembles another and diseases are deemed concrete entities to be dealt with by the "best evidence." Doctors sometimes forget that much more of their time outside a hospital setting is spent caring for patients who feel and suffer and fear, and for that intuition and emotion are needed. The right hand of fellowship, the close relationship of physician and patient, and, in this existential crisis of cancer, faith in caretaker or Creator, all help to relieve pain and suffering and to reduce anxiety. A myriad of writers remind us that we "health care" professionals treat diseases, but we care for people.

Let me explain those quotation marks in the preceding. Nurses and physicians and other caretakers have been denominated by that new category, but one can wonder whether we confer good health or more likely simply eliminate disease some of the time. Health may be a gift from the Creator. Here let me also observe how much I prefer the word "person" to "patient," for the stereotypical patient does not exist, any more than the much-abused "case." Both are jargon terms, useful as shorthand but threatening to lose the person in his or her disease.

Indeed, people with cancer risk losing their identity in the over-whelming portentousness of that diagnosis, a label that changes everything. To call someone a "recovered cancer patient" affixes a label which ignores the person. It's like the stamp of schizophrenia: one never shakes the adjective "schizophrenic" which arouses so much skepticism in caretakers . Once so labeled, a "cancer patient" – a doctor even cannot exchange that tag for a nicer one at "Lands' End." Physicians with cancer have complained that they are never again regarded as wholly healthy, always a suspicion that they may not be available in an emergency. Such opprobrium is rarely discussed, yet it adds to the burden of those who have survived cancer, the young woman with breast cancer far more than the elderly man with prostate cancer.

Such observations are not far from the idea which motivates this book, that culture plays a crucial role in the transactions of medicine, whether the doctor/patient relationship, the sick person's response to therapy, or the cultivation of valetudinarianism. Thanks to our postmodern diversity, women now are free to prefer female gynecologists, African-Americans justly choose a physician of their own background, and as a physician looking at 80, I like to think that I have special understanding of the problems and opinions of sick people over 65. The powerful drugs with which cancer can be assailed should not blind physicians to the importance of cultural background, and individual experience, in the care of people with cancer. That is the focus of this book that you are about to read. Empathy counts. And it helps.

"God writes straight with crooked lines," is the way Pope John 23 described the ebb and flow of customs and ideas. Over the past two centuries, mainstream medicine with its reliance on science and reason has gained sway, and rightly so because the nostrums of alternative ways could not challenge the very real cures of science. In the past few decades, however, even mainstream physicians have begun to confess that these triumphs conquer diseases but do not much relieve the disabilities and symptoms that come from sorrow, stress, or the daily events of life on earth. Our victories do not set straight passions gone awry. Antidepressants may cure sadness, but they do not relieve sorrow, nor is it likely that antioxidants can cure love. With newfound diversity has come the recognition that many people come to their practitioners for reassurance, the right hand of fellowship, advice and consolation from an experienced expert. They come for comfort and not always for cure.

It is sad that modern physicians have made so little use of their own powers of persuasion, the powers of comforting words to help their patients, the power of the placebo response in the patient–physician encounter. Here the editors and writers prefer the phrase "context effect" as a stand-in for placebo, but they have much to say, explicit and implicit, about the importance of the placebo-response in people with cancer. Placebos do help, and sometimes in controlled trials almost as much as the agent under study. As the authors realize, more than pills, placebos are procedures, diagnostic studies, the routines of diagnosis that provide certainty. But they are also words of comfort, rhetoric as well as potions and pills.

Pain is part of life, and does not always rattle along the C-fibers to yield to anodynes. Pain may come from the wounds of cancer, but it has many other wellsprings, and among them are bitterness, tribulation, and anger. Medical measuring and counting and the ever-growing attention to statistics and to evidence – based medicine, run the risk of failing to give enough attention to that phenomenon, to teach it to our students. They need to learn how much culture as well as heredity, the mindset as well as the molecular disposition, play in the management of the sick. Such matters and more are brilliantly discussed in this powerful book that emphasizes the humanity of our patients and strengthens us as physicians, nurses, and – yes – as "health-care" workers.

HOWARD SPIRO M.D.
Professor Emeritus, Yale School of Medicine
New Haven, Connecticut

Acknowledgments

The completion of a book is never an individual endeavor. Others always assist along the way. At this time we thank those individuals who were supportive of this edited volume. We begin by thanking our collaborators for their enthusiasm, commitment, and support of this project. We could not have completed this edited volume without your fine insight and the wisdom of your words. We thank Mariclaire Coutier, Mary Panarelli, Joe Zito, Herman Makler, and Bill Tucker of Kluwer Academic/Plenum Publishers. Their words of encouragement made this dream a reality.

As a postdoctoral fellow at the University of Texas M.D. Anderson Cancer Center, I (R.M.) could not have completed this edited volume without the support of a National Cancer Institute (NCI) Cancer Prevention fellowship, Grant # 3R25 CA5770-8S2. I gratefully acknowledge the support of Dr. Sonya Springfield, Belinda Locke, and Bobby Rosenfeld at the NCI. I am also indebted to the encouragement of my mentors Fadlo R. Khuri, MD, Professor of Hematology, Oncology, Medicine, Pharmacology, and Otolarygngology, Biomeyer Chair in Translational Cancer Research, Winship Cancer Institute, Emory University, and Robert M. Chamberlain, PhD, Deputy Chair, Epidemiology Department at the University of Texas M.D. Anderson Cancer Center (MDACC). I am especially grateful to Fadlo for allowing me access to enhance my clinical expertise in the department of Thoracic/Head and Neck Medical Oncology at MDACC. I also thank the many patients with cancer and their families who allowed me to share and learn more about their lives before cancer, their explanatory models of illness, death, survival, and victory. This volume is a promise kept and is dedicated to you all. I also thank Sherry Widdoes, Aretha Johnson, Roxanne Dolan, Wes Browning, and April Bennington from the Research Medical Library at the University of Texas MDACC in Houston, Texas, for their support for this endeavor. Last and certainly not least, I thank David Spiegel, MD, for his mentoring in the past as a postdoctoral fellow in the

Department of Psychiatry and Behavioral Sciences at Stanford Medical School, and now, which includes his commitment to this edited volume. I thank Howard Spiro, MD, for his sincerity and words of kindness. I also thank my mum, and my friends, including SKYY, Dorota A. Doherty, PhD (Perth, Australia), Gloria Valentine of the Hoover Institution (Stanford, CA), CKO Williams, MD (BC Cancer Center), C. Wilson, and Richard M. Hirshberg, MD (Houston, Texas) for their friendship and care all these years.

As coeditor of this book, I (D.S.) thank Rhonda Moore for her initiative, enthusiasm, and boundless energy in bringing this project to fruition. I also thank many colleagues around the world for finding a common ground of shared purpose in helping cancer patients and their families. I am indebted to many such patients and their families for their willingness to share their lives and deaths in the hopes of helping others navigate the same course more smoothly. The many dedicated faculty and staff associated with our Center on Stress and Health have worked long and hard to devise and evaluate better interventions for cancer patients and their families, and to understand mind/body interactions that link stress and support to health. Work on this book was made possible by generous research support from the National Institute of Mental Health (MH17280), (MH47226), (MH52134), (MH54930), (MH60556), (MH66366), with special support from the AIDS branch, the NCI (CA61309), the National Institute on Aging (AG18784), The California Breast Cancer Research Program (93-18851), (1 FB-0383), (1FB-0490), (6AB-1100), (7BB-2400), the Mind/Body Network of the John D. and Catherine T. MacArthur Foundation, the Charles A. Dana Foundation, the Nathan S. Cummings Foundation, the Fetzer Institute, and numerous private donors to the Stanford Center on Stress and Health.

RHONDA J. MOORE
DAVID SPIEGEL

Contents

Chapter 5
Children with Cancer: Cultural Differences in Communication
between the United States and the United Kingdom 109
Edward J. Estlin and Javier R. Kane

Chapter 6
Cancer Risk Assessment: Clinically Relevant Information is Key 127
Patricia T. Kelly

PART III: SYMPTOMS AND THEIR MANAGEMENT ACROSS CULTURES

Chapter 9
The Cultural Experience of Cancer Pain 187
Judith A. Paice and Joseph F. O'Donnell

Chapter 10
Complementary and Alternative Medicine in Patients with Cancer   221
Edzard Ernst and Clare Stevinson

Cancer, Culture, and Communication

CHAPTER 1

Introduction

Rhonda J. Moore and David Spiegel

The importance of the cultural context to health outcomes has only recently become a central concern and a part of the biomedical literature.[1-3] A medical encounter is an interpersonal interaction occurring in and influenced by one or more cultural contexts. Ideally, this communication is the seed from which the relationship between the clinician and patient develops. It begins when the patient comes to the clinician with a problem, the patient is diagnosed, the appropriate therapy is administered, the patient is treated, and the clinician has rendered a valuable service. The underlying cultural assumption is that the development of a common language facilitates an easy flow of medical care, serving to fortify the relationship between the clinician and the patient. In the West, the strong cultural assumption is that this biomedical dialogue of exchange is based on the presumption of the autonomy of the individual patient, presupposes that patient and clinician come from similar cultural worlds and, therefore, interpret life experiences through the matching cultural and cognitive frameworks. In an ideal world, the model works. However, the efficacy of this dialogue and, therefore, the effectiveness of the medical encounter, including the ability to communicate in increasingly diverse cultural and biomedical contexts, can be especially problematic in the field of oncology.[1-3]

Difficulties in clinician-patient communication have been increasingly observed in both Western and non-Western cultural contexts.[3-9] This is probably so because, despite clinical advances, cancer remains a life-threatening disease that is heavily invested with meaning. Cancer and its related symptoms have meant death, pain, shame, social isolation, and loss of meaning in life across the cultural divide.[3,5,10,11] It also challenges the prevailing Western biomedical assumption that all diseases are potentially curable, and that any patient's death is a failure rather than an inevitable part of human life. The crisis caused by the delivery of a diagnosis of cancer by the clinician, the arduous treatments, and, in advanced-stage disease, the repeated confrontations with recurrence, physical limitations, and treatment side effects contributes to this breakdown in language. Age, socioeconomic status (SES), nationality, ethnicity, and sex differences also mediate the cultural context of care, which can also adversely impact oncology care outcomes, particularly in minority, elderly, female, and other underserved individuals.[12-17] These populations all continue to suffer disproportionately from decreased survival rates from cancer, and substandard treatments for related symptoms such as pain and suffering in the global context of Western oncology care.[18-29] This suffering, as Cassell[30] has observed, is related to the severity of the affliction. An affliction, measured in the patient's terms, expressed in the distress they are experiencing, their assessment of the seriousness or threat of their problem, and how impaired they feel themselves to be.[30,31] The life narratives of patients with advanced cancers perhaps best highlight this experience. Here, the limits of modern medical technologies to both extend and enhance the quality of the patient's life can also contribute to a breakdown in language, as clinicians attempt to find the words to rationally communicate some of the dire consequences of cancer to the patient and their own limitations.

Throughout the history of medicine, clinicians have long understood that placebo effects are relevant to both the therapeutic context and to clinician-patient communication.[32-37] Yet, our ability to directly harness such effects for maximum therapeutic benefit has not been resolved, even though such effects have been shown to improve subjective and objective measures of disease in up to at least 40% of patients with a wide range of clinical conditions and cultural contexts.[34,38-42]

Clinician-patient communication does not operate outside the context of culture. Yet, the actual significance of cultural differences—its influence on the beliefs, expectations, and experiences of clinicians, significant others, and patients with cancer—in the therapeutic encounter has only recently begun to be evaluated.[3-6,38,43-46] The goal of this multidisciplinary edited volume is to draw on the expertise of clinicians, anthropologists, geneticists, psychologists, and supportive care professionals to create a cross-disciplinary dialogue. This text offers a description of the relevance of culture as a context effect that influences clinician-patient communication in the Western context of oncology care. We maintain that the impact of these context effects is bidirectional: They may be positive and beneficial, or negative and adverse.[32-34,45,47-50] Finally, because context effects are intertwined with placebo effects, we use these terms interchangeably in the text, thereby situating our discussion in light of this vibrant ongoing debate.[32,34,39,45,48-54] In this manner, we hope to add to an ongoing discussion, while, at the same time, beginning to address some of the major concerns in the field of clinician-patient communication in oncology.

Given the need to understand and characterize the underlying mechanisms of the context effect and the desire to harness such effects to maximize therapeutic benefit, scholars from a variety of fields have come together to discuss these possibilities.[33,55,56] As a consequence of these and other analyses, the reputation of the placebo effect is undergoing considerable reinterpretation.[33,40,42,53,55] This includes the expansion of the definition to encompass not only context effects but also to ascribe more positive connotations, in terms of healing properties.[33] Ongoing discussions in oncology trials highlight this, showing that while tumor responses are rare following treatment with placebo and have not historically been associated with extended survival, placebo effects remain common in oncology and they could potentially explain many of the effects attributed to active agents (specific effects).[38] Other evidence provided by analyses of the placebo arms of trials have also noted statistically significant improvements in qualitative traits, including appetite, weight gain, pain, anxiety and depression, performance status, and other dimensions of quality of life in cancer patients.[38]

Administration of placebo is not absence of treatment, just an absence of active medication, and patient and clinician beliefs and expectations have been shown to influence outcomes of both placebo and active treatment in life and in clinical settings.[33,42] Indeed, as Hahn and Kleinman[57] assert, what is especially needed is an understanding of the underlying cultural framework. The breadth of such an understanding could incorporate the neglected systems of beliefs and expectations of patients and clinicians, their meanings, the systems of socialization by which these are incorporated, and the social cultural situations in which they are called forth.[57] Insight into the underlying cultural framework would certainly aid in understanding the who, what, when, where, and how of the context effect since certain medical conditions are more susceptible to context effects. These include afflictions that have a strong psychological component that lack identifiable physiologic correlates, chronic conditions with a fluctuating course often influenced by selective attention, and affective disorders such as fatigue, arthritis, headache, allergies, heart disease including hypertension, sleep disorders like insomnia, asthma, chronic digestive disorders (eg, duodenal ulcer), pain, anxiety, depression, and Parkinson disease.[37,42,45,58-63]

There have been numerous attempts to differentiate the underlying mechanisms of the context effect. However, transducing the actual mechanisms whereby context effects convert meaning into modifications of physiological responses is only beginning to be characterized.[56,64] Three components, however, are necessary: (1) positive beliefs and expectations on the part of the patient; (2) positive beliefs and expectations on the part of the physician or health care professional; and (3) a good relationship between both parties.[34,38,47-49,51,56,64] Belief, operant conditioning, and suggestibility are also all thought to play important roles in the placebo effect. Indeed, two alternative theories have traditionally been proposed in the attempt to understand the underlying mechanisms: expectation and conditioning.[33,56,64,65] Context effects, as we have previously stated, are not always positive. The term *nocebo* from the Latin *nocere* meaning *to harm*, was initially coined to distinguish it from the generally positive effects of the placebo.[45,47,48,66].

Finally, and perhaps most significant, both the cultural and biomedical contexts in which these symptoms are experienced remain central to understanding the import of the context effect. It is now well known that different beliefs and expectations produce different effects on bodily function. Clinical analgesia, for instance, is dependent not only on the physiological action of the treatment but also on the expectations of the clinician and the patient.

To summarize, we propose that clinician-patient communication in oncology does not operate outside of the context of culture. We also suggest that beliefs and expectations can hurt or heal. From our daily encounters with patients, to correspondences with friends and colleagues around the world, to our cultural experience and practice of oncology care, we began to understand the relevance of culture and cultural differences as context effects that impact oncology care. In the often otherworldly and disembodied space that is often part of cancer care, we know that more effective communication skills that take advantage of context effects for therapeutic benefit are necessary to enhance oncology care. Therefore, the origins of this book began with a need to do our best to care for the patients we serve across cultural, linguistic, national, and ethnic lines. This book is an attempt to address some of these concerns. We also believe that the information provided here can begin to provide the reader with a sense of the issues that face the field of clinician-patient communication in oncology.

No text answers all questions, and this book is certainly no exception. The contributors share personal insights as well as present empirical data that have formed the basis of their understandings of how to effectively tailor care to deal with the cultural differences which impact clinician-patient communication. For these reasons, varied personal styles of discussion reflect the preference of each contributor as well as the particular aspect or ranges of the subject area they chose to write on. Also, several who were invited to contribute could not do so. Thus, for these reasons, certain regions of the world are perhaps not adequately represented, while others may appear to be overrepresented. The reader is asked to understand these limitations with the knowledge that future volumes that will perhaps address their concerns on this subject may be forthcoming.

The book is organized as follows: in Chapter 2, the broad goal of Moore and Butow is to provide a review of the literature regarding culture as a context effect that impacts clinician-patient communication, primarily in the Western context. In the first section, they explore the importance of culture as a context effect that shapes the environment in which individual and social experiences and responses to health, illness, and disease occur. The relevance of context is also apparent in barriers to effective care, including race, gender, and SES. This section also discusses the relevance of migration and translation issues that impact the effective unification of care to patients across cultural, national, and linguistic boundaries, and also briefly discusses the role of the family as cultural mediators of clinician-patient communication and oncology care. The third section briefly describes the various methodologies that have been used in the attempt to understand these cultural differences in the clinical context. The fourth and final section discusses what we have learned and then provides some guidelines of what might be done to better incorporate cultural considerations in clinician-patient communication in oncology. Finally, they provide a list of helpful websites, selected readings, and resources. In Chapter 3, Gotay defines the meaning of quality of life, and goes on to review the literature on how to effectively assess quality of life in culturally diverse cancer patients. In Chapter 4, Balducci, Johnson, and Beghe review the literature on cancers in children with a particular emphasis on peadiatric cancers in the United Kingdom and in the United States. In Chapter 5, Estlin and Kane attempt to establish a conceptual frame of reference in which different experiences of aging may be accommodated by exploring the following questions: What questions are unique to aging in the prevention and management of cancer? Are there aspects of aging that are unique and common to the whole aging population? And, finally, do different cultures react to aging in different ways?

Studies have shown that Americans misunderstand their risk for cancer, overemphasizing hereditary factors at the expense of risk factors like age. In Chapter 6, Kelly, using breast cancer as a model, highlights certain problems in communicating risk about cancer to patients. The first part of the chapter defines what "risk" for cancer actually means, and how to adequately communicate cumulative risk for cancer, including individual risk over time to patients. The second part includes discussion of the individual's relative risk for disease, hereditary risk for cancer, clinical relevance of statistical significance, the emotional toll of being a high-risk person, and barriers to effective communication about risk. The third part draws on the expertise of the medical geneticist, from working with high-risk patients, in terms of how to appropriately address and correct certain misperceptions, including those that affect the management of distress of patients and family members. Chapter 7, Weisburger explores the relationship between lifestyle and cancer prevention strategies. Using the techniques of geographic pathology, be provides a detailed review regarding the import of lifestyle factors, including diet as a cause of many types of diverse cancers. Chapter 8 details psychosocial aspects of care, including, have been linked to enhanced quality and increased survival time in cancer patients. In this chapter, Ho, Saltel, Machavoine, Rapoport, and Spiegel evaluate cultural approaches to communicating cancer fear, anxiety, depression, and existential pain and distress. The effectiveness of a supportive/expressive model of helping cancer patients cope with their illness developed in the United States is examined through experience of its application in two different cultures—China and France—as a means of illustrating principles of support that apply across cultures, and those that need to be tailored to specific cultural differences. Finally, this chapter offers suggestions on how clinicians can enhance their practice. Chapter 9 considers that Ethnic, racial, and gender differences have also been observed in the medical assessment and treatment of patients with cancer pain. Paice and O'Donnell provide a broad overview of the cultural and biomedical context in terms of the organization of health care systems in the United States and the United Kingdom. They then explore the prevalence of cancer pain, including cancer pain in minorities, barriers to cancer pain management, and cancer pain syndromes. They detail the measurement, assessment, and communication regarding cancer pain, treatment of cancer pain including pharmacogenetics, cancer therapies and other treatment options, and nonpharmacologic therapies. They then summarize their findings and also offer some useful websites and resources for learning more about cancer pain. There has been a great deal of debate regarding the efficacy of complementary medicine and its effectiveness in extending and enhancing the quality of life of patients. Most recently there has been some concern regarding toxicity related to treatments. In Chapter 10, Ernst first defines what is meant by complementary and alternative medicine (CAM), and then provides a brief overview of those factors that inform this debate in the Western biomedical context. Using data from randomized controlled clinical trials, he then evaluates toxicity issues in CAM treatments of patients with cancer. Finally, he suggests how better communication among the clinician, the patient, and the biomedical team can prevent adverse health outcomes. In Chapter 11, Penson examines cultural issues related to bereavement and the family in oncology. He first explores cultural approaches to understanding bereavement and family care, including carer quality of life, caregiver support, and collusion as these factors impact clinician-patient communication. The final section offers the clinician some suggestions of how he or she may better attend to family issues in the cross-cultural context of oncology care. Chapter 12 is entitled, "The Unmet Need: Addressing Spirituality and Meaning Through Culturally Sensitive Communication and Intervention". While we often treat cancer as if it has only physiological or mental component, the experience of cancer also has a spiritual component. Questions of why me? Who am I? And what is the meaning of life—all come to the fore as individuals survive cancer. The purpose of Chapter 12 by Breitbart and Gibson is to affirm the different aspects of being human in health and in chronic illness. This chapter gives the clinician guidelines on how to communicate with culturally and ethnically diverse patients about spirituality. It also describes the current interventions aimed at enhancing the role of spirituality and meaning in patients' lives in the face of their illnesses.

Communication encompasses many aspects of the clinician-patient relationship, including the provision of information, support from the clinician and the biomedical team, and the freedom to discuss a variety of concerns or problems. Nevertheless, while the words, attitudes, and nonverbal behaviors used by clinicians and the biomedical team certainly affect the patterning of communication in the medical encounter, and related clinical outcomes, they are not the only instigators of context effects, since culture mediates the individual and social contexts where changing interpretations, expectations and evaluations of life events, in states of health, illness, disease, and potentially death occur. Indeed, the quality of care of the patients with cancer also depends on the quality and duration of the clinician-patient relationship, on their trust, attitude, belief, and expectations that these individuals have of their clinicians.

For these reasons, the ways communication is shared between the patient, their significant others, the clinician, and the biomedical team, directly and indirectly, shapes the cultural context of oncology care. The chapters in this volume show us that culture imbues every aspect of the experience of living with and dying of cancer, from the social implications of a cancer diagnosis (shame, stigma, fear, isolation, secondary gain) through the nature of communication between the clinician and patient (hope for care vs cure, placebo vs nocebo, hope vs despair) through concerns about age, cost of care, pain, and other treatment side effects, through the best means of providing psychosocial support, to cultural ceremonies surrounding death and bereavement. These chapters also offer suggestions regarding the reinterpretation of the meaning of life after cancer, in terms of using the medical context and encounter as a way of affirming the different aspects of being human.

In summary, the patients' and their significant others' hopes are associated with the level of trust in the relationship with their clinicians, which is also reflected in their patterns of communication. Images of healing and hopes for a cure certainly do affirm trust and inspire hope, however, when this reality fails to be realized, particularly in the advanced stages of disease, the patients and their significant others may feel that their trust has been betrayed. This is because similar to hope, the trust between the patient and the clinician reflects not only the promise of care, understanding, and concern, but also of a future. A future is not promised to anyone. Cancer is a socially loaded experience, so cultural differences are amplified. A better understanding of the common problems across cultures as well as the salient cultural differences can only improve the standard of cancer care in many cultures.

REFERENCES

1. Van Baalen M, Jansen VA. Common language or Tower of Babel? On the evolutionary dynamics of signals and their meanings. *Proc R Soc Lond B Biol Sci.* 2003;270(1510):69-76.
2. Lakoff 2000. *Metaphors we Choose.*
3. Surbone A, Zwitter M (eds). Communication with the cancer patient: information and truth. *Ann NY Acad Sci.* 1997;809. New York Academy of Sciences.
4. Huang X, Butow PN, Meiser M, Clarke S, Goldstein D. Communicating in a multi-cultural society: the needs of Chinese cancer patients in Australia. *Austr NZJM.* 1999;29:207-213.
5. Harris JJ, Shao J, Sugarman J. Disclosure of cancer diagnosis and prognosis in Northern Tanzania. *Soc Sci Med.* 2003;56(5):905-913.
6. Delvecchio Good MJ, Good BJ, Schaffer C, Lind SE. American oncology and the discourse on hope. *Cult Med Psychiatr.* 1990;14(1):59-79.
7. Buckman R. Communication skills in palliative care: a practical guide. *Neurol Clin.* 2001;19(4):989-1004.
8. Fallowfield LJ, Jenkins VA, Beveridge HA. Truth may hurt but deceit hurts more: communication in palliative care. *Palliat Med.* 2002;16(4):297-303.
9. Baile WF, Lenzi R, Parker PA, Buckman R, Cohen L. Oncologists' attitudes toward and practices in giving bad news: an exploratory study. *J Clin Oncol.* 2002;20(8):2189-2189.
10. Spiegel D. Effects of psychotherapy on cancer survival. *Nat Rev Cancer.* 2002;2(5):383-389.
11. Sontag S. *Illness as Metaphor.* New York: Picador, 2001.
12. Peake MD, Thompson S, Lowe D, Pearson MG. Ageism in the management of lung cancer. *Age Ageing.* 2003;32(2):171-177.
13. Taylor SE, Repetti RL, Seeman T. Health psychology: what is an unhealthy environment and how does it get under the skin? *Annu Rev Psychol.* 1997;48:411-447.
14. Dedier J, Penson R, Williams W, Lynch T. Race, ethnicity, and the patient-caregiver relationship. *Oncologist.* 2002;7(90002):43-49.
15. Ferguson WJ, Candib LM. Culture, language, and the doctor-patient relationship. *Fam Med.* 2002;34(5):353-361.

16. Cioffi J. Communicating with culturally and linguistically diverse patients in an acute care setting: nurses' experiences. *Int J Nurs Stud.* 2003;40(3):299-306.
17. Toms FD, Hodge FS, Pullen-Smith B. Cultural diversity and the delivery of health care services. *Cancer.*1998;83:1843-1848.
18. Hall JA, Roter DL, Katz NR. Meta-analysis of correlates of provider behavior in medical encounters. *Med Care.* 1988;26(7):657-675.
19. Anderson KO, Richman SP, Hurley J, et al. Cancer pain management among underserved minority outpatients: perceived needs and barriers to optimal control. *Cancer.* 2002;94(8):2295-2304.
20. Todd KH. Pain assessment and ethnicity. *Ann Emerg Med.* 1996;27(4):421-423.
21. Cleeland CS, Gonin R, Baez L, Loehrer P, Pandya KJ. Pain and treatment of pain in minority patients with cancer. The Eastern Cooperative Oncology Group Minority Outpatient Pain Study. *Ann Intern Med.* 1997;127(9):813-816.
22. Sheiner EK, Sheiner E, Shoham-Vardi I, Mazor M, Katz M. Ethnic differences influence care giver's estimates of pain during labour. *Pain.* 1999;81(3):299-305.
23. Gordon NH. Socioeconomic factors and breast cancer in black and white Americans. *Cancer Metastasis Rev.* 2003;22(1):55-65.
24. Jack RH, Gulliford MC, Ferguson J, Moller H. Geographical inequalities in lung cancer management and survival in South East England: evidence of variation in access to oncology services? *Br J Cancer.* 2003;88(7):1025-1031.
25. Morris K. Cancer? In Africa? *Lancet Oncol.* 2003;4(1):5.
26. Ayinde OA, Omigbodun AO. Knowledge, attitude and practices related to prevention of cancer of the cervix among female health workers in Ibadan. *J Obstet Gynaecol.* 2003;23(1):59-6.
27. Michelozzi P, Perucci CA, Forastiere F, Fusco D, Ancona C, Dell'Orco V. Inequality in health: socioeconomic differentials in mortality in Rome, 1990-95. *J Epidemiol Commun Health.* 1999;53(11):687-693.
28. Higginson IJ, Jarman B, Astin P, Dolan S. Do social factors affect where patients die: an analysis of 10 years of cancer deaths in England. *J Public Health Med.* 1999;21(1):22-28.
29. Brunswick N, Wardle J, Jarvis MJ. Public awareness of warning signs for cancer in Britain. *Cancer Causes Control.* 2001;12(1):33-37.
30. Cassell EJ. Diagnosing suffering: a perspective. *Ann Intern Med.* 1999;131(7):531-534.
31. Frank A. *The Wounded Storyteller.* Chicago: University of Chicago Press; 1995.
32. Balsham M. *Cancer in the Community: Class and Medical Authority.* Smithsonian Press; 1991.
33. Gregg J, Curry RH. Explanatory models for cancer among African-American women at two Atlanta neighborhood health centers: the implications for a cancer screening program. *Soc Sci Med.* 1994;39(4):519-526.
34. Barsky AJ, Saintfort R, Rogers MP, Borus JF. Nonspecific medication side effects and the nocebo phenomenon. *JAMA.* 2002;287(5):622-627.
35. Chvetzoff G, Tannock IF. Placebo effects in oncology. *J Natl Cancer Inst.* 2003;95(1):19-29.
36. Schofield PE, Butow PN, Thompson JF, Tattersall MH, Beeney LJ, Dunn SM. Psychological responses of patients receiving a diagnosis of cancer. *Ann Oncol.* 2003;14(1):48-56.
37. Hahn RA. The nocebo phenomenon: concept, evidence, and implications for public health. *Prev Med.* 1997;26(5 Pt 1):607–611.
38. Spiegel H. Nocebo: the power of suggestibility. *Prev Med.* 1997;26(5 Pt 1):616-621.
39. Di Blasi Z, Harkness E, Ernst E, Georgiou A, Kleijnen J. Influence of context effects on health outcomes: a systematic review. *Lancet.* 2001;357(9258):757-762.
40. Brody H. Placebo.
41. Balint M. *Doctor His Patient and the Illness.* International Universities Press; 2000.

42. Benson H, Friedman R. Harnessing the power of the placebo effect and renaming it "remembered wellness." *Annu Rev Med.* 1996;47:193-199.
43. Benedetti F. How the doctor's words affect the patient's brain. *Eval Health Prof.* 2002;25(4):369-386.
44. Benson H. The nocebo effect: history and physiology. *Prev Med.* 1997;26(5 Pt 1):612-615.
45. Pollo A, Vighetti S, Rainero I, Benedetti F. Placebo analgesia and the heart. *Pain.* 2003;102(1-2):125-133.
46. Chaput de Saintonge DM, Herxheimer A. Harnessing placebo effects in health care. *Lancet.* 1994;344(8928):995-998.
47. Moerman DE. The meaning response and the ethics of avoiding placebos. *Eval Health Prof.* 2002;25(4):399-409.
48. Gracely RH, Dubner R, Deeter WR, Wolskee PJ. Clinicians' expectations influence placebo analgesia. *Lancet.* 1985;1(8419):43.
49. Ernst E, Herxheimer A. The power of placebo. *BMJ.* 1996;313(7072):1569-1570.
50. Spiro, H. *The Power of Hope: A Doctor's Perspective.* Yale University Press; 1998.
51. Spiro HM. Hope helps: placebos and alternative medicine in rheumatology. *Rheum Dis Clin North Am.* 1999;25(4):855-860.
52. Enserink M. Can the placebo be the cure? *Science.* 1999;284(5412):238-240.
53. Beecher, H.K.: The powerful placebo. *J Amer Med Assoc* 1955;159:1602-1606.
54. Hrobjartsson A, Gotzsche PC. Is the placebo powerless? An analysis of clinical trials comparing placebo with no treatment. *N Engl J Med.* 2001;344(21):1594-1602.
55. Kaptchuk TJ. The placebo effect in alternative medicine: can the performance of a healing ritual have clinical significance? *Ann Intern Med.* 2002;136(11):817-825.
56. Shapiro AK, Morris LA. Placebos in psychiatric therapy. *Curr Psychiatr Ther.* 1977;17:157-163.
57. Harrington A (ed.). *The Placebo Effect.* Harvard University Press; 1997.
58. *The American Heritage® Dictionary of the English Language.* 4th ed. 2000.
59. Mayberg HS, Silva JA, Brannan SK, Tekell J, Mahurin R, McGinnis S, Jerabek P. The functional neuroanatomy of the placebo effect. *Am J Psychiatr.* 2002;159(5):728-737.
60. World Medical Association. Declaration of Helsinki. Ethical principles for medical research involving human subjects. *JAMA.* 2000;284:3043-3045.
61. Andrews G. Placebo response in depression: bane of research, boon to therapy. *Br J Psychiatr.* 2001;178:192-194.
62. Miller FG, Brody H. What makes placebo-controlled trials unethical? *Am J Bioeth.* 2002;2(2):3-9.
63. Guest H, Kleinman A. *Science of the Placebo.* BMJ Publishing Group; 2002.
64. Hahn R. Kleinman A. Belief as pathogen, belief as medicine. *Med Anthropol Quart.* 1983;14(4):16-19.
65. Petrovic P, Kalso E, Petersson KM, Ingvar M. Placebo and opioid analgesia—imaging a shared neuronal network. *Science.* 2002;295(5560):1737-1740.
66. Amanzio M, Pollo A, Maggi G, Benedetti F. Response variability to analgesics: a role for non-specific activation of endogenous opioids. *Pain.* 2001;90(3):205-215.
67. Pollo A, Amanzio M, Arslanian A, Casadio C, Maggi G, Benedetti F. Response expectancies in placebo analgesia and their clinical relevance. *Pain.* 2001;93(1):77-84.
68. Rainville P, Carrier B, Hofbauer RK, Bushnell MC, Duncan GH. Dissociation of sensory and affective dimensions of pain using hypnotic modulation. *Pain.* 1999;82(2):159-171.
69. Goetz CG, Leurgans S, Raman R, Stebbins GT. Objective changes in motor function during placebo treatment in PD. *Neurology.* 2000;54(3):710-714.
70. Goetz CG, Leurgans S, Raman R. Placebo-associated improvements in motor function. *Mov Disord.* 2002;17(2):283-288 (Brody H 2000:37).

71. Eskandari F, Sternberg EM. Neuroendocrine mechanisms of the placebo effect. In: Guest, H et al eds. Science of the Placebo. *BMJ Publishing*; 2002.
72. Kirsch I. How expectancies shape experience. *Am Psychol Assoc* (APA). 1999.
73. Pollo A, Torre E, Lopiano L, Rizzone M, Lanotte M, Cavanna A, Bergamasco B, Benedetti F. Expectation modulates the response to subthalamic nucleus stimulation in Parkinsonian patients. *Neuroreport.* 2002;13(11):1383-1386.
74. Amanzio M, Benedetti F. Neuropharmacological dissection of placebo analgesia: expectation-activated opioid systems versus conditioning-activated specific subsystems. *J Neurosci.* 1999;19(1):484-494.
75. West AF, West RR. Clinical decision-making: Coping with uncertainty. *Postgrad. Med.* 2002;78(920):319-321.
76. Von Roenn JH, von Gunten CF. Setting goals to maintain hope. *J Clin Oncol.* 2003;21(3):570-574.
77. Strohle A. Increased response to a putative panicogenic nocebo administration in female patients with panic disorder. *J Psychiatr Res.* 2000;34(6):439-442.
78. Leor J, Poole WK, Kloner RA. Sudden cardiac death triggered by an earthquake. *N Engl J Med.* 1996;334:413-419.
79. Sternberg EM, Walter B. Cannon. Voodoo. Death: a perspective from 60 years on. *Am J Public Health.* 2002;92(10):1564-1566.
80. Cannon W Voodoo. Death. *Am Anthropologist.* 1942;44(new series):169-181.
81. Meador CK. Hex death: Voodoo magic or persuasion? *South Med J.* 1992;85(3):244-247.
82. Phillips DP, Liu GC, Kwok K, Jarvinen JR, Zhang W, Abramson IS. The Hound of the Baskervilles effect: natural experiment on the influence of psychological stress on timing of death. *BMJ.* 2001;323:1443-1444.

PART I

Cancer across Cultures

CHAPTER 2

Culture and Oncology

Impact of Context Effects

Rhonda J. Moore and Phyllis Butow

> *Caring can be learned by all human beings, can be worked into the design of every life, meeting an individual need as well as a pervasive need in society.*
> Mary Catherine Bateson

> *The placebo effect or for that matter the nocebo effect will only work if one believes that something positive or negative will happen.*
> J. H. Benson 1997. *Preventive Medicine*. 26:612

> *What I'm saying is that a lot of behavior that you are talking about is a direct response of people not having a future, or feeling that they don't have a future.*
> William Julius Wilson, *The New York Times,*
> December 4, 1994, p. 77

Clinician-patient communication in oncology does not operate outside of the context of culture. Culture can be defined as the socially transmitted body of values, beliefs, behaviors, social and political institutions, arts, crafts, and science that are shared by a given group of people.[1] This concept of culture can also be applied to groups who share characteristics other than geography or ethnicity. For instance, groups defined by sexual preference, gender, occupation (eg, the culture of Science), class and socioeconomic status (SES) have, and share cultural characteristics, including a group identity, elements of a world view, uses of a specialized language and a shared history.[2] For the purposes of this chapter, we employ this broader definition of culture.[2-8]

Culturally determined perceptions and responses are, largely, so innate for an individual that the role of culture in determining them is largely unconscious and "invisible." Thus, one tends to experience one's own perceptions and responses as innately true, coherent, meaningful, and obvious.[2] This can make it difficult to question our own perceptions and responses, or to value different responses in others. For these reasons, we are likely to ascribe other people's "different" responses to "culture," and assume that our own are innately correct. The culture of others is also much more apparent, as is the influence of their culture on specific beliefs and behaviors. Furthermore, we may be "blind" to culturally specific needs, if they are in an area that is seemingly absent or different from our own cultural experience and culture. Thus, provision of accessible, appropriate, and helpful services to all patients is challenging, and requires particular attention to cultural issues.

Culture influences most relations and day-to-day behaviors. It is also intricately linked to social interactions, affecting the transmission of belief systems, the sharing of common systems of symbols, symptoms, gestures, language and signals that convey information and meaning, responses (eg, to pain), and attitudes toward illness, disease, death and health care services.[3-8]

For these reasons, insight into the cultural worlds of the patient with cancer, their significant others, and the clinician represents an important starting point for mutual understanding of the experience of illness and better communication, leading to more effective oncology care.[9-18] However, while an understanding of cultural may be of great benefit to clinicians and other health professionals, an important proviso is awareness of the diversity that exists even within the same culture context. Moreover, generalizations concerning a group linked by cultural factors can lead to stereotyping, rigid rules, and a lack of tailoring to individual differences. Thus, information about beliefs and practices within particular cultures and ethnic groups never obviates the need for exploring individual preferences and needs.

In what follows, we review the relevance of culture as a context effect on clinician-patient communication in oncology.[13,19-22] We begin with the premise that the human healing process can be substantially influenced in actual medical practice by context effects including appropriate kinds of understanding, trust, and caring, as these are crucial to effective communication.[13,14,17,18,23-25] Additionally, when we speak of understanding the medical context, including the roles played by context in the effectiveness of clinician-patient communication, we are talking about the placebo effect (see also Chapter 1, this volume).[10,13,20,23,26-32] Context effects, as we previously stated, are intertwined with placebo effects and are thus bidirectional. They can be positive and beneficial, or negative and adverse.[13,26-32] As such we situate our discussion in light of this vibrant ongoing debate.[10,13,18,20,21,26,30-32]

In the first section, we explore the importance of culture as a context effect that shapes the environment where individual and social experiences and responses to health, illness, and disease occur. The distinction between disease and illness is well documented in the literatures.[33-35] Disease refers to a pathophysiologic process. Defined by the individual, illness represents an individual's unique, biopsychosocial experience of being unwell.[33,35,36] The relevance of context is also apparent in barriers to effective care, including race, gender, and SES.[13,37-39] This section will also discuss the significance of migration and translation issues that impaet the effective communication of care of patients across cultural, national, and linguistic boundaries, and will also briefly discuss the role of the family as cultural mediators of clinician-patient communication. The second section offers an overview of beliefs about cancer causation and discusses the importance of language and words, truth telling and disclosure on the interaction between the clinician and the patient. The third section will briefly describe the various methodologies that have been used in the attempt to understand these cultural differences in the clinical context. The fourth and final section will provide some guidelines of what clinicians can do to better address the problems in clinician-patient communication in oncology in culturally diverse populations. Finally, we will provide a list of websites, suggested readings, and resources.

THE IMPORTANCE OF CULTURE IN ONCOLOGICAL CARE

It is sometimes assumed that medical encounters are objective and culturally neutral spaces where issues of culture, age, SES, ethnic, or gender differences fail to permeate. Certainly, there are common ethical principles governing medical practice, which comes from the equal rights of any human being to life and dignity,[40] and which have led to the Universal Declaration of Human Rights.[41] These rights are shared and are cross-cultural. However, medical encounters are also cultural performances through their constitutive gestures and responses.[42] Thus, the ways these rights are performed, expressed, communicated, and acted upon are profoundly influenced by the cultural context.[42-57] Ethnic, social, and economic factors have all been shown to both directly and indirectly affect equity and access to health care and interactions between patients and clinicians.[42-57]

Environmental Effects: Influence of SES and Social Suffering on Health

The relevance of environmental factors such as SES and social suffering to health in general, and to cancer outcomes in particular, has been well described in the oncology literature. SES, a broad term describing economic and social circumstances, is difficult to measure directly and studies have previously used a number of proxy measures to indicate different socioeconomic groups.[58-62] SES may be determined by background and by early and late life experiences. Social suffering refers to what is done to and by people through their involvement with processes of political, economic, and institutional power. It also influences personal levels of distress, the potential context of care in terms of what is available, accessible, and realizable, and if the patients communicate their concerns to the clinician.[63-67] Disparities, such as SES and social suffering, in health occur because privilege and power remain unequal in racially and ethnically stratified societies. Indeed, the globalization of complex chronic diseases seems to confirm the view that all populations are susceptible and that variation in rates can be understood as the result of differential exposure to environmental causes. Put more succinctly, systematic variations in health and mortality across the range of income, ethnicity and education, collectively referred to as SES and social suffering, contribute to the negative consequences of cancer and adversely impact clinician-patient communication.[68-85]

In both sociological and epidemiological terms, cancer has been characterized as a disease of both poverty and affluence. Yet, while affluence elevates the risks associated with cancer both in individuals and in nations, low SES is also associated with a variety of adverse health outcomes. For instance, minority, poor, elderly, and other underserved patients continue to disproportionately suffer from decreased survival rates from cancer, compared to their upper- and middle-class counterparts, often due to delays in time to diagnoses, in referrals for treatment, and in actual treatments offered.[44-85]

Another important outcome is a lack of adequate medical care. Individuals from minority, elderly, culturally, and linguistically diverse and low SES communities are least likely to have adequate medical insurance or to receive appropriate medical care. Low SES patients from the United States, for instance, due to an inability to afford adequate medical coverage, often use emergency room services to obtain care for chronic conditions including cancer.[51-54,89,90] As a consequence, many are diagnosed with advanced stage tumors. There is also evidence that certain medical therapies, particularly invasive medical techniques, are under-utilized in the treatment of African American, elderly, female, and poor patients with chronic conditions including coronary artery disease and cancer, who do use US medical facilities.[63-84,90-98] Such instances are also found in other cultural contexts. In the United Kingdom, for instance, despite socialized medicine, older lung cancer patients are less likely to be offered surgery and more likely to die prematurely compared to younger patients.[89]

A recent study in Turkey, where there is no private health insurance program, found that cancer patients who covered their own health expenses not only played a greater role in the treatment decision-making process, but were also more satisfied with their care. These patients had more choices, and were better able to explore alternative treatment options, than the majority of patients who used the public health system.[85,88]

The influence of race, ethnicity, and sex on health outcome is also recognized by medical students. For example, a recent study of medical students in the United States reported lower utility values for the health state described by an African American female patient actor than for a White male patient actor. This was the case, even though the African American female patient actor was viewed as friendlier, a better communicator, and as having a more positive affect than the White male patient actor. All the same, the African American female patient actor was perceived to be less likely to obtain adequate followup care.[85,88-94] These studies highlight the need for sensitivity to and awareness of the particular difficulties faced by those with few resources, and people who have migrated to a new country.[81-94]

One body of research has explored the possibility that SES, stress, and other culturally determined characteristics, may more directly influence health and disease.[10,27,31,37-39,46,63-108] The body's principal adaptive responses to psychophysiological stress (eg, poverty, discrimination, social stress, perceptions, and responses to pain, etc.) are mediated by an intricate stress system, which includes the hypothalamic-pituitary-adrenocortical (HPA) axis and the sympathoadrenal system (SAS).[99-108] Dysregulation of the system, caused by the cumulative burden of repetitive or chronic environmental stress challenges (allostatic load) may contribute to the development of a variety of illnesses including hypertension, atherosclerosis, the metabolic syndrome, as well as certain disorders of immune function, including cancer. Moreover, while little is known about the mechanisms that convert psychosocial and environmental stress into monocellular activation,[237] and the underlying mechanisms of these effects remain uncertain, it is clear that both adverse and health-resiliency promoting factors related to SES and health influence the developmental process and start early in life.[72,89-106,237] Early in life, various interactions between social and environmental factors and genetic susceptibilities lead to large individual differences in susceptibility to stress and disease. The SAS plays a crucial role, since alterations in sympathoadrenal function due to exposures in early life aid in the development of a phenotype that is adapted to the challenges of the local environment. Social and environmental exposures at crucial points in development have been shown to permanently alter sympathoadrenal function in mammals.[106,107,109,110] For example, very low birth-weight that is often found in low SES and minority women has been shown to elevate the relative risk of developing diabetes, asthma, respiratory problems, heart disease, and cancer as the child grows older.[102-104] Under these circumstances, adaptations in early life prove maladaptive in adulthood and, as a consequence, might provide a basis for developmental origins of pediatric and adult diseases or in the permanent impairments in neural regulatory pathways. In addition, even though the SAS is capable of responding to stressors during fetal life, the long-term effects of such exposures on the adult organism are relatively unknown. What we do know is that the HPA axis is fundamental for long-term survival and protection from the ravages of autoimmune disease. However, in response to long-term chronic stress over the life course, physiological and psychological systems fluctuate, in the attempt to meet the taxing demands of an ever-changing environment. Exposure to many types of physical and psychological stressors *over time* initiates a cascade of neuroendocrine events in the HPA axis. Recently Bierhaus and associates[237] identified adrenergic signaling pathway that explained the rapid increase in activation of the transcription factor NF-κB observed in PBMC shortly after exposure to psychosocial stress, thus linking psychosocial stress to mononuclear cell activation and subsequent changes in the immune system. This extends previous work showing a role of catecholamines in the mechanism for atherosclerosis and others which implicate the sequential release of corticotrophin releasing hormone (CRH) from the hypothalamus, adrenocorticotropic hormone (ACTH) from the anterior pituitary and, ultimately, glucocorticoids (cortisol in primates and corticosterone in rodents) from the adrenal cortex. Indeed, the observation that mental stress in humans and rodents results in nuclear translocation of NF-κB and changes in transcriptional activity thus closes an important gap in understanding the cellular consequences of stress. Induction of NF-κB is in part dependent on the interaction of NA with x_1- and β-adrenergic receptors. The NA-dependent adrenergic signal transduction is mediated by Ptx-sensitive G proteins inducing P13-kinase and Ras/Raf signaling that results in MAPK activation and subsequent NF-κB induction. The observation that binding activity of NF-κB, but not a Oct-1, was altered further confirms that psychosocial stress elicits a receptor-dependent specific signal rather than a nonspecific cell activation. NF-κB activation is supposed to contribute to the pathophysiology of lifestyle-related diseases such as diabetes mellitus, cardiovascular disease, and atherosclerosis, implicating stress-dependent NF-κB activation in the cumulative burden that finally leads to morbidity and mortality.[237] Similarly, the stress-induced persistent genetic instability in the context of carcinogenesis may also be a general response of tumor cells to a wide range of stress conditions.[105-110]

This state of fluctuation, as severe variation from homeostasis, has been termed allostasis, and over time, allostatic load builds up. Allostatic load defined as the physiological and psychological costs of chronic exposure to fluctuating or heightened neuroimmune or neuroendocrine responses results from repeated or chronic environmental challenges that an individual reacts to as stressful. As such, poverty or affluence are merely two of the more important environmental factors, which can adversely impact allostatic load, including the individual and social experience of suffering from chronic stress which then enhances susceptibility to disease, or decreased risk for survival once diagnosed with cancer.[72,99-110]

Impact of Culture on Patient and Clinician Roles

Cultural values and structures also play a major role in determining the roles played by patients and clinicians. The "sick" are expected to behave within certain parameters, as are clinicians. This scenario is perhaps best exemplified by the model of Parsons, who posits that clinicians and patients are drawn together through shared values, affect, and role commitment, while at the same time, being pushed apart by social structure.[111] The role of the clinician is paradoxical, in that they must show compassion toward those who seek help, yet be on guard against those who may abuse the sick role. Patients, especially the chronically ill, face a similar contradiction, since they must consistently present themselves as "sick," while at the same time projecting an image of wanting to get well. Affect in the form of emotional expression is also essential to this particular model since patients and clinicians share a similar attachment to cultural values underpinning the sick role, modern medical practice, and a commitment that is derived from emotional gratification. The sick role is always embedded in social relations, thus the making of meaning in such cultural contexts is always in constant tension.[6] In addition, the relationship continues to function due to the clinician's professional practice in terms of affective neutrality, functional specificity, an orientation toward universals, and the patient's acceptance of the limits of this role. It is these factors, at least according to Parsons, which protect clinicians from an overwhelming emotion present in their roles but also sustains a social distance (ie, objectivity) between clinicians and patients.[111]

Expectations regarding patient and clinician roles vary in different cultures, and this can create tension. For instance, patients of Chinese descent often have great respect for the expertise of the clinician. Thus, any ambiguity or uncertainty in presenting the diagnosis or treatment recommendations is viewed as reflecting a lack of expertise.[112] As such, communication in accordance with the current Western emphasis on informed consent and active patient involvement in decision-making may be interpreted as incompetence by patients from this population. The sick role also has different faces in different cultures; for example, the degree of overt expression of cancer-related symptoms including suffering varies considerably cross-culturally.[112-117]

Impact of Culture on Behavior and Mutual Understanding

For these reasons, the cultural assumptions, expectations, and interpretations of the patient also influence how they behave in the medical consultation, what they understand, how they feel, and if they adhere to the treatment afterwards.[118,119] Patients bring beliefs about the causes of diseases, knowledge and beliefs concerning body structure and functions, and beliefs surrounding the use of alternative therapies (see Chapter 10, this volume).[118] Religious and spiritual beliefs and practices affect how patients respond to bad news (see Chapter 11, this volume), medical treatments such as transfusions, quality of life (see Chapter 3, this volume) and end of life issues (see Chapters 11 and 12, this volume). Personal or historical experiences of discrimination, violence or racism may influence level of trust in health professionals, institutions, and the practice of medical research. For example, Gonzalez[120] presents a case study of a mother who delayed taking her ill child (appendicitis) to hospital for 4 days, in part because of harsh treatment she had received as an immigrant and her embarrassment at not speaking good English.[88,120]

Such issues can also affect patterns of adherence. Adherence can also serve as a surrogate marker for a patient's own contribution to the activation of context effects.[87,111] Alternatively, it may also provide an explanation for patterns of non-adherence and delay, particularly in low SES, linguistically diverse, and other high-risk patients.[118,119,121] Moreover, if the patient's and clinician's belief systems are not the same, difficulties can ensue. For instance, the relatively widespread practice in Asia of self-medication, which arises from a strong tradition of self-care,[121] can conflict with clinicians' beliefs in evidence-based medicine. The ways these important issues are discussed (or avoided) may determine much about the future relationship between patient and clinician and the way in which treatment progresses.

In the ideal scenario, however, the relationship between clinician and patient is a straightforward dialogue that ends with a clear resolution. A common language, or a significant degree of resemblance between the clinician and the patients' thoughts and feelings, facilitates this process enormously.[3,42,111] In other words, when there is cultural similarity between communicators, messages about health and illness are more likely to be conveyed efficiently and with less ambiguity.[3,96-98,122-124]

When the participants come from different cultural backgrounds, however, special care is needed to bridge potential gaps and barriers.[89,91-98,122-127]

An example is seen in the treatment of pain. Several studies have shown that ethnic minority and female patients (with and without cancer) are undertreated for pain. The expression of pain is a form of communication, and cultural differences in emotional expression and stereotypes about pain also influence the clinician's interpretation and expectations regarding pain severity. This is possibly due to conscious and unconscious bias on the part of the clinician and patient, or subtle differences in cultural expressive cues (ie, body language), since an individual can more readily recognize emotions expressed in the style to which they are accustomed.[91-126]

Language translation issues can also lead to difficulties in adequately matching an addresser to a receiver.[88,93,94] For example, clinicians' use of medical language with patients who do not share it, may result in serious misunderstanding. One instance of this problem is in the field of genetics, where patients who are told that their genetic test results are positive (signaling that a mutation has been found) may interpret this statement to mean the outcome is good (signaling that a mutation has *not* been found).[93,94]

Cancer: A Particular Threat

In the West, public discourses about cancer have changed from those that associate a diagnosis of cancer with death, to those that claim that cancer is potentially curable and definitely treatable.[88,143] On the one hand, particularly in the Western context, open disclosure not only of the cancer diagnosis, but also of available treatment options and the statistical likelihood of survival and death from cancer is now increasingly promoted.[7,143-144] Nonetheless, such disclosure is always culturally mediated even within various Western contexts. In North America, for instance, there is great emphasis on patient autonomy, immediacy of action, and a shared decision-making model for health. Yet, in France (and in many other European societies, Japan, the Middle East. Africa, for that matter), relationships with patients are much more hierarchical, protective, and paternalistic. Indeed, patients who come from cultures where the doctor is revered may mistrust or devalue doctors who try directly to involve the patient in their care.[7,15-16,27,88,132-134,143]

Still, the fact remains that cancer still remains curable for only half the patients who get it. The remainder seek to be cured but require care. Medical progress has rendered many forms of cancer chronic rather than terminal illnesses, but the treatments are often arduous, and the anxieties of patients and their families are continuous. Consequently, studies show that lay populations in both Western and non-Western contexts still have a universal dread of cancer. The stigma associated with cancer has not (in many instances) decreased.[15-16,138,143-144] Cancer remains an illness heavily invested with symbolic meaning, where cancer and related symptoms threaten irreparable destruction of the patient's body/self, death, pain, and loss of previous sources of meaning in life. As such, it presents perhaps the greatest challenge to clinician-patient communication of any illness. In advance-stage disease in particular, clinicians are presented with the task of finding words to rationally communicate some of the more dire consequences of cancer and their own limitations to patients, and to assist patients in adjusting to this news.[123–146]

These contradictions and realities are the core of many of the difficulties incurred in clinician-patient communication in oncology.[127–143]

The Impact of Migration on Cancer Outcomes and Access

The demographic composition of people in the West also continues to grow and change. With this ever-increasing diversity, there are more patients from culturally diverse backgrounds with cancer. While people moving to a new country may adopt new ways and customs, in critical situations, such as the diagnosis of cancer, they also often return to the ways and customs of their childhood, as do the people around them.[147–153] Chinese Americans, but not Whites, for example, have been shown to die significantly earlier than normal if they have a combination of disease (lymphatic cancer) and birth year which Chinese astrology and medicine consider ill-fated. The intensity of this effect has been correlated with "the strength of commitment to traditional Chinese culture."[148–155] Others, upon migration to the United States from cultures with pluralistic medical systems, like India, where there is a widespread use of Ayurvedic medicine, may find that Western medicinal practices remain alien despite a growing familiarity with them.[154] Similarly, in Nigeria, some patients rely on traditional healers for the cure of cancer when they perceive that Western biomedicine has failed them. The plurality of the health care system that exists in Nigeria, particularly among the Igbo, encourages health-seeking behaviors that enable people to switch from one system to another in search of the most affordable and accessible means of care.[155] For these reasons, the need to find ways of communicating effectively from one culture to another will only increase over time.[147,155,156]

Communication with Cancer Patients

The ability to effectively communicate with cancer patients and significant others has been linked to patient satisfaction, reduced psychological morbidity, enhanced health outcomes,[157-207] and reduced clinician "burn-out."[162,163] Yet, despite what we now "know" about the benefits of effective communication between patients and clinicians, cancer clinicians did not, until recently, receive effective training in the psychosocial and emotional aspects of cancer patient care.[167,172-175] Nor did they receive training in how to cope with the increasing cultural complexities that mediate the experience of care. As a consequence, they often rate their skills as deficient in terms of communicating bad news, or dealing with unrealistic expectations for cure on the part of patients, in both mono-ethnic and in culturally diverse patient populations.[88,175,184] Audit studies have provided objective evidence for deficiencies in these areas.[88,112,169]

Many studies have examined clinician-patient communication in oncology; however, the majority tends to emphasize phenomena such as *history taking* and *breaking bad news* as focal points of inquiry.[7,15,16,125,126,143,156-192] Such studies have been helpful in identifying aspects of clinician-patient communication that are particularly difficult, and strategies that are more or less effective in these situations, but have been less successful in exploring over-arching issues such as the cultural context. Furthermore, the majority of these studies has been conducted in the Western world and have excluded non-English-speaking patients and clinicians to facilitate data collection and reduce costs.[156] Thus, their ability to throw light on cultural issues is inherently limited.[156-192]

These studies have also identified barriers to effective clinician-patient communication that are likely to be relevant to the experience of patients from different cultures.[88,175] Clinician-related barriers include: (1) an inability or unwillingness to deal with patients' emotional concerns[167-174,207]; (2) over-involvement with patients and denial, leading to a mutual collusion with patients in sustaining unrealistic expectations for cure; (3) time constraints, which leads to inability to adequately address patients' informational and emotional concerns and fears[164-167,176,179-182,188]; (4) the use of ambiguous words to convey the diagnosis, treatment, and prognosis.[176-180,188] For example, the clinician's failure to employ accurate terminology often squanders an ideal opportunity to correct misconceptions about the disease.[180,181] Patient-related barriers include vulnerability and high emotion at the time of diagnosis, lack of familiarity with the medical setting, and perceptions of the patient role as passive and compliant. Such factors can also prevent patients from actively interacting in medical consultations, asking questions, expressing their needs and feelings, and participating in decisions.[88,155,157,159-175] These barriers are also likely to be present for patients from culturally and linguistically diverse backgrounds, and such patients are also likely to have additional difficulties.[88,175]

People of a different culture to the dominant one, also often report that health professionals do not understand them, which adversely affects their psychological and physiological well-being.[13,16,88,96-98,112,183-191,208,209,211,214-221]

Indeed, given a consistent lack of cross-cultural understanding, patients may tend to try to offset these barriers by either avoiding the biomedical context until a condition is chronic, or by preferring clinicians of their own race.[32,44,175] For example, in a recent study of Greeks living in Australia, participants (particularly those who were of lower levels of acculturation) noted that they would prefer to see Greek physicians, with whom they shared language and culture. One woman reported "A Greek doctor, I feel as if he is my husband or my father, as if he one of mine."[189] In addition, patients living in a new culture may have greater difficulty understanding information presented to them, and in having their treatment preferences (including for alternative therapy) understood and respected.[189] Some participants in the Australian study reported above, felt that a Greek doctor would be less likely to make the Greek person feel "inferior" because of his/her poor language skills. In addition, such patients may also have problems accepting information presented to them, given that many patients, when they fear that their prognosis is rather poor, do not ask for precise information and do not hear it if it is provided by the clinician.[179,180] Finally, these patients might also have much difficulty in having their treatment preferences (including for alternative therapy) understood and respected.[88,194,203]

Communication Crisis in Oncology

One important consequence of all these issues is that there is much public and private dissatisfaction with clinician-patient communication in oncology, which has led to a cultural crisis in communication in this field. The word *cancer* with all its connotations and meanings, remains stressful for both patients and clinicians alike, and the context of oncology practice exacerbates this crisis because delivering news about diagnosis, treatments, and metastases is complex and difficult. In addition, while good communication skills are essential for all aspects of effective medical care, a lack of understanding of cultural differences can cause the communication between patients and clinicians to falter.[88,143-214,208-226] And though much of the research has assessed the effects of training in communication skills, these studies have not adequately highlighted the relevance of culture as a context effect that influences the patient's health. Nor have they properly evaluated the underlying mechanisms by which clinicians can appropriately harness context effects for therapeutic benefit.[3,13-22,26-32,35,163-191,204]

This crisis in communication can also be understood as a problem of language, meaning, and context since medical treatments and the language used reflects not only words in reference to the linguistic properties of a group, but also the various meanings that different persons attribute to these same words.[3,13-22,88,226-229] Then again, language is not the only way cultural meanings are embodied and conveyed. The previously mentioned: touch, words, eye contact, gestures, tone, listening, the clinician's uniform, and the ambience of the consultation are all meaningful and all play a role in conveying a clinician's confidence in a treatment, empathy with the patient, and professional status. The responses of the patient to the clinician, affect both bodily and mental states, since these messages work after a fashion to alter the meaning of states of heath or illness.[13-22,227,228] For example, a recent analysis showed that a breast cancer survivor's perceptions of their physician's behavior during the consultation might influence long-term psychologic adjustment, in terms of state anxiety levels. In this study, enhanced compassion was shown to be an effective tool in decreasing anxiety.[160] Similarly, Street and Voigt examined the relationship between perceptions of control over treatment decisions in early breast cancer patients, and subsequent health-related quality of life. Patients who reported more involvement in their consultation later believed they had received more of a choice of treatment, and reported higher levels of quality of life than did the patients who perceived they had less decisional control.[193] For these reasons, as Ernst suggests, context effects to the remedy itself have a powerful influence; and the more actively they involve the patient, and their social worlds, the larger the effect.[13-22,195]

BELIEFS ABOUT CANCER CAUSATION AND THE IMPORTANCE OF LANGUAGE AND WORDS, TRUTH TELLING, AND DISCLOSURE ON THE INTERACTION BETWEEN THE CLINICIAN AND THE PATIENT

When cancer strikes, the individual often attributes a multitude of causes and meanings to why it happened.[13-16,88,213] These include: the disapproval of ancestral spirits, the embodiment and projection of others' negativity, actions of jealousy, or the nonobservance of a taboo.[198-206] Additional reasons include: sorcery, bad behaviors, high-blood pressure, bad blood, worms, incestuous acts, adultery, bad diet, seeding of tumor by surgery, exposure to "wind or air," lack of balance, improper ritual of planting or harvesting, a dirty womb, too much hot food, miasmas, microbes, bad luck, stress in relationships, stepping on poison, crossing an evil line, worry, lump cannot be cancer if it is not painful, heartbreak, bad genes, fate, the devil.[15-16,88,211,212,214-221,224,225] Such variation is also reflected in the meanings and understandings attributed to cancer causation within different cultural groups, including among those who are now live in Western countries. A study in Australia within the Italian community revealed a common belief that tumors "with roots" (metastatic cancer) are always fatal, because it is impossible to remove all of the roots. The women interviewed also believed that an operation could be dangerous and cause one to die more quickly, because it might let air into the body causing the roots to grow more quickly.[202] In another study amongst the Australian Greek community, several participants mentioned the causal role of "microvia" or microbes in the development of cancer, which could originate from within the body or in the air, while others believed that fatigue, interpersonal conflict, and stress could cause cancer.[189] Studies of African American women in North America suggest that many believe that only a "chosen few" survive breast cancer.[203-205] Others state that tumors could be caused by being hit in the breast during an act of violence, that cancer was a condition of the mind and could be cured by prayer, that breast cancer was caused by repeated heartbreak or that it is a disease of White women.[203-205,218] In other studies on South African cancer patients, patients with cancer, teachers, and secondary school students often still believe that a special witchcraft causes cancer and, therefore, their first priority is to reverse the sorcery before presenting to hospital to be treated by modern medicine methods.[200,201,211,218] The patient sought help first from a traditional healer as a way of dealing with the cause of the disease and, in their view, this did not imply delay in medical treatment. If the treatment fails then it is concluded that the patient did not follow the instructions given by the healer because the *inyanga* is never wrong.[200,201,211] Similarly, while many traditional Native American healers believe that cancer is a White man's disease and therefore the treatment needs to include Western medicine, urban Native American breast carcinoma patients may refuse to initiate treatment until they participate in traditional Indian ceremonies. These ceremonies often require many months of preparation.[206] Thus, despite apparent advances in medical science that have led to effective treatments for cancer, such myths and perceptions can adversely influence beliefs about causation, expectations regarding the meanings and the course of illness, treatment, and act as barriers to early detection, treatment, and recovery. Reinforcing this point are negative attitudes toward cancer or the environment where cancer is treated, which can create barriers to effective communication, between patients and clinicians and may influence decision-making about referrals and treatments.[6,13-18,26-32,183-191,198,201,207] These beliefs are often culturally specific, and reinforce the importance of eliciting and addressing patient beliefs so that they do not cause unnecessary distress, nor reduce the chance of a clear and agreed decision about treatment.

The Meaning of Cancer and Causation

Such rich cultural variation can also be found in the meanings (or lack of meaning) associated with the word "cancer" across the different cultural groups. A fascinating comment on the influence of language and culture on beliefs about cancer causation is provided by Bezwoda and colleagues.[211]

They note that in only three of the nine ethnic Black languages (Zulu, Swazi, and Xhosa) is there a word for cancer at all, and that the reactions of patients to these words do not include any concept of a disease that may spread to other sites of the body, or that requires any special treatments to effect cure. Mirroring this fact is the finding that the majority (65%) of 100 African women presenting for the first time with breast cancer surveyed by the authors were found to have advanced disease at the time of referral.[88,212] Cancer, generally defined as loss of genomic stability, comes from the Latin word for crab, a clawed creature that reinforces the idea of a fierce, unstoppable force creeping relentlessly through the body. This one word, *cancer*, is generally used to describe cancer in most Western contexts. However, in Nigeria, there is no common name for cancer among traditional healers (*dibias*). Indeed, often more than one word is used to describe cancer and there is usually more than one etiology. For instance, certain cultures also use local terms to describe cancer as a disease of the breast (*mbubu ara*), or as ulcers (*onya*) at various locations on the body. Healers may also believe that the causes of cancer lie outside the body, others may note that it exists inside the body, and still others claim it is both outside and inside. What this means it that the treatment of patients is highly influenced by individual subjective perceptions of the healer about the causes of the cancer. It also raises additional questions and concerns, as to whether or not cancer is a foreign illness not known in *Igbo* terminology or if it is a new disease that has not yet been classified by the *Igbo*.[200,201,221]

Other studies highlight the power of negative thoughts given that an angry or jealous person with enough power can "send cancer" to another person. In South Africa, for instance, an evil *sangoma* (sorcerer) is believed to poison the cancer patient by placing the cancer in their food, taking it to them when they are sleeping, or leaving it on the ground for the individual to walk over. Once this poison enters the body, it moves to a specific site and unless the cancer is drawn out through indigenous medicines and healing rituals (*imbizas*), it will kill the patient.[201] Other studies also emphasize this point since many women believe that once diagnosed only a "chosen few" actually survive breast cancer. Others claim to "know" that tumors are caused by air since cancer spreads when the air hits it (surgery), and that it cancer a condition of the mind and could be cured by prayer.[203-205] Of particular relevance is the belief that if the individual has enough mindfulness, faith, and hope, they can alter the course of the disease in the body. Such beliefs express fundamentally North American notions of personhood, autonomy, and the power of thought for good or ill to transform body function.[7] Yet, beliefs such as these can lead to demoralization, depression, and self-blame when (given advanced stage at diagnoses in these patients) if or when the cancer does return.[7,213] Likewise, a study in Northeast Thailand found that *mot luuk* problems (translated literally as cancer in the mouth of the uterus) has a wide range of causes and a variety of events that occur over time to make a woman more susceptible to cervical cancer. Women with recurrent symptoms, for instance, see these problems as resulting from failing to follow traditional postpartum practices including "staying by the fire" or *yuu fai*, germs, an injury, working too hard in youth, a difficult pregnancy or abortion or sterilization.[214]

Culture, Causation, and Cancer Prevention: Western and Non-Western Contexts

Still other investigations assess perceptions that breast cancer is a disease of White people.[204,205] Research using narrative analysis, for instance, found that African-American women often perceived that cancer as a disease of White women and not African-American women. These women also report that oncology care and treatments are designed to enhance the care of White women, but not African-American women.[203-205] Comparable studies on rural women in the United States and Xhosa women in South Africa also note that there is the underlying belief that breast cancer is still a fatal disease and thus one should abscond from treatment since there is really no point in having conventional medical treatment.[201,220–21,215-221] Wood, for instance, in a study of womb cancer in Colored and Black South African women, found that the cancer was described as eating away the womb and that the womb first gets tired, then it become loose, and then it gets eaten. This leads to an itchy discharge and terrible pains. It is also perceived to be terminal since no one could recall anyone who had survived it, even if the women had consulted with doctors or traditional healers in the attempt to be cured.[210] Likewise, in other rural communities in South Africa, indigenous healers are perceived to be the only legitimate and successful healers of cancer given their expert knowledge of the causes and cures of cancer.[15,16,200,201,217-219] In other situations, the failure of curative efforts represents a sign, which then is used to reinforce a reliance on traditional therapies, at the expense of the use of conventional Western biomedical treatments. This can also lead to doubts regarding the efficacy of Western biomedical treatments, if prevention is truly worthwhile, or if the cancer can actually be cured using Western biomedical tools.[15,16,88,144,145,200,201,203-205] For example, in both Nigeria and Tanzania, the failure of Western medicine to obtain a cure for advanced stage cancer is often perceived as a signal to initiate other health care services.[15,200,201,217-221] For these reasons, many patients and families request a discharge, perhaps even against medical advice to seek the care of traditional healers. These cultural beliefs and associated practices, often termed *cancer fatalism* in the oncology literatures, are enduring, working, against cancer detection and prevention efforts in the global setting, since why would anyone endure cancer screening tests that to them seem to serve only as heralds of a disease that will ultimately kill them.[144,145,149,200,201,203-205]

Similar findings regarding the impact of cultural beliefs on health prevention is in testing for sexually transmitted disease and genetic testing, where a positive result has implications not only for the individual but also for the family. McCaffery[231] in a recent analysis of White British, African Caribbean, Pakistani, and Indian attitudes toward HPV testing noted that many of the women were not fully aware of the sexually transmitted nature of cervical cancer and expressed anxiety, confusion, and stigma about HPV as a sexually transmitted infection. Testing positive for HPV raised important issues for women's relationships in terms of trust, blame, fidelity, and protection through safer sex. In addition, testing had the potential to communicate unwanted messages to one's partner, family, and the wider community about trust and sexual behaviors. Concerns were expressed by women from all of the ethnic groups, but appeared to be particularly pertinent for some of the Indian and Pakistani women, for whom sex outside marriage can be strongly proscribed. In such circumstances, HPV infection (or perceived risk of infection) would have more significant consequences, and these findings have serious implications particularly among some South Asian women, whose chosen sexual lifestyle may directly impact on their family and wider community.[231] Similarly, in Cambodia, Africa, Japan, and China, there is an emphasis on family reputation, lineage, and privacy. In these contexts, the shame associated with cancer or even cancer testing (genetics or screening) is a polluting force since its affects are not only inflicted on the individual by their diagnosis, but also on the family.[15,16,125,126,211,214,225,226] A recent study highlighting cultural variations in genetic testing, for instance, found that chiefly the male line of descent from a common ancestor defines the kindred. Thus, a disease "running in the family" may be construed as being derived directly from a common ancestor and this belief may adversely impact help seeking behaviors.[149,226]

Such differences are also apparent within the Western context. In studies on cervical cancer, for instance, Spanish-speaking Latinas and women of Asian descent in North America endorse fatalistic beliefs and misconceptions, which lead to delays in care including screening as primary cancer prevention.[228] Gregg and colleagues, in their study, found that the cancer models those African-American women in North America held were very different from those held by their clinicians.[144,145] The women attending the clinics often endured cancer-screening tests that to them seemed to serve only as a messenger of a disease that would kill them.[145] While the women in this particular study were not cancer survivors, they held quite negative impressions of breast and cervical cancer screenings as primary cancer prevention, since no one they knew seemed to survive cancer. This research study parallels what medical anthropologist Balsham[144] found in her study on cancer in a community of working class Whites; that to think about cancer, to try to prevent it, was to tempt fate. Put differently: "cancer testing is looking for trouble."[144,145] As a consequence, often talking about or even thinking about cancer (or about prevention) conjured this disease, bringing it into existence, in a social, economic, and biomedical context where cancer generally means death.[144,145,149,226]

In sum, despite apparent advances in medical science that have led to effective treatments for cancer, such myths influence beliefs about causation, expectations regarding the meanings and the course of illness, treatment can serve as barriers to early detection, treatment, and recovery. Reinforcing these points are negative attitudes toward cancer or the environment where cancer is treated, which can also perpetuate cultural barrier to communication between patients and clinicians and may influence decision-making about referrals and treatments.

Truth Telling, Disclosure, and Hope

Amidst a decline in public trust in the medical profession, cultural norms regarding clinician-patient communication have significantly changed.[143,222] As a consequence, open disclosure of the cancer diagnosis, and discussions of available treatment options and the statistical likelihood of survival and death from cancer, have become common in the war on cancer waged by oncology clinicians and patients alike[128-135] (see also Chapter 6 by Kelly, this volume). Nonetheless, the ways risk and treatment decisions are evaluated even within the Western context is also culturally mediated. In the North American context, for instance, there is great emphasis on patient autonomy, immediacy of action, and a shared decision-making model for health. Yet in France (and in many other European societies, Japan, the Middle East, Africa), relationships with patients are much more hierarchical, protective, and paternalistic (see also Chapter 8 by Spiegel, this volume). In these cultures, truth may be culturally interpreted and valued in terms of patient protection.[7,13,15,16,88,132,167]

Truth telling evolves in interactions over time and the synchrony of time between clinician and patient shapes the biomedical objectives and the cultural context of care.[88,198] What the patient believes about time has a great deal to do with underlying beliefs and expectations about health, illness, and disease.[88,198] A patient's readiness to hear a poor prognosis or discuss end of life issues may very much depend on his/her own assessment of the time they have left. There are two dimensions of truth in medicine that are equally important: the patient's subjective perception of disease and the context which varies according to the historical, cultural, and spiritual background of the patient and clinician (see also Chapter 11 by Penson and Chapter 12 by Gibson et al., this volume).[7,88,198]

An important study of US oncologists highlights these findings, noting that patient concerns are managed over time and in the context of an evolving relationship.[7] At each stage of an extended process of disclosure, consideration is given to the level of hope patients and families should be encouraged to maintain. As with disclosure, hope is staged, given in calibrated, achievable, and realistic bits.[7,223] Hope, for these reasons, is Janusfaced with caring conveyed through the contexts of treatments, through the offering of new therapeutic, potentially beneficial treatment options and through the holding out of hope for the development of new treatments and hopes for a cure.[7] Nevertheless, while hope is associated with heightened activation of the autonomic nervous system, personal animation, and social connectedness,[7,22] it is also mediated by cultural, ethnic, and socioeconomic concerns. As we have noted, minority, elderly, culturally and linguistically diverse, and medically underserved patients in many societies in both Western and non-Western contexts are least likely to have adequate access to care.[22,27,37-39,51-57,63-72] Often they might not even have a longstanding relationship with their primary caregiver. Others either have nonexistent social networks or networks that have limited resources or they cannot respond adequately to the challenges of their illness. It is often quite difficult to have "hope" in such circumstances, and patients and family members may eventually feel demoralized by inadequate care and adverse prognoses and outcomes.[37-39] Demoralization as the opposite of hope in such contexts is associated with contrary effects. In addition, the negative messages from the health care environment and from the patient's social and economic milieu can reinforce these adverse context effects. Such profound demoralization can also lead to what Engel has described as the *giving up/giving up complex*, where following a stressful situation the person feels unable to cope and has no expectation that any change will possibly help.[233]

In contrast, in disclosing a cancer diagnosis in Tanzania, clinicians may invoke *therapeutic privilege*.[16] They factor in issues such as treatment availability, age, stigma associated with cancer that would adversely affect the family, prognosis about time left to live, and patient poverty, as moral justifications for withholding diagnostic and prognostic information from patients with cancer. Direct disclosure is seen in these instances to harm the patient, to strip them of hope, and clinicians even encourage patients with advanced stage disease to consult alternative healers to seek comfort for their disease.[16] Similarly, Ethiopian immigrants' preference for nondisclosure of terminal illness arises from cultural beliefs regarding appropriateness of space, time, and familial support. Direct disclosure of cancer status is considered "cruel," "inconsiderate," and even damaging since it is deemed as a failure to properly care for the patient, give them hope, or protect them from harm. Indeed, direct action against the patient's beliefs may distress patients, leading to a deterioration of their health.[7,16,88] Likewise, the Issan people of Northeast Thailand also believe that cancer is an incurable and painful disease, the direct result of a *kamma* that is feared by all. Thus, a person experiencing a long and painful cancer is considered a victim of his own *kamma* and the term *modbun* or finishing one's merit is frequently used as a metaphor for death.[225] Nonetheless, cancer is not the same as a tumor (which can be cured). Similar to other studies in non-Western contexts, clinicians and village people alike believe that telling the truth to a person with cancer robs them of hope and will *(kamlancai)*, and is likely to provoke rapid decline and death.[7,16,88,225] For these reasons, if the disclosure is made, clinicians will often tell the patient that they have a tumor that is curable, while informing the family that the person has cancer.[225] Thus, when the clinician tells a patient with few resources the truth about their cancer, without understanding the underlying cultural meanings, they may inadvertently demoralize the patient by extinguishing their hope. This can unintentionally impede progress of patients, and in the long term affect the health behaviors of patients and other members in their communities.[7,15,16,22,225,231]

Impact on the Family

A diagnosis of cancer often causes great suffering to patients and families.[7,15,88,225] A major source of differences in truth-telling practice lies in the degree to which the individual or family is seen as the primary focus for medical communication.[15-17,149,156] As we previously mentioned, in many Western and non-Western cultures, relationships with patients are often much more hierarchical, protective, and paternalistic than in the North American culture, and the family remains the central organizing structure, particularly when an individual is ill.[7,15,16,88,125,126,198] As a consequence, when time is in short supply, and the cancer and related symptoms become unbearable, the family often becomes important in managing the disease (see Chapter 11, this volume).[125–126,198] For example, in a survey of Chinese cancer patients and carers living in Australia, the majority said that the family should advise the doctor how much information to give to the patient, and in what manner, as they knew the patient very well.[112] Most patients indicated a preference for the family to be fully informed about issues relating to the illness to allow each family member to contribute as much as possible to the support of the patient.[112] Participants expressed the view that full disclosure of information was important so that the responsibilities of the sick person could be assumed by others, and appropriate planning for the future could be undertaken. This familial support is seen as a coping mechanism whereby members provide mutual economic and emotional support, with the members relying on social ties created and maintained in such groups.[15-17,88,112,125,126]

In Japan, family members are informed of the cancer patient's diagnosis, condition, and treatment, before the cancer patient is told the truth.[125,126,232] Then all family members, except the patient, discuss whether the cancer diagnosis should be disclosed and the entire family makes a final decision about the truth-telling policy. A survey in Japan of 1918 family caregivers who had recently cared for a cancer patient who died was undertaken in 1992. All family caregivers reported that the physician informed them of the condition and treatment, although only 22.5% of the cancer patients were informed.[234] Similarly, in Saudi Arabia, the patient is viewed as one member of the larger family, and the family is responsible for the patient. The consent for the patient's treatment is usually a substitute consent given by the family, who aims to avoid emotional disturbance to the patient.[235]

In South Africa, patients with cancer (particularly in rural areas) are also not necessarily the key decision-makers with regard to the different therapeutic choices available.[217-200-201,218] Care and help seeking is collaborative involving family members and sometimes elders of the community. Given the role of these individuals in decision-making, it is still, often, suggested that patient's abscond from further Western treatment and visit the traditional healers.[201] African patients living in the milieu of an urban community, with exposure to Western medical standards of care and where there are fewer tribal ties, however, may have the necessary freedom of action and choice to obtain available medical attention. Nevertheless, in general, patients tend to conform to cultural and familial norms since in most cases, it is more important to please the family, given that patients fear rejection and a lonely death.[200,201,218]

These cultures differ from the Western context where the individual is generally seen as the unit of care, and familial needs for information are secondary to those of the patient. Furthermore, in some Western centers it is still considered unethical practice to disclose anything to relatives without the patient's permission. This may mean that relatives are actually denied information about diagnosis or prognosis if the patient so wishes, forming a very different practice to that pursued in family-centered cultures, and potentially causing great angst if the family culture emphasizes different values.[88,200,201,218]

METHODOLOGIES

Exploring cultural issues in cancer communication and strategies to optimize outcome is not easy. One common and useful strategy has been to compare results of similar surveys/audits across different cultures.

Exploration of patient and doctor preferences for information and involvement in decision-making, has been undertaken in many countries[112] and when similar methodologies have been used to elicit these preferences, cross-cultural comparisons are not difficult. This however assumes that the measuring instruments have been validated in each setting, which is not always the case. It may be that patients surveyed in different settings or times might respond similarly but actually mean something different. For instance, one might expect cultural variation in the meanings associated with this illness to be somewhat different in the patient who has just learned that they have cancer or metastasis to the brain, as compared with a long-term disease-free individual. Furthermore, attitudes to completing surveys may vary across cultures. Indigenous Australians, for example, prefer to present a group view, reached after discussion and consultation with elders, rather than an individual response. Thus, questionnaires in this setting are likely to produce missing or invalid responses.

For these reasons, qualitative or ethnographic studies have dominated this field (see also Cross-Cultural Resources section, end of this chapter). As there may be some pressure to produce socially desirable responses, in-depth interviewing or observation by a person trusted by the community who speaks the language and understands the subtext are likely to produce more valid data, useful to the clinician who is trying to communicate effectively within different cultures. Such a person may be difficult to find and may take a long time to reach a position of trust. Once the data are collected, translation may be required. This needs to be done by a trained, accredited translator. Ideally, the data should be translated and back-translated to check for accuracy and meaning.[235,236] The final report can be brought back to the people who generated the data, to check that it accords with their understanding.

The impact of acculturation has been rarely explored. While several studies have explored attitudes and behaviors in groups of migrants,[88,112] these have not been directly compared with people of similar ethnic background in their country of origin. In several qualitative studies in which the level of acculturation of participants was measured, acculturation was associated with degree of interest in traditional medicines, but with no other attitudes, suggesting either that in sickness people revert to traditional views, or that there are fewer differences between cultures than might be expected.[88]

Much remains to be learned about context effects in health, and methods for providing effective cross-cultural health care. Most studies have focused on single ethnic groups, and have not taken into account complexities such as level of acculturation, mixed ethnocultural heritage, interactions between ethnicity and other group characteristics such as sexual orientation and age, and the match between patient, health professional, and system factors. Thus, future work in this area needs to increase in complexity and sophistication.[88,235,236] The following guidelines, resources, websites, and references may also assist in communicating with culturally diverse patients with cancer.

GUIDELINES FOR CULTURALLY COMPETENT CARE

1. Become aware of your own ethnocultural history, identity and world view, of your preconceptions and stereotypes of other cultures, and of ways in which you may benefit from inequities of power and resources.
2. Find out the ethno-religious-cultural groups to which your patients belong.
3. Build your knowledge of important beliefs, attitudes, and preferences common in such groups. The References section provides a starting point for suitable reading.
4. Attendance at churches, festivals and films, and reading novels are other ways of gaining familiarity with cultural views. There may also be ethnocultural education materials available through your institution (or through the websites listed at the end of this chapter).
5. Build on your knowledge of what health means to the individual in other cultural contexts. Remember that the ways that cancer and treatment are prioritized in individual decision-making in the West are not always the ways that patients and family members cope with such concerns. Such information represents an important starting point for understanding the patient's explanatory models of illness and disease.
6. Build your knowledge of cultural and socioeconomic barriers to optimal health care experienced by different groups and consider taking action to overcome these barriers (eg, extended clinic hours, satellite clinics, reimbursement for travel expenses for clinical visits [ie, clinical trial], use of interpreters; the production of culturally specific educational materials and programs).
7. Spend time at the beginning of the consultation establishing the ethno-cultural context from which your patient (and their family) comes, the language and words that they use to convey their understanding of the disease (which may contrast Western biomedical reasoning and words), their reason for referral and clinic procedures. Note and be prepared for the fact that this cultural insight tends to occur *over time* rather than in this initial consultation.

8. If appropriate, acknowledge that communication problems could potentially occur, and the importance of both parties checking understanding and sharing views and values.
9. Explicitly explore preferences for information, involvement in decision-making, and preferred mode of information delivery (initially to cancer patient or through the family). This is preferably done with all parties present. You could share your own views and their rationale, but indicate your willingness to allow the patient and family to determine the course of action.
10. Employ professional interpreters when language is a barrier; avoid using family or friends as interpreters if possible, as they can act as gate-keepers, misunderstand, and pass on incorrect information or cause suppression of important issues (such as sexual dysfunction, spirituality, death and dying, and palliative care).
11. Avoid stereotyping about cultural groups since there is always variation in preferences. As such, the clinician must always remain open to individual differences within cultural groups.

CROSS-CULTURAL RESOURCES

Websites

- Multi-Cultural Resource Centre (Northern Ireland)
  www.mcrc-ni.org
- North West Ethnic Health (UK)
  www.ethnichealth-northwest.net
  http://www.health.qld.gov.au/hssb/hou/links.htm
  http://mhcs.health.nsw.gov.au/
  http://medicine.ucsf.edu/resources/guidelines/culture.html
  http://www.culturediversity.org
- EthnoMed: Ethnic Medicine Guide
  http://ethnomed.org/
- Conversations in Care: web book on cancer communication
  http://www.conversationsincare.org/web_book/
- Culture Clues™: Culture Clues© are tip sheets for clinicians designed to increase awareness of cultural diversity. Currently there are seven cultures represented, such as Albanian, African American, Chinese, Korean, Latino, Russian, and Vietnamese
  http://depts.washington.edu/pfes/culturalclues.html

- Cross-Cultural Health Care Program: Cultural Diversity and Cultural Competency Training, Interpreter Training, and Translation Services. Profiles of Ethnic Communities
  http://xculture.org
- Diversity Rx: Promoting language and cultural competence to improve the quality of health care for minority, immigrant, and ethnically diverse communities
  http://www.diversityrx.org
- Office of Minority Health, Department of Health and Human Services
  http://www.omhrc.gov
- UICC International Directory of Cancer (Internationale Contre le Cancer)
  http://www.uicc.org/publ/directory
- People Living With Cancer
  http://www.plwc.org/plwc/
- American Cancer Society
  www.acs.org
- National Institutes of Health (US)
  www.nih.gov
- University of California, San Francisco, School of Medicine, Department of Medicine
  http://medicine.ucsf.edu/resources/guidelines/culture.html
- CancerBACUP (United Kingdom)
  http://www.cancerbacup.org.uk/
- Cancer Black Care (UK)
  www.cancerblackcare.org
- Race Equality in the Department of Health, United Kingdom Department of Health
  www.doh.gov.uk/race_equality/index.htm
- Cancer Research UK
  http://www.cancerresearchuk.org/
- Research into ageing (UK)
  www.ageing.com
- Cancer Services Collaborative
  www.modern.nhs.uk
- MacMillan Cancer Relief
  www.macmillan.org.uk
- Cancer Support UK
  www.cancersupportuk.nhs.uk
- National Cancer Institute, Usability.gov: a resource for improving the communication of cancer research
  http://usability.gov/lessons/index.html

- Office of Cancer Information, National Cancer Institute
  http://www.health.gov/NHIC/
- Gillette Cancer Connection
  http://www.gillettecancerconnect.org/
- Agency for Toxic Substances and Disease Registry, Health Risk Communication Primer
  http://www.atsdr.cdc.gov/HEC/primer.html
- Centers for Disease Control and Prevention, Epidemiology Program Office
  http://www.cdc.gov/epo/index.htm
- Centers for Disease Control and Prevention, Office of Communication
  http://www.cdc.gov/od/oc/media/index.htm
- Communication Initiative
  http://www.comminit.com/index.html/
- Mitretek Systems, "Criteria for Assessing the Quality of Health Information on the Internet"
  http://hitiweb.mitretek.org/docs/criteria.html
- Refugee experience: psychosocial training module
  http://earlybird.qeh.ox.ac.uk/rfgexp/start.htm

SUGGESTED READINGS

Apanovitch AM, McCarthy D, Salovey P. Using message framing to motivate HIV testing among low-income, ethnic minority women. *Health Psychol.* 2003;22(1):60-67.

Aruguete MS, Roberts CA. Participants' ratings of male physicians who vary in race and communication style. *Psychol Rep.* 2002;91(3 Pt 1):793-806.

Baile WF, Lenzi R, Parker PA, Buckman R, Cohen L. Oncologists' attitudes toward and practices in giving bad news: an exploratory study. *J Clin Oncol.* 2002;20(8):2189-2196.

Bakker LJ, Cavender A. Promoting culturally competent care for gay youth. *J Sch Nurs.* 2003;19(2):65-72.

Baty BJ, Kinney AY, Ellis SM. Developing culturally sensitive cancer genetics communication aids for African Americans. *Am J Med Genet.* 2003; 118A(2):146-155.

Bean DL, Rotheram-Borus MJ, Leibowitz A, Horwitz SM, Weidmer B. Spanish-language services assessment for children and adolescents (SACA): reliability of parent and adolescent reports. *J Am Acad Child Adolesc Psychiatr.* 2003;42(2):241-248.

Betancourt JR, Green AR, Carrillo JE. The challenges of cross-cultural healthcare—diversity, ethics, and the medical. *Bioethics Forum.* 2000;16(3):27-32.

Bruce J, Link Jo Phelan. Social conditions as fundamental causes of disease. *Health Soc Behav.* 1995; extra issue:80-94.

Buckman R. Communication skills in palliative care: a practical guide. *Neurol Clin.* 2001;19(4):989-1004.

Burr JA, Mutchler JE. English language skills, ethnic concentration, and household composition: older Mexican immigrants. *J Gerontol B Psychol Sci Soc Sci.* 2003;58(2):S83-S92.

Chrystal K, Allan S, Forgeson G, Isaacs R. The use of complementary/alternative medicine by cancer patients in a New Zealand regional cancer treatment centre. *N Z Med J.* 2003;16(1168):U296.

Cioffi RN. Communicating with culturally and linguistically diverse patients in an acute care setting: nurses' experiences. *Int J Nurs Stud.* 2003;40(3):299-306.

Chloe E Bird, Patricia P Rieker. Gender matters: an integrated model for understanding men's and women's health. *Soc Sci Med.* 1999;48:745-755.

Costalas JW, Itzen M, Malick J, et al. Related Articles, Links Abstract Communication of BRCA1 and BRCA2 results to at-risk relatives: a cancer risk assessment program's experience. *Am J Med Genet.* 2003;119C(1):11-18.

Cram F, Smith L, Johnstone W. Mapping the themes of Maori talk about health. *N Z Med J.* 2003;116(1170):1p following U353.

Dean RA. Native American humor: implications for transcultural care. *J Transcult Nurs.* 2003;14(1):62-65.

Diaz VA Jr. Cultural factors in preventive care: Latinos. *Prim Care.* 2002;29(3):503-517, viii.

Dunckley M, Hughes R, Addington-Hall J, Higginson IJ. Language translation of outcome measurement tools: Views of health professionals. *Int J Palliat Nurs.* 2003;9(2): 49-55.

Fleming DA. Cultural sensitivity in end-of-life discussions. *Mo Med.* 2003;100(1):69-75.

Geller G, Tambor ES, Bernhardt BA, Fraser G, Wissow LS. Related Articles, Links Abstract Informed consent for enrolling minors in genetic susceptibility research: a qualitative study of at-risk children's and parents' views about children's role in decision-making. *J Adolesc Health.* 2003;32(4):260-271.

Greer AL, Goodwin JS, Freeman JL, Wu ZH. Bringing the patient back in. Guidelines, practice variations, and the social context of medical practice. *Int J Technol Assess Health Care.* 2002;18(4):747-761.

Hantho A, Jensen L, Malterud K. Mutual understanding: a communication model for general practice. *Scand J Prim Health Care.* 2002;20(4):244-251.

Ishii K, Reyes JA, Kitayama S. Spontaneous attention to word content versus emotional tone: differences among three cultures. *Psychol Sci.* 2003;14(1):39-46.

Jejeebhoy SJ. Convergence and divergence in spouses' perspectives on women's autonomy in rural India. *Stud Fam Plann.* 2002;33(4):299-308.

Jeppsson A, Ostergren PO, Hagstrom B. Restructuring a ministry of health—an issue of structure and process: a case study from Uganda. *Health Policy Plan.* 2003;18(1):68-73.

Kagawa-Singer M, Wellisch DK. Breast cancer patients' perceptions of their husbands' support in a cross-cultural context. *Psychooncology.* 2003;12(1):24-37.

Karakiewicz PI, Kattan MW, Tanguay S, et al. Cross-cultural validation of the UCLA prostate cancer index. *Urology.* 2003;61(2):302-307.

Kearns CJ, Meehan NK, Carr RL, Park LI. Using cross-cultural definitions of health care. *Nurse Pract.* 2003 Jan;28(1):61-62.

Kelly, PT. Hereditary breast cancer: risk assessment is the easy part. *Breast J.* 1999;52-58.

Krieger N. Embodying inequality: A review of concepts, measures, and methods for studying health consequences of discrimination. *Int J Health Serv.* 1999; 29(2):295-352.

Lin Y, Rancer AS. Sex differences in intercultural communication apprehension, ethnocentrism, and intercultural willingness to communicate. *Psychol Rep.* 2003;92(1):195-200.

Luffy R, Grove SK. Examining the validity, reliability, and preference of three pediatric pain measurement tools in African-American children. *Pediatr Nurs.* 2003;29(1):54-59.

Mak MH. Awareness of dying: an experience of Chinese patients with terminal cancer. *Omega* (Westport). 2001;43(3):259-279.

Maly RC, Leake B, Silliman RA. Health care disparities in older patients with breast carcinoma: informational support from physicians. *Cancer.* 2003;97(6):1517-1527.

Marshall MN, Shekelle PG, McGlynn EA, Campbell S, Brook RH, Roland MO. Can health care quality indicators be transferred between countries? *Qual Saf Health Care.* 2003;12(1):8-12.

Maund T, Espinosa JA, Kosnik LK, Scharf J. Video-storytelling: a step-by-step guide. *Jt Comm J Qual Saf.* 2003;29(3):152-155.

Mclean C, Campbell C, Cornish F. African-Caribbean interactions with mental health services in the UK: Experiences and expectations of exclusion as (re)productive of health inequalities. *Soc Sci Med.* 2003;56(3):657-669.

Mill JE, Ogilvie LD. Establishing methodological rigour in international qualitative nursing research: a case study from Ghana. *J Adv Nurs.* 2003;41(1):80-87.

Narayanasamy A. Transcultural nursing: how do nurses respond to cultural needs? *Br J Nurs.* 2003;12(3):185-194.

Newell S, Edelman L, Scarbrough H, Swan J, Bresnen M. 'Best practice' development and transfer in the NHS: The importance of process as well as product knowledge. *Health Serv Manage Res.* 2003;16(1):1-12.

Ngo-Metzger Q, Massagli MP, Clarridge BR, et al. Linguistic and cultural barriers to care. *J Gen Intern Med.* 2003;18(1):44-52.

Ohlinger J, Brown MS, Laudert S, Swanson S, Fofah O. Development of potentially better practices for the neonatal intensive care unit as a culture of collaboration: communication, accountability, respect, and empowerment. *Pediatrics.* 2003;111(4 Pt 2):e471-e481.

Olesen F. A framework for clinical general practice and for research and teaching in the discipline. *Fam Pract.* 2003;20(3):318-323.

Parsons LC. Transcultural communication: the cornerstone of culturally competent care. *SCI Nurs.* 2002;19(4):160-163.

Post DM, Cegala DJ, Marinelli TM. Teaching patients to communicate with physicians: the impact of race. *J Natl Med Assoc.* 2001;93(1):6-12.

Randhawa G, Owens A, Fitches R, Khan Z. Communication in the development of culturally competent palliative care services in the UK: a case study. *Int J Palliat Nurs.* 2003;9(1):24-31.

Rudan VT. The best of both worlds: a consideration of gender in team building. *J Nurs Adm.* 2003;33(3):179-186.

Stone J. Race and healthcare disparities: Overcoming vulnerability. *Theor Med Bioeth.* 2002;23(6):499-518.

Sweeney C, Bruera E. Communication in cancer care: recent developments. *J Palliat Care.* 2002;18(4):300-306.

Thomas EJ, Sexton JB, Helmreich RL. Discrepant attitudes about teamwork among critical care nurses and physicians. *Crit Care Med.* 2003;31(3):956-959.

Volpp KG, Grande D. Residents' suggestions for reducing errors in teaching hospitals. *N Engl J Med.* 2003;348(9):851-855.

Wass V, Roberts C, Hoogenboom R, Jones R, Van der Vleuten C. Effect of ethnicity on performance in a final objective structured clinical examination: Qualitative and quantitative study. *BMJ.* 2003;12;326(7393):800-803.

Watters EK. Literacy for health: An interdisciplinary model. *J Transcult Nurs.* 2003;14(1):48-54.

Williams-Brown S, Baldwin DM, Bakos A. Storytelling as a method to teach African American women breast health information. *J Cancer Educ.* 2002;17(4):227-230.

Williams DR. Race, socioeconomic status, and health. The added effects of racism and discrimination. *Ann N Y Acad Sci.* 1999;896:173-188.

Wireman JR, Long GC. Communicating risk in diverse communities. *Toxicol Ind Health.* 2001;17(5-10):298-301.
Witt D, Brawer R, Plumb J. Cultural factors in preventive care: African-Americans. *Prim Care.* 2002;29(3):487-493.
Worsley P. Non-Western medical systems. *Annu Rev. Anthropol.* 1982;11:315-348.
Young, A. The anthropologies of illness and sickness. *Annu Rev Anthropol.* 1982;11:257-285.

RECOMMENDED BOOKS

Aguilar L, Stokes L. *Multicultural Customer Services: Providing Outstanding Service Across Cultures.* Chicago, IL: Irwin Professional Publishing/Mirror Press; 1996.
Aguirre-Molina M, Molina CW, Zambrana RE. *Health Issues in the Latino Community.* John Wiley & Sons; 2001.
American Cancer Society. *Good for You: Reducing Your Risk of Developing Cancer.* 2002.
American Cancer Society. *Cancer: What Causes It, What Doesn't* 2003.
Baker S. *Managing Patient Expectations: The Art of Finding and Keeping Loyal Patients.* Jossey Bass; 1998.
Beck U. *The Risk Society and Beyond: Critical Issues for Social Theory.* Sage Publications; 2000.
Becker H. *Outsiders: Studies in the Sociology of Deviance.* Free Press; 1985.
Berkman L, Kawachi I. *Social Epidemiology.* Oxford University press; 2000.
Borkan JM, Reis S, Medalie JH, Steinmetz D. *Patients and Doctors: Life-Changing Stories from Primary Care.* Univ of Wisconsin Press; 1999.
Brislin RW, Yoshida, T. *Improving Intercultural Interactions: Modules for Cross-Cultural Training Programs.* Newbury Park, CA: Sage Publications, 1994.
Broyard A. *Intoxicated by My Illness and Other Writings on Life and Death.* Fawcett Books; October 1998.
Buckman R, Kason Y. *How to Break Bad News: A Guide for Health Care Professionals.* Johns Hopkins Univ Press; 1992.
Byock I. *Dying Well: Peace and Possibilities at the End of Life.* Riverhead Books; 1998.
Campo R. *Education in Empathy, Identity, and Poetry.* W.W. Norton & Company; 1998.
Carey JW. *Communication As Culture: Essays on Media and Society (Media and Popular Culture 1).* Unwin Hyman; December 1988.
Charon R, Montello M. *Stories Matter: The Role of Narrative in Medical Ethics.* Routledge; 2002.
Coles R, Testa R, O'Donnell J. *A Life in Medicine: A Literary Anthology.* New Press; 2002.
Conrad P, Gabe J. *Sociological Perspectives on the New Genetics (Sociology of Health and Illness).* Blackwell Publishers; 1999.
Desmond J, Copeland L. *Communicating with Today's Patient: Essentials to Save Time, Decrease Risk, and Increase Patient Compliance.* San Francisco, CA: Jossey-Bass, 2000.
DiClemente RJ, Crosby RA, Kegler MC. *Emerging Theories in Health Promotion Practice and Research: Strategies for Improving Public Health.* John Wiley & Sons; 2002.
Doak CC, Doak, LG, Root, JH. *Teaching Patients With Low Literacy Skills.* Philadelphia, PA: J.B. Lippincott Company; 1985.
Eliason, M. *Who Cares? Institutional Barriers to Healthcare for Lesbian, Gay, and Bisexual Persons.* New York: National League for Nursing Press; 1996.
Fadiman A. *The Spirit Catches You and You Fall Down.* Farrar Straus & Giroux; 1998.
Farmer P. *AIDS and Accusation: Haiti and the Geography of Blame (Comparative Studies of Health Systems and Medical Care, No 33).* University of California Press; 1993.

Farmer P, Connors M, Simmons J, eds. *Women, Poverty and AIDS: Sex, Drugs and Structural Violence (Series in Health and Social Justice).* Common Courage Press; 1996.

Frank A. *The Wounded Storyteller: Body, Illness, and Ethics.* University of Chicago Press; 1997.

Frank A. *At the Will of the Body: Reflections on Illness.* Mariner Books; 1992.

Galanti GA. *Caring for Patients from Different Cultures: Case Studies from American Hospitals.* Philadelphia, PA: University of Pennsylvania Press; 1992.

Garrett, L. *Betrayal of Trust: The Collapse of Global Public Health.* Hyperion; 2001.

Gerteis M, Edgman-Levitan S, Daley J, Delbanco T, eds. *Through the Patient's Eyes: Understanding and Promoting Patient-Centered Care.* Jossey-Bass, 1993.

Gawande A. *Complications: A Surgeon's Notes on an Imperfect Science.* Picador; 2003.

Goffman E. *Stigma: Notes on the Management of a Spoiled Identity.* Touchstone Books; 1986.

Groopman J. *Second Opinions: Stories of Intuition and Choice in a Changing World of Medicine.* Viking Press; 2000.

Grealy L. *Autobiography of a Face.* New York, NY: HarperCollins; 2003.

Groopman J. *The Measure of Our Days: A Spiritual Exploration of Illness.* Penguin; 1998.

Gropper RC. *Culture and the Clinical Encounter: An Intercultural Sensitizer for the Health Professions.* Yarmouth, ME: Intercultural Press, Inc, 1996.

Hollingsworth A. *The Truth About Breast Cancer Risk Assessment.* National Writers Press; 2000.

Henderson G. *Women at Risk: The Hpv Epidemic and Your Cervical Health.* Avery Penguin Putnam; 2002.

Komaromy C. *Dilemmas in UK Health Care (Health and Disease).* Open Univ Pr; 2001.

Kawachi I, Berkman L. *Neighborhoods and Health.* Oxford University Press; 2003.

Kawachi I, Kennedy BP, Wilkinson R eds. *The Society and Population Health Reader: Income Inequality and Health.* New Press; 1999.

Kelly PT. *Assess Your True Risk of Breast Cancer.* New York, NY: Henry Holt and Company; 2000.

Kleinman A. *Writing at the Margins: Discourse Between Anthropology and Medicine.* University of California Press; 1997.

Kleinman A. *Patients and Healers in the Context of Culture.* University of California Press; 1981.

Kreps GL, Kunimoto EN. *Effective Communication in Multicultural Health Care Settings.* Thousand Oaks CA: Sage Publications, 1994.

Kus R, ed. *Keys to Caring: Assisting Your Gay and Lesbian Clients.* Boston, MA: Alyson; 1990.

LaVeist T. *Race, Ethnicity, and Health: A Public Health Reader.* Jossey-Bass; 2002.

Lupton D. *Medicine as Culture: Illness, Disease and the Body in Western Societies.* Sage Publications; 1994.

Mattingly C, Garro L. *Narrative and the Cultural Construction of Illness and Healing.* University of California Press; 2000.

Morris D. *Culture of Pain.* University of California Press; 1993.

Morris D. *Illness and Culture in the Postmodern Age.* University of California Press; 2000.

Nelson HL. *Stories and Their Limits: Narrative Approaches to Bioethics.* Routledge; 1997.

Nuland S. *How We Die: Reflections on Life's Final Chapter.* Vintage Books; 1995.

Scarry E. *The Body in Pain.* Oxford University Press; 1985.

Silverman J, Kurtz SM, DraperJ. *Skills for Communicating With Patients.* Radcliffe Medical Pr Lt, 1998.

Spiro HM. *Empathy and the Practice of Medicine.* Yale Univ Press; 1993.

Spiro HM. *The Power of Hope: A Doctor's Perspective.* Yale University Press; 1998.

Vogel V. *Management of Patients at High Risk for Breast Cancer.* Blackwell Science Inc; 2001.

Weisman J. *As I Live and Breathe: Notes of a Patient-Doctor.* North Point Press; 2002.

Wright P, Treacher A. *Problem of Medical Knowledge.* Edinburgh Univ Press; 1982.

REFERENCES

1. Randall-David E. *Strategies for Working with Culturally Diverse Communities and Clients, Comprehensive Hemophilia Program, Bowman Gray School of Medicine.* Bethesda, MD: Association for the Care of Children Health; 1989.
2. Weil J. Multicultural education and genetic counseling. *Clin Genet.* 2001;59:143-149.
3. Van Baalen M, Jansen VA. Common language or Tower of Babel? On the evolutionary dynamics of signals and their meanings. *Proc R Soc Lond B Biol Sci.* 2003;270(1510):69-76.
4. Moore RJ. African American women and breast cancer: notes from a study of narrative. *Cancer Nurs.* 2001 Feb;24(1):35-42.
5. Morris D. *Culture and Pain.* Berkeley: University of California Press; 1999.
6. Kleinman A. *Patients and Healers in the context of culture.* Berkeley, CA: University of California Press; 1980.
7. Delvecchio Good MJ, Good BJ, Schaffer C, Lind SE. American oncology and the discourse on hope. *Cult Med Psychiatry.* 1990;14(1):59-79.
8. Lakoff G. *Metaphors We Live by.* Chicago: University of Chicago Press; 2003.
9. Plato. In: *Plato Complete Works.* Cooper JM ed. Hackett Pub Co, 1997.
10. Balint M. *The doctor, his Patient and the Illness.* London: Pitman; 1957.
11. Roter D. The medical visit context of treatment decision-making and the therapeutic relationship. *Health Expect.* 2000;3(1):17-2.
12. Hall JA, Stein TS, Roter DL, Rieser N. Inaccuracies in physicians' perceptions of their patients. *Med Care.* 1999;37(11):1164-1168.
13. Di Blasi Z, Harkness E, Ernst E, Georgiou A, Kleijnen J. Influence of context effects on health outcomes: a systematic review. *Lancet.* 2001;357(9258):757-762.
14. Spiro HM. *The Power of Hope: A Doctor's Perspective.* New Haven, CT: The Yale University Press; 1998.
15. Harris JJ, Shao J, Sugarman J. Disclosure of cancer diagnosis and prognosis in Northern Tanzania. *Soc Sci Med.* 2003;56(5):905-913.
16. Beyene Y. Medical disclosure and refugees. Telling bad news to Ethiopian patients. *West J Med.* 1992;157(3):328-332.
17. Moerman DE, Jonas WB. Deconstructing the placebo effect and finding the meaning response. *Ann Intern Med.* 2002;136(6):471-476.
18. Moerman DE. The meaning response and the ethics of avoiding placebos. *Eval Health Prof.* 2002;25(4):399-409.
19. Spiro HM. Hope helps: placebos and alternative medicine in rheumatology. *Rheum Dis Clin North Am.* 1999;25(4):855-860.
20. Benson H, Friedman R. Harnessing the power of the placebo effect and renaming it "remembered wellness". *Annu Rev Med.* 1996;47:193-199.
21. Benson H. The nocebo effect: history and physiology. *Prev Med.* 1997;26(5 Pt 1):612-615.
22. Hahn R, Kleinman A. Belief as Pathogen, Belief as Medicine. *Med Anthropology Q* 1983; 14(4):16-19.
23. Sobo, E.J. Inner-City Women and AIDS: The Psycho-social Benefits of Unsafe Sex. *Cul Med Psychiatr.* 1993;17(4):455-485.
24. Mechanic D, Meyer S. Concepts of trust among patients with serious illness. *Soc Sci Med.* 2000 Sep;51(5):657-668.
25. Brody H, Brody D. *The Placebo Response: How You Can Release the Body's Inner Pharmacy for Better Health.* Cliff Street Books; 2001.
26. Benedetti F. How the doctor's words affect the patient's brain. *Eval Health Prof.* 2002;25(4):369-386.

27. Barsky AJ, Saintfort R, Rogers MP, Borus JF. Nonspecific medication side effects and the nocebo phenomenon. *JAMA*. 2002;287(5):622-627.
28. Hahn RA. The nocebo phenomenon: concept, evidence, and implications for public health. *Prev Med*. 1997;26(5 Pt 1):607-611.
29. Spiegel H. Nocebo: the power of suggestibility. *Prev Med*. 1997;26(5 Pt 1):616-621.
30. Pollo A, Vighetti S, Rainero I, Benedetti F. Placebo analgesia and the heart. *Pain*. 2003;102(1-2):125-133.
31. Chaput de Saintonge DM, Herxheimer A. Harnessing placebo effects in health care. *Lancet*. 1994;344(8928):995-998.
32. Gracely RH, Dubner R, Deeter WR, Wolskee PJ. Clinicians' expectations influence placebo analgesia. *Lancet*. 1985;1(8419):43.
33. Helman C. *Culture, Health and Illness*. Butterworth-Heinemann; 1985.
34. Kleinman A. *The Illness Narratives: Suffering, Healing, and the Human Condition*. New York: Basic Books; 1989.
35. Engel GL. The need for a new medical model: a challenge for biomedicine. *Science*. 1977;196(4286):129-136.
36. Kleinman A. Social violence: research questions on local experiences and global responses. *Arch Gen Psychiatry*. 1999;56(11):978-979.
37. Kawachi I, Berkman LF. Social ties and mental health. *J Urban Health*. 2001;78(3):458-467.
38. Marmot M, Wilkinson R. Social Determinants of Health. Oxford university press, 1999.
39. Taylor SE, Repetti RL, Seeman T. Health psychology: what is an unhealthy environment and how does it get under the skin? *Annu Rev Psychol*. 1997;48:411-447.
40. Thompson IE. Fundamental ethical principles in health care. *Br Med J*. 1987;295:1461-1465.
41. General Assembly of the United Nations. *Universal Declaration of Human Rights*, Geneva: United Nations; 1948.
42. Monk JA. Talk as Social Suffering. *Anthropology & Medicine*. 2000;7(1):15-38.
43. Laveist TA, Nuru-Jeter A. Is doctor-patient race concordance associated with greater satisfaction with care? *J Health Soc Behav*. 2002;43(3):296-306.
44. Hall JA, Horgan TG, Stein TS, Roter DL. Liking in the physician-patient relationship. *Patient Educ Couns*. 2002;48(1):69-77.
45. Kawachi I, Berkman LF. Social ties and mental health. *J Urban Health*. 2001;78(3):458-467.
46. Levy B, Ashman O, Dror I. To be or not to be: the effects of aging stereotypes on the will to live. *Omega (Westport)*. 1999-2000;40(3):409-420.
47. Hess TM, Auman C, Colcombe SJ, Rahhal TA. The impact of stereotype threat on age differences in memory performance. *J Gerontol B Psychol Sci Soc*. 2003;58(1):3-11.
48. Corley MC, Goren S. The dark side of nursing: impact of stigmatizing responses on patients. *Sch Inq Nurs Pract*. 1998;12(2):99-118.
49. Roter DL, Hall JA, Aoki Y. Physician gender effects in medical communication: a meta-analytic review. *JAMA*. 2002;288(6):756-764.
50. Krieger N, Sidney S. Racial discrimination and blood pressure: the CARDIA Study of young black and white adults. *Am J Public Health*. 1996;86(10):1370-1378.
51. Krieger N. Epidemiology, racism, and health: the case of low birth weight. *Epidemiology*. 2000;11(3):237-239.
52. Krieger N. Is breast cancer a disease of affluence, poverty, or both? The case of African American women. *Am J Public Health*. 2002;92(4):611-613.
53. Schulman KA, Berlin JA, Harless W, Kerner JF, Sistrunk S, Gersh BJ, Dube R, Taleghani CK, Burke JE, Williams S, Eisenberg JM, Escarce JJ. The effect of race and sex on physicians' recommendations for cardiac catheterization. *N Engl J Med*. 1999;340(8):618-626.
54. Shih M, Ambady N, Richeson JA, Fujita K, Gray HM. Related Articles, Links Abstract Stereotype performance boosts. *J Pers Soc Psychol*. 2002;83(3):638-647.

55. Elfenbein HA, Ambady N. Predicting workplace outcomes from the ability to eavesdrop on feelings. *J Appl Psychol.* 2002;87(5):963-971.

56. Matsumoto D. Cross cultural influences on the perception of emotion. *J Cross-cult psychology* 1989;20:95-105.

57. Dallabetta GA, Miotti PG, Chiphangwi JD, et al. High socioeconomic status is a risk factor for human immunodeficiency virus type 1 (HIV-1) infection but not for sexually transmitted diseases in women in Malawi: implications for HIV-1 control. *J Infect Dis.* 1993;167(1):36-42.

58. Newell J, Senkoro K, Mosha F, et al. A population-based study of syphilis and sexually transmitted disease syndromes in north-western Tanzania. 2. Risk factors and health seeking behaviour. *Genitourin Med.* 1993;69(6):421-426.

59. Sack WH, McSharry S, Clarke GN, Kinney R, Seeley J, Lewinsohn P. The Khmer Adolescent Project. I. Epidemiologic findings in two generations of Cambodian refugees. *J Nerv Ment Dis.* 1994;182(7):387-395.

60. Jansen HA, Morison L, Mosha F, et al. Geographical variations in the prevalence of HIV and other sexually transmitted infections in rural Tanzania. *Int J STD AIDS.* 2003;14(4):274-280.

61. Fylkesnes K, Musonda RM, Kasumba K, et al. The HIV epidemic in Zambia: socio-demographic prevalence patterns and indications of trends among childbearing women. *AIDS.* 1997;11(3):339-345.

62. Kleinman A, ed. *Social Suffering.* Berkeley, CA University of California Press, 1997.

63. Cooper RS, Kaufman JS, Ward R.Race and genomics. *N Engl J Med.* 2003;348(12): 1166-1170.

64. Catalano RA, Satariano WA, Ciemins EL. Unemployment and the detection of early stage breast tumors among African Americans and non-Hispanic whites. *Ann Epidemiol.* 2003;13(1):8-15.

65. Stoll BA. Obesity, social class and Western diet: a link to breast cancer prognosis. *Eur J Cancer.* 1996;32A(8):1293-1295.

66. Govindarajan R, Shah RV, Erkman LG, Hutchins LF. Racial differences in the outcome of patients with colorectal carcinoma. *Cancer.* 2003;97(2):493-498.

67. Lochner KA, Kawachi I, Brennan RT, Buka SL. Social capital and neighbourhood mortality rates in Chicago. *Soc Sci Med.* 2003;56(8):1797-1805.

68. Claussen B, Davey Smith G, Thelle D. Impact of childhood and adulthood socioeconomic position on cause specific mortality: the Oslo Mortality Study. *J Epidemiol Community Health.* 2003;57(1):40-45.

69. Hall SA, Rockhill B. Race, poverty, affluence, and breast cancer. *Am J Public Health.* 2002;92(10):155.

70. Stoll BA. Affluence, Obesity, and Breast Cancer. *Breast J.* 2000;6(2):146-149.

71. Dula A, Goering S. *It Just Ain't Fair: the Ethics of Health Care for African Americans.* Westport, CT: Praeger; 1994.

72. McEwen BS, Wingfield JC. The concept of allostasis in biology and biomedicine. *Horm Behav.* 2003;43(1):2-15.

73. Adler N, Boyce WT, Chesney, M, Folkman S, Syme L. Socioeconomic inequalities in health: no easy solution. *JAMA.* 1993;3140-3145.

74. Bobak M, Marmot M. East-West mortality divide and its potential explanations: proposed research agenda. *BMJ.* 1996;312(7028):421-425.

75. Cannon W. The wisdom of the body. *Physiol Rev.* 1929;9:399-431.

76. DeVasa SS, Diamond, EL. Association of breast cancer and cervical cancer incidences with income and education among whites and blacks. *J Natl Cancer Inst.* 1980;65:515-528.

77. Felitti V, Anda RF, Nordenberg F, et al. Relationship of childhood abuse and household dysfunction to many of the leading causes of death in adults. *Am J Prev Med.* 1998;14:245-258.

78. Marmot MG, Davey G, Smith S, et al. Health inequalities among British civil servants: the Whitehall II study. *Lancet.* 1991;337:1387-1393.

79. McEwen BS. Protective and damaging effects of stress mediators. *N Engl J Med.* 1998;33:171-179.

80. McEwen BS, Stellar E. Stress and the individual: mechanisms leading to disease. *Arch Intern Med* 1993;153:2093-2101.

81. Einbinder LC, Schulman KA. The effect of race on the referral process for invasive cardiac procedures. *Med Care Res Rev.* 2000;57(suppl 1):162-180.

82. Rathore SS, Berger AK, Weinfurt KP, et al. Race, sex, poverty, and the medical treatment of acute myocardial infarction in the elderly. *Circulation.* 2000;102(6):642-648.

83. Bach PB, Cramer LD, Warren JL, Begg CB. Racial differences in the treatment of early-stage lung cancer. *N Engl J Med.* 1999;341(16):1198-1205.

84. Bradley CJ, Given CW, Roberts C. Disparities in cancer diagnosis and survival. *Cancer.* 2001;91(1):178-178.

85. Freeman HP. Cancer in the socioeconomically disadvantaged. *CA Cancer J Clin.* 1989;39(5):266-288.

86. Sen M. Communication with cancer patients; the influence of age, gender, education and health insurance status. In: Surbone and Zwitter eds. *Communication with the Cancer Patient; Information and Truth.* New York, NY: The NY Academy of Sciences; 1997: 514-524.

87. Austin D, Russell EM. Is there ageism in oncology? *Scott Med J.* 2003;48(1):17-20.

88. Surbone A, Zwitter M, eds. *Communication with the Cancer Patient: Information and Truth.* New York: New York Academy of Sciences; 1997. Annals of the New York Academy of Sciences; Vol 809.

89. Peake MD, Thompson S, Lowe D, Pearson MG. Ageism in the management of lung cancer. *Age Ageing.* 2003;32(2):171-177.

90. Rathore SS, Lenert LA, Weinfurt KP, et al. The effects of patient sex and race on medical students' ratings of quality of life. *Am J Med.* 2000;108(7):561-566.

91. Bennett KJ, Torrance GW. Measuring health preferences and utilities: rating scale, time trade-off and standard gamble methods. In: Spliker B, ed. *Quality of Life and Pharmacoeconomics in Clinical Trials.* Philadelphia, PA: Lippincott-Raven Publishers; 1996:235-265.

92. Dedier J, Penson R, Williams W, Lynch T. Race, Ethnicity, and the Patient-Caregiver Relationship. *Oncologist.* 2002;7(90002):43-49.

93. Selby M. Ethical dilemma: dealing with racist patients. *BMJ.* 1999;318(7191):1129.

94. Ferguson WJ, Candib LM. Culture, language, and the doctor-patient relationship. *Fam Med.* 2002;34(5):353-361.

95. Cioffi J. Communicating with culturally and linguistically diverse patients in an acute care setting: nurses' experiences. *Int J Nurs Stud.* 2003;40(3):299-306.

96. Saha S, Komaromy M, Kopsell TD, Bindman AB. Patient-physician racial concordance and the perceived quality and use of health care. *Arch Intern Med.* 1999;159:997-1004.

97. Cooper-Patrick L, Gallo JJ, Gonzales JJ, et al. Race, gender, and partnership in the patient-physician relationship. *JAMA.* 1999;282:583-589.

98. Toms FD, Hodge FS, Pullen-Smith B. Cultural diversity and the delivery of health care services. *Cancer.* 1998;83:1843-1848.

99. Eskandari F, Sternberg EM. Neural-immune interactions in health and disease. *Ann N Y Acad Sci.* 2002;966:20-27.

100. Webster JI, Tonelli L, Sternberg EM. Neuroendocrine regulation of immunity. *Annu Rev Immunol.* 2002;20:125-163.

101. Lupien SJ, Lepage M. Stress, memory, and the hippocampus: can't live with it, can't live without it. *Behav Brain Res.* 2001;127(1-2):137-158.

102. Sandhu MS, Luben R, Day NE, Khaw KT. Self-reported birth weight and subsequent risk of colorectal cancer. *Cancer Epidemiol Biomarkers Prev.* 2002;11(9):935-938.
103. Bernstein L. Epidemiology of endocrine-related risk factors for breast cancer. *J Mammary Gland Biol Neoplasia.* 2002;7(1):3-15.
104. Jaing TH, Hung IJ, Lin JN, Lien RI, Hsueh C, Lu CS. Hepatoblastoma in a child of extremely low birth weight. *Am J Perinatol.* 2002;19(3):149-153.
105. Harbuz M. Neuroendocrinology of autoimmunity. *Int Rev Neurobiol.* 2002;52:133-161.
106. Young JB. Programming of sympathoadrenal function. *Trends Endocrinol Metab.* 2002;13(9):381-385.
107. Seals DR, Esler MD. Human ageing and the sympathoadrenal system. *J Physiol.* 2000;528(Pt 3):407-417.
108. Kee F, Wilson R, Currie S, Sloan J, Houston R, Rowlands B, Moorehead J. Socioeconomic circumstances and the risk of bowel cancer in Northern Ireland. *J Epidemiol Community Health.* 1996;50(6):640-644.
109. Sternberg EM. Does stress make you sick and belief make you well? The science connecting body and mind. *Ann N Y Acad Sci.* 2000;917:1-3.
110. Eskandari F, Sternberg EM. Neural-immune interactions in health and disease. *Ann N Y Acad Sci.* 2002;966:20-27.
111. Parsons T. *The Social System.* London: Routledge and Kegan Paul; 1951.
112. Huang X, Butow PN, Meiser M, Clarke S, Goldstein D. Communicating in a multi-cultural society: The needs of Chinese cancer patients in Australia. *Aust N Z J Medicine,* 1999;29:207-213.
113. Todd KH. Influence of ethnicity on emergency department pain management. *Emerg Med (Fremantle).* 2001;13(3):274-278.
114. Todd KH, Deaton C, D'Adamo AP, Goe L. Ethnicity and analgesic practice. *Ann Emerg Med.* 2000;35(1):11-16.
115. Todd KH. Pain assessment and ethnicity. *Ann Emerg Med.* 1996;27(4):421-423.
116. Anderson KO, Richman SP, Hurley J, et al. Cancer pain management among underserved minority outpatients: perceived needs and barriers to optimal control. *Cancer.* 2002 Apr 15;94(8):2295-2304.
117. Cleeland CS, Gonin R, Baez L, Loehrer P, Pandya KJ. Pain and treatment of pain in minority patients with cancer. The Eastern Cooperative Oncology Group Minority Outpatient Pain Study. *Ann Intern Med.* 1997;127(9):813-816.
118. Kaptchuk TJ. The placebo effect in alternative medicine: can the performance of a healing ritual have clinical significance? *Ann Intern Med.* 2002;136(11):817-825.
119. Horwitz RI, Horwitz SM. Adherence to treatment and health outcomes. *Arch Intern Med.* 1993;153:1863-1868.
120. Gonzalez G. Health care in the United States; A perspective from the front line. In: Surbone and Zwitter, eds. *Communication with the Cancer Patient; Information and Truth.* New York, NY: The NY Academy of Sciences; 1997:211-222.
121. Anderson JN. Health and illness in Philippino immigrants. *West J Med.* 1983;139(6):811-819.
122. Lange JW. Methodological concerns for non-Hispanic investigators conducting research with Hispanic Americans. *Res Nurs Health.* 2002;25(5):411-419.
123. Race, Ethnicity, and Medical Care. A Survey of Public Perceptions and Experiences. Washington, DC: Henry J. Kaiser Family Foundation; 1999.
124. Hochschild AR. *The Managed Heart: Commercialization of Human Feeling.* Berkley, CA: University of California Press; 1985.
125. Elfenbein HA, Ambady N. Is there an in-group advantage in emotion recognition? *Psychol Bull.* 2002 Mar;128(2):243-249.

126. Long So, Long BD. Curable cancers and fatal ulcers. Attitudes toward cancer in Japan. *Soc Sci Med.* 1982;16(24):2101-2108.

127. Kakai H. A double standard in bioethical reasoning for disclosure of advanced cancer diagnoses in Japan. *Health Commun.* 2002;14(3):361-376.

128. Domino G, Regmi MP. Attitudes towards cancer; A cross cultural comparison of Nepalese and US students. *J Cross cult Psychol.* 1993;24:389-398.

129. Bailar JC 3rd, Bailer AJ. Risk assessment—the mother of all uncertainties. Disciplinary perspectives on uncertainty in risk assessment. *Ann N Y Acad Sci.* 1999;895:273-285.

130. Wingo PA, Ries LA, Giovino GA, et al. Annual report to the nation on the status of cancer, 1973-1996, with a special section on lung cancer and tobacco smoking. *J Natl Cancer Inst.* 1999;91(8):675-690.

131. Solomon A. The politics of breast cancer. *Camera Obscura.* 1992;28(1)29.

132. Middlebrook C. *Seeing the Crab: A Memoir of Dying.* New York: Basic Books; 1996.

133. Eisinger F, Geller G, Burke W, Holtzman NA. Cultural basis for differences between US and French clinical recommendations for women at increased risk of breast and ovarian cancer. *Lancet.* 1999;353(9156):919-920.

134. Nathan D, Benz EJ. Comprehensive cancer centres and the war on cancer. *Nat Rev Cancer.* 2001;1(3):240-245.

135. Sporn MB. The war on cancer. *Lancet.* 1996;347(9012):1377-1381.

136. Sontag S. *Illness as Metaphor.* Picador; 2001.

137. Mayer M. *Examining Myself: One Woman's Story of Breast Cancer Treatment and Recovery.* New York, NY: Faber & Faber; 1994.

138. Frank A. *At the Will of the Body.* Chicago: University of Chicago Press; 1995.

139. Broyard A. *Intoxicated by My Illness.* Fawcett Books; 1998.

140. De Beauvoir S. *A Very Easy Death.* New York: Pantheon; 1965

141. Grealy L. *Autobiography of a Face.* Boston: Houghton Mifflin; 1994.

142. Raz H (ed.). *Living on the Margins: Women Writers on Breast Cancer.* New York: Persea; 1999

143. Fallowfield L, Ratcliffe D, Souhami R. Clinicians' attitudes to clinical trials of cancer therapy. *Eur J Cancer.* 1997;33(13):2221-2229.

143. Daugherty CK. The "cure" for cancer: can the media report the hope without the hype? *J Clin Oncol.* 2002;20(18):3761-3764.

144. Balshem M. *Cancer in the Community: Class and Medical Authority* Washington D.C.: Smithsonian Institution Press; 1993. Smithsonian Series in Ethnographic Inquiry.

145. Gregg J, Curry RH. Explanatory models for cancer among African-American women at two Atlanta neighborhood health centers: the implications for a cancer screening program. *Soc Sci Med.* 1994;39(4):519-526.

146. Foucault M. *The Birth of the Clinic: An Archaeology of Medical Perception.* Vintage Books; 1994.

147. Surbone, Zwitter M. Learning from the world; the Editor's Perspective. In: Surbone and Zwitter eds. *Communication with the Cancer Patient; Information and Truth.* New York, NY: The NY Academy of Sciences; 1997:1-6.

148. Phillips DP, Ruth TE, Wagner LM. Psychology and survival. *Lancet.* 1993;342:1142-1145.

149. Meiser B, Eisenbruch M, Barlow-Stewart K, Tucker K, Steel Z, Goldstein D. Cultural aspects of cancer genetics: setting a research agenda. *J Med Genet.* 2001;38(7):425-429.

150. Thang NM, Swenson I. Variations in Vietnamese marriages, births and infant deaths by months of the Julian calendar and years of the Vietnamese and Chinese astrological calendars. *J Biosoc Sci.* 1996;28:367-371.

151. Goodkind DM. New zodiacal influences on Chinese family formation: Taiwan, 1976. *Demography.* 1993;30:127-142.

152. Phillips DP, Liu GC, Kwok K, Jarvinen JR, Zhang W, Abramson IS. The Hound of the Baskervilles effect: natural experiment on the influence of psychological stress on timing of death. *BMJ* 2001;323:1443-1444.

153. Keng Ho Pwee. *4 is inauspicious too. BMJ.* 2002;325:1443.

154. Ramakrishna J, Weiss MG. Health, illness, and immigration. East Indians in the United States. *West J Med.* 1992 Sep;157(3):265-270.

155. Nwoga IA. Traditional healers and perceptions of the causes and treatment of cancer. *Cancer Nursing* 1994;17(6):470-478.

156. Haffner L. Translation is not enough. Interpreting in a medical settings. *West J Med.* 1992 Sep;157(3):255-259.

157. Stewart MA. Effective physician-patient communication and health outcomes: a review. *CMAJ.* 1995;152(9):1423-1433.

158. Baile WF, Buckman R, Lenzi R, Glober G, Beale E. Kudelka A. SPIKES—A six step protocol for delivering bad news: application for the patient with cancer. *Oncologist.* 2000;5:302-311.

159. Baile WF, Lenzi R, Parker PA, Buckman R, Cohen L. Oncologists' attitudes toward and practices in giving bad news: an exploratory study. *J Clin Oncol.* 2002;20(8):2189-2196.

160. Fogarty LA, Curbow BA, Wingard JR, McDonnell K, Somerfield MR. Can 40 seconds of compassion reduce patient anxiety? *J Clin Oncol.* 1999 Jan;17(1):371-379.

161. McPhail G, Wilson S. Women's experience of breast conserving treatment for breast cancer. *Eur J Cancer Care.* 2000 Sep;9(3):144-150.

162. Ong LM, Visser MR, Lammes FB, de Haes JC. Doctor-patient communication and cancer patients' quality of life and satisfaction. *Patient Educ Couns.* 2000 Sep;41(2):145-148.

163. Ramirez AJ, Graham J, et al. Mental health of hospital consultants: the effects of stress and satisfaction at work. *Lancet.* 1996;347(9003):724-728.

164. Peters J, McManus IC, Hutchinson A. Good Medical Practice: comparing the views of doctors and the general population. *Med Educ.* 2001;35(suppl 1):52-59.

165. Zachariae R, Pedersen CG, Jensen AB, Ehrnrooth E, Rossen PB, Von Der Maase H. Association of perceived physician communication style with patient satisfaction, distress, cancer-related self-efficacy, and perceived control over the disease. *Br J Cancer.* 2003;88(5):658-665.

166. Bredart A, Robertson C, Razavi D, et al. Patients' satisfaction ratings and their desire for care improvement across oncology settings from France, Italy, Poland and Sweden. *Psycho-Oncology.* 2003;12(1):68-77.

167. Fallowfield LJ, Jenkins VA, Beveridge HA. Truth may hurt but deceit hurts more: communication in palliative care. *Palliat Med.* 2002;16(4):297-303.

168. Leighl N, Gattellari M, Butow P, Brown R, Tattersall MHN. Discussing adjuvant cancer therapy. *JCO.* 2001;19(6):1768-1778.

169. Gattellari M, Voigt K, Butow P, Tattersall MHN. When the treatment goal is not cure: are cancer patients equipped to make informed decisions? *JCO.* 2002;20(2):503-513.

170. DiMatteo MR, Taranta A, Friedman HS, Prince LM. Predicting patient satisfaction from physicians' nonverbal communication skills. *Med Care.* 1980;18(4):376-387.

171. Buckman R. *How to Break Bad News: A Guide for Health Care Professionals.* Baltimore, MD: Johns Hopkins University Press; 1992.

172. Lind SE, DelVecchio Good MJ, Seidel S, Csordas T, Good BJ. Telling the diagnosis of cancer. *JCO.* 1989;7(5):583-589.

173. Hogbin B, Fallowfield L. Getting it taped: the 'bad news' consultation with cancer patients. *Br J Hosp Med.* 1989;41(4):330-333.

174. Fallowfield L, Ford S, Lewis S. No news is not good news: information preferences of patients with cancer. *Psycho-Oncology* 1995;4(3):197-202.

175. Chambers T. Cross-cultural issues in caring for patients with cancer. *Cancer Treat Res.* 2000;102:23-37.
176. Christakis NA. Death foretold: prophecy and prognosis in medical care. Chicago, IL: University of Chicago Press; 2000.
177. Rainey LC. Effects of preparatory patient education for radiation oncology patients. *Cancer.* 1985;56(5):1056-1061.
178. Christakis NA, Iwashyna TJ, Zhang JX. Care after the onset of serious illness: a novel claims-based dataset exploiting substantial cross-set linkages to study end-of-life care. *J Palliat Med.* 2002;5(4):515-529.
179. McCague K. Collusion in doctor-patient communication. Doctors should adopt patient's perspective. *BMJ.* 2001;322(7293):1063.
180. Anne-Mei The, Tony Hak, Gerard Koëter, Gerrit van der Wal. A Collusion in doctor-patient communication about imminent death: an ethnographic study. *BMJ.* 2000;321:1376-1381.
181. Meredith C, Symonds P, Webster L, et al. Information needs of cancer patients in west Scotland: cross sectional survey of patients' views. *BMJ.* 1996;313:724-726.
182. Kirwan JM, Tincello DG, Lavender T, Kingston RE. How doctors record breaking bad news in ovarian cancer. *Br J Cancer.* 200324;88(6):839-842.
183. Ayanian JZ, Cleary PD, Weissman JS, Epstein AM. The effect of patients' preferences on racial differences in access to renal transplantation. *N Engl J Med.* 1999;341:1661-1669.
184. Berger JT. Culture and ethnicity in clinical care. *Arch Intern Med.* 1998;158(19):2085-2090.
185. Cassel EJ. The nature of suffering and the goals of medicine. New York: Oxford University Press; 1991.
186. Cassell EJ. The 'student doctor' and a wary patient. Commentary. *Hastings Cent Rep.* 1982;12(1):28.
187. Balsa AI, McGuire TG. Prejudice, clinical uncertainty and stereotyping as sources of health disparities. *J Health Econ.* 2003;22(1):89-116.
188. Christakis, NA, Lamont,EB. Extent and determinants of error in doctors' prognosis in terminally ill patients: prospective cohort study. *BMJ.* 2000;320:469-473.
189. Goldstein D, Thewes B, Butow P. Communicating in a multicultural society II: Greek community attitudes towards cancer in Australia. *Intern Med J* 2002;32:289-296.
190. Rosner F. Principles and Practice Concerning the Jewish Patient. *J Gen Intern Med.* 1993;11:486-489.
191. Loustaunau MO, Sobo EJ, eds. *The Cultural Context of Health, Illness, and Medicine.* Westport, CT: Bergin & Garvey; 1997.
192. Chapman CR, Gavrin J. Suffering: the contributions of persistent pain. *Lancet.* 1999;353(9171):2233-2237.
193. Street RL, Voigt B: Patient participation in deciding breast cancer treatment and subsequent quality of life. *Med Decision Making.* 1997;17:298-306.
194. Bruner, J. *Acts of meaning.* Cambridge: Harvard University Press; 1990.
195. Ernst E, Herxheimer A. The power of placebo. *BMJ.* 1996;313(7072):1569-1570.
196. Hodes RM. Cross cultural medicine and diverse health belief - ethiopians abroad. *West J Med.* 1997;166:29-36.
197. Harrington A, ed. *The Placebo Effect: An Interdisciplinary Exploration.* Cambridge: Harvard University press; 1997.
198. Spiro H. Compliance, adherence, and hope. *J Clin Gastroenterol.* 2001;32(1):5.
199. Lee RV. Doctoring to the music of time. *Ann Intern Med.* 2000;132(1):11-17.
200. Hacking A. Breast cancer in Xhosa women. *SA Journal of CME.* 1998;6:57-62.
201. Wright SV. An investigation into the causes of absconding among black African breast cancer patients. *S Afr Med J.* 1997;87(11):1540-1543.

202. Gifford SM. The change of life, the sorrow of life: menopause, bad blood and cancer among Italian-Australia working class women. *Cult Med Psychiatry*. 1994;18:1-21.

203. Lannin DR, Mathews HF, Mitchell J, Swanson MS, Swanson FH, Edwards MS. Influence of socioeconomic and cultural factors on racial differences in late-stage presentation of breast cancer. *JAMA*. 1998;279(22):1801-1807.

204. Phillips JM. Breast cancer and African American women: moving beyond fear, fatalism, and silence. *Oncol Nurs Forum*. 1999;26(6):1001-1007.

205. Moore RJ. African American women and breast cancer: notes from a study of narrative. *Cancer Nurs*. 2001;24(1):35-44.

206. Burhansstipanov L. Urban native American health issues. *Cancer*. 2000;88(S5):1207-1213.

207. Kearney N. Oncology health care professionals' attitudes to cancer: a professional concern. *Ann Oncol*. 2003;14:57-61.

208. Eisenbruch M, Handelman L. Cultural consultation for cancer: astrocytoma in a Cambodian adolescent. *Soc Sci Med*. 1990;31:1295-1299.

209. Ananth S, Amin M. Implantation of oral squamous cell carcinoma at the site of a percutaneous endoscopic gastrostomy: a case report. *Br J Oral Maxillofac Surg*. 2002;40(2):125-130.

210. Wood K, Jewkes R, Abrahams N. Cleaning the womb: constructions of cervical screening and womb cancer among rural black women in South Africa. *Soc Sci Med*. 1997;45(2):283-294.

211. Bezwoda W, Colvin H, Lehoka J. Transcultural and language problems in communicating with cancer patients in Southern Africa. In: Surbone and Zwitter, eds. *Communication with the Cancer Patient; Information and Truth*. New York, NY: The NY Academy of Sciences; 1997: 211-222.

212. Spiegel D. Effects of psychotherapy on cancer survival. *Nat Rev Cancer*. 2002;2(5): 383-389.

213. Boonmongkon P, Nichter M, Pylypa J. Mot luuk problems in Northeast Thailand: why women's own health concerns matter as much as disease rates. *Soc Sci Med*. 2001;53(8):1095-1112.

214. Mayne L, Earp J. Initial and repeat mammography screening: different behaviors/different predictors. *J Rural Health*. 2003;19(1):63-71.

215. Pillay AL. Rural and urban South African women's awareness of cancers of the breast and cervix. *Ethn Health*. 2002;7(2):103-114.

216. Cummings DM, Whetstone LM, Earp JA, Mayne L. Disparities in mammography screening in rural areas: analysis of county differences in North Carolina. *J Rural Health*. 2002;18(1):77-83.

217. Santora LM, Mahoney MC, Lawvere S, Englert JJ, Symons AB, Mirand AL. Breast cancer screening beliefs by practice location. *BMC Public Health*. 2003;3(1):9.

218. Hoffman M, de Pinho H, Cooper D, et al. Breast cancer incidence and determinants of cancer stage in the Western Cape. *S Afr Med J*. 2000;90(12):1212-1216.

219. Nzarubara RG. Control of breast cancer using health education. *East Afr Med J*. 1999;76(12):661-663.

220. Odusanya OO. Breast cancer: knowledge, attitudes, and practices of female schoolteachers in Lagos, Nigeria. *Breast J*. 2001;7(3):171-175.

221. Njah M, Hergli R, Gloulou J, Bent Ahmed S, Marzouki M. Knowledge, attitude and behavior of Tunisian women apropos of gynecological cancers. *Soz Praventivmed*. 1994;39(5):280-286.

222. Von Roenn JH, von Gunten CF. Setting goals to maintain hope. *JCO*. 2003;21(3):570-574.

223. Moore RJ, Spiegel D. Uses of guided imagery for pain control by African-American and white women with metastatic breast cancer. *Integr Med*. 2000;21;2(2):115-126.

224. Hira K, Fukui T, Endoh A, Rahman M, Maekawa M. Influence of superstition on the date of hospital discharge and medical cost in Japan: retrospective and descriptive study. *BMJ.* 1998;317(7174):1680-1683.

225. Bennett E. Soft truth. *Anthropol Med.* 1999;6(3):395-404.

226. Koehly LM, Peterson SK, Watts BG, Kempf KK, Vernon SW, Gritz ER. A social network analysis of communication about hereditary nonpolyposis colorectal cancer genetic testing and family functioning. *Cancer Epidemiol Biomarkers Prev.* 2003;12(4):304-313.

227. Ambady N, Laplante D, Nguyen T, Rosenthal R, Chaumeton N, Levinson W. Surgeons' tone of voice: a clue to malpractice history. *Surgery.* 2002;132(1):5-9.

228. Corley MC, Goren S. The dark side of nursing: impact of stigmatizing responses on patients. *Sch Inq Nurs Pract.* 1998;12(2):99-118.

229. Ambady N, Koo J, Rosenthal R, Winograd CH. Physical therapists' nonverbal communication predicts geriatric patients' health outcomes. *Psychol Aging.* 2002;17(3):443-445.

230. Griffith Charles H, Wilson John F, Langer Shelby Haist SA. House staff nonverbal communication skills and standardized patient satisfaction. *J. Gen Intern Med.* 2003;18(3):170-174.

231. McCaffery K, Forrest S, Waller J, Desai M, Szarewski A, Wardle J. Attitudes towards HPV testing: A qualitative study of beliefs among Indian, Pakistani, African-Caribbean and white British women in the UK. *Br J Cancer.* 2003;88(1):42-46.

232. Nelson K, Geiger AM, Mangione CM. Effect of health beliefs on delays in care for abnormal cervical cytology in a multi-ethnic population. *J Gen Intern Med.* 2002;17(9):709-716.

233. Engel GL. A life setting conducive to illness. The giving-up—given-up complex. *Bull Menninger Clin.* 1968;32(6):355-365.

234. Uchitomi Y, Yamawaki S. Truth-telling practice in cancer care in Japan. In Surbonne and Zwitter, 290-300.

233. Younge D, Moreau P, Ezzat A, Gray A. Communicating with cancer patients in Saudi Arabia. In: Surbone and Zwitter, eds. *Communication with the cancer patient.* New York, NY: The NY Academy of Sciences; 1997:309-316.

234. Charlton RC. Breaking Bad News. *Med J Aust.* 1992;157:615-621.

235. Cella D, Hernandez L, Bonomi AE, et al. Spanish language translation and initial validation of the functional assessment of cancer therapy quality-of-life instrument. *Med Care.* 1998;36(9):1407-1418.

236. Hilton A, Skrutkowski M. Translating instruments into other languages: Development and testing processes. *Cancer Nurs.* 2002;25(1):1-7.

237. Bierhaus A, Wolf J, Andrassy M, Rohleder N, Humpert PM, Petrov D, Ferstl R, von Eynatten M, Wendt T, Rudofsky G, Joswig M, Morcos M, Schwaninger M, McEwenB, Kirschbaum C, Nawroth PP. A mechanism converting psychosocial stress into mononuclear cell activation. 237. *Proc Natl Acad Sci USA.* 2003 Feb 18;100(4): 1920–5.

CHAPTER 3

Quality of Life in Culturally Diverse Cancer Patients

Carolyn Cook Gotay

INTRODUCTION

The increased ethnic diversity of many countries around the world, telecommunications technologies facilitating global information exchange, and international research collaborations are among the factors that have led to an enhanced appreciation of the importance of cultural factors in all aspects of life, including quality of life (QOL) in cancer patients and their families. In fact, the World Health Organization (WHO) has defined QOL as "an individual's perception of their position in life, in the context of the culture and value systems in which they live and in relation to their goals, expectations, standards, and concerns."[1,2] This definition embeds individual QOL squarely within the setting of a person's heritage and environment and implies that QOL may differ according to cultural factors.

There are many reasons why culture may affect cancer-related QOL. These include patterns of cancer diagnosis and treatment, historical factors, and cultural beliefs and values. Cancer rates also vary considerably internationally. In many parts of the world, there are few resources devoted to early cancer detection, and as a consequence, cancers are diagnosed late. According to Stjernsward and Teoh,[3] "for a long time to come, as many as 80%-90% of cancer patients in the developing countries will probably continue to be diagnosed with far-advanced, incurable cancer, if they are diagnosed at all." In countries and cultures where cancer is inevitably linked with pain and death (especially considering that pain is inadequately managed in most parts of the world),[3] it seems likely that the distress associated with such a diagnosis, and its deleterious effects on QOL, may be considerable and greater than in an environment where pain can be controlled, nausea can be prevented, and hope for a cure can be provided.

Different cultural groups have distinct histories, and it is important to consider political and historical contexts in understanding reactions to cancer. For example, part of QOL assessment frequently includes asking patients to state if they have family members or others who provide them with social support, and how many people make up their social network. This line of questioning may be threatening for someone who has fled an oppressive political regime where naming one's family and friends led to their imprisonment. Several Israeli investigators have investigated how a major 20th century event—the Holocaust—has affected Holocaust survivors' coping with cancer. Mark and Roberts[4] discuss how shaved heads and loss of hair during cancer treatment, coupled with hospital identification bracelets and gowns, may trigger flashbacks to Holocaust experiences. Holocaust survivors who are subsequently diagnosed with cancer experience much higher levels of stress, compared to cancer patients who have not been through the Holocaust and healthy Holocaust survivors.[5] Such increased distress has been found among second generation Holocaust survivors diagnosed with breast cancer.[6]

Other cultural factors including views of cancer etiology and family structure are also likely to have profound influences on QOL in cancer patients and survivors. For example, many Asian and Polynesian cultures stress the harmony between physical, mental, and spiritual well-being[7] and its role in disease etiology. QOL issues in cancer survivors from such traditions may differ from those of Anglos who see cancer as a "disease" which is treated and eradicated. Thus, the implications of and problems associated with "recovery" and "re-entry" on QOL may differ in cancer survivors from diverse ethnic groups.

Family structure also varies culturally. For example, the most critical family axis differs, with the husband-wife, parent-child, and brother-sister bonds being most important for Anglos, Asians, and Micronesians, respectively.[8] This may imply that a cancer that leads to impaired sexual functioning (eg, as is often the case for prostate cancer) may affect Anglo prostate survivors more acutely, given the centrality of the husband-wife relationship, compared to Asians and Micronesians. However, cancers that affect fertility (such as cervical, uterine, or testicular cancer) could have more profoundly negative implications for many aspects of QOL in cultural groups where the parent-child bond is pre-eminent, such as among the Asians.

Despite all these fascinating speculations about the link between culture and QOL in cancer, much of what has been written to date remains just that: speculation. Empirical data to affirm cultural differences in cancer-related QOL are scarce. In this chapter, we provide a summary of the state-of-the-art in this area of study by reviewing relevant empirical research using different methodologies: studies of individual cultural groups, comparisons with normative data, and comparative studies. Each of these methods has strengths and weaknesses, as will be discussed. We will also review current cross-cultural approaches to measuring QOL using self-administered questionnaires, which is currently the most common approach to QOL assessment. For the purposes of this chapter, we define QOL as patient-reported levels of physical, psychological, social, and/or spiritual/existential well-being. Other domains that are often included as part of cancer-related QOL including pain, will not be discussed here as they are addressed elsewhere in this volume, for instance, in chapter 9, 8, and 4 by Paice and ODonnell. Spiegel et al. (psychosocial support and cancer care),[7] Balducci et al. (cultural differences in aging), respectively. We are drawing on literature from around the world that investigates cultural influences in cancer patients in different countries, or racial/ethnic groups or subgroups.

STUDIES OF SPECIFIED CULTURAL GROUPS

Some research focuses on individuals, or groups of individuals, all from the same culture. While many small-scale case studies rely on qualitative data collected through semi-structured and unstructured interviews, other reports use quantitative methods to address their research questions. Such methodologies have been used to address a number of questions, including how QOL is defined in specific cultures, and how individuals in a particular cultural group experience the effects of cancer on their QOL. We will provide some illustrative examples.

How Is QOL Defined in Different Cultures?

Chaturvedi[9] asked a sample of Indian cancer patients ($N = 18$), family members ($N = 20$), and caregivers ($N = 12$) how important 10 factors were to QOL. She found that individual functioning was the least important: 58% said that level of individual functioning was "not important," whereas 60% or more rated "peace of mind," "spiritual satisfaction," "satisfaction with religious acts," and "happiness with family" as "very important." This finding contrasts markedly with the content of many current questionnaires used to assess QOL in cancer patients, which have the most items related to physical functioning and a patient's ability to act independently.[10] This may not be surprising, since researchers in North America and Europe, where the dominant culture highly values autonomy and the individual, developed most of these scales.

Juarez and colleagues[11] conducted qualitative interviews with 17 Spanish-speaking patients of Mexican ancestry who had cancer pain. The patients' responses to the question "What does QOL mean to you?" included positive affect ("being happy"), being able to maintain an active lifestyle, and having family interaction. The study examined how pain affected QOL and found confirmation of a QOL definitional framework previously developed by these investigators in non-Hispanic cancer patients, that includes physical, psychological, social, and spiritual well-being. The authors conclude that spiritual beliefs and social support seem to be relatively more important in Hispanics.

Freedman[12] investigated one aspect of QOL—the impact of hair loss associated with cancer chemotherapy—in relation to cultural factors in 32 (30 White and 2 African American) patients who were receiving treatment for breast cancer. This study does not address the question of defining QOL as directly as the two previous studies, but we are including it here because it illustrates another important point: cultural factors are important to understand in every patient, even those from the "dominant culture." Freedman found that hair loss was one of the most feared and distressing aspects of the women's cancer experience, and its impact extended to self-concept, loss of privacy in social interactions, and isolation. These negative consequences stemmed from the American culture's emphasis on hair as an indicator of personality, attractiveness, sexuality, and femininity. Loss of hair endangered all of these positive attributes, as well as invoked societal notions of punishment (associated with the shaved heads of prisoners and internees) and general negative attributions (reflected in expressions such as "bald as a cue ball"). QOL in these breast cancer patients was linked to the meaning of hair loss in American culture.

How Does Cancer Affect QOL in Individuals in a Particular Culture?

A number of investigators have investigated this question through qualitative and quantitative research on groups within the United States, such as African Americans,[13-15] and in other parts of the world such as China[16,17] and India.[18]

Moore[13] conducted open-ended semi-structured interviews with 23 African American breast cancer survivors to understand their "lived experience"; QOL was one of a number of aspects of areas that was included in the interview schedule. Results indicated that QOL was lower in social and psychological domains due to social isolation and stress. Some of the interviewees' concerns stemmed from racial/cultural factors, such as a lack of African American breast cancer survivor role models, and the unavailability of skin color-matched prostheses. Moore[13] makes the important observation that the ethnicity of the researcher—an African American woman—may have affected the candor that the women felt in expressing their concerns and their comfort in bringing up issues related to racism. It is unclear if the women would have been comfortable exploring such themes had the interviewer been of a different racial background.

Northouse et al.[14] also studied African American breast cancer survivors ($N = 98$) using quantitative methods. They used the FACT-G, a validated cancer-specific QOL questionnaire[19] and found that the survivors were doing well in all areas of QOL. Lowered QOL was linked to disease and treatment related variables (symptoms and having breast cancer recurrence), lower family functioning, and negative perspectives about the effect of illness on their lives. Interestingly, while the Moore[13] and Northouse et al.[14] studies give completely different perspectives on the experience of African American breast cancer survivors, they both agree that more exposure to African American breast cancer survivors with high QOL, including in the media, would be inspiring to African Americans confronted with a breast cancer diagnosis. Perhaps participants on Northouse et al.[14] could talk with the participants on Moore's study![13]

Pandey and colleagues[18] studied 50 breast cancer patients in India using linear analog scales. While the sample included patients with both early and advanced disease, most had advanced disease, consistent with the stage of disease most common on presentation in India, which does not have active breast cancer detection programs in effect. They found that patients reported problems in a number of areas, particularly recreation, social life, mobility, physical activity, and sleep and attitude. The study concluded that until there is a change in health care in India, such that early detection of breast cancer is prevalent, women will be diagnosed with advanced disease that needs intensive treatment, and QOL will continue to be compromised.

Advantages and Disadvantages of Single Culture Studies

Studies in a single culture can provide a rich picture of the nuances in a given group. With the use of a common language, issues of cultural equivalence do not arise, and items can be tailored to the understanding and communication style of particular individuals or groups of individuals. However, as Navon[20] has pointed out, there is the potential for misinterpretation with such designs as well. For example, results found in such a study might be attributed to culture, when in fact they are due to other variables, such as socio economic factors or lack of medical care. The low QOL expectations and experiences associated with Indian cancer patients that Pandey et al.[18] report might change rapidly once early cancer detection and associated medical care result in better biomedical outcomes, such as increased survival. And conclusions based on a particular cultural group may be over-attributed to that cultural group. For example, the study of Hispanic cancer patients[11] concludes that "It is important to recognise that QOL is influenced by cultural background, life experiences, religion, and family."[11(p323)] This statement seems applicable to all cancer patients (and all human beings, including those without cancer). Appropriately, Juarez et al[11] urge studies of other cultures, a suggestion that is echoed here.

COMPARISONS WITH NORMATIVE DATA

Another approach to understanding QOL differences across ethnic and cultural groups is to utilize normative data against which the QOL of any given population can be compared. Such a strategy requires an approach to measuring QOL that has been validated in all groups to be compared, as well as normative samples that are matched on characteristics thought to be relevant to QOL; for example, sex, age, and socioeconomic status (SES). Meeting such criteria is often difficult, which is why not many such comparisons have been reported to date.

Table 1 provides an example of the comparative approach to QOL assessment in breast cancer. In this case, a common QOL assessment questionnaire, the Quality of Life-Cancer-30 items questionnaire (QLQ-C30), was available. This questionnaire was developed by the European Organization for Research and Treatment of Cancer for use in multicenter clinical trials, and it been validated in many European countries, including Sweden and Norway,[21] and Gotay et al.[22] validated the questionnaire in their primarily Asian and Pacific Islander cancer patient population in Hawaii and found that the factor structure was largely confirmed, construct validity was supported, and the subscales were internally consistent.[22] Gotay et al.[23] collected QLQ-C30 data on American women with breast cancer in Hawaii ($N = 230$), Carlsson and Hamrin[24] with Swedish breast cancer patients ($N = 362$), and Hjermstad et al.[25] with a large probability sample ($N = 2892$) of Danish residents. The data were reported by sex and 10-year age increments. This enabled a comparison between groups of similar sex and age.

TABLE 1. Comparison between Two Breast Cancer Studies and Population Norms on the QLQ-C30[a]

QLQ-C30 subscale[b]	Gotay et al.[c]	Carlsson and Hamrin[d]	Population Norms[e]
PF	86.1 (17.6)	82.3 (21.4)	82.9
RF	86.9 (24.6)	85.0 (26.1)	90.7
EF	79.6 (18.8)	84.2 (19.9)	81.3
CF	84.7 (18.1)	89.8 (15.6)	86.2
SF	84.1 (22.2)	91.9 (17.5)	83.7
QL	80.6 (14.7)	77.0 (21.2)	71.1
FA	24.0 (17.9)	21.6 (23.6)	31.4
NV	5.7 (14.9)	2.9 (10.7)	3.7
PA	16.4 (17.0)	14.7 (23.6)	28.9
DY	10.6 (18.2)	17.0 (24.1)	15.4
SL	23.0 (25.8)	19.9 (27.2)	28.9
AP	8.2 (17.7)	3.4 (13.3)	4.8
CO	11.6 (21.2)	6.6 (17.5)	15.2
DI	4.5 (12.9)	4.9 (14.8)	10.2
FI	18.0 (27.5)	5.1 (16.1)	12.1

[a]QLQ-C30 refers to the Quality of Life-Cancer-30 items questionnaire.[21]
[b]QLQ-C30 subscales are as follows: PF = Physical functioning, RF = Role functioning, EF = Emotional functioning, CF = Cognitive functioning, SF = Social functioning, QL = Global quality of life, FA = Fatigue, NV = Nausea and vomiting, PA = Pain, DY = Dyspnea, SL = Insomnia, AP = Appetite loss, CO = Constipation, DI = Diarrhea, FI = Financial difficulties. Numbers reflect means and standard deviations in parentheses.
[c]Gotay et al.[23] US sample with 75% Asians and Pacific Islanders.
[d]Carlsson and Hamrin[24] Swedish sample.
[e]Hjermstad et al.[25] General Norwegian population sample. Reported data were combined from women 50 to 59 and 60 to 69 for comparison with breast cancer patients.

As can be seen in Table 1, QOL was similar in all three groups, leading to the tentative conclusions that breast cancer survivors report QOL similar to women in the population at large, and that breast cancer patients in the US report similar QOL to breast cancer patients in Sweden. One difference across the three groups can be seen in the Financial (FI) subscale, where higher numbers mean more problems. The US patients reported more problems, consistent with the personal expense that is more likely associated with medical expenses in the United States compared to Scandinavia, where health care and social services are more widely available.

Advantages and Disadvantages of Normative Comparisons

While comparisons using normative data can be quite informative, there are limitations to such approaches. For example, there are a number of differences between the United States, Sweden, and Norway, and across the specific samples, that should also be considered in comparisons. Information on SES would be particularly useful, although equivalent indicators of SES can be difficult to define cross-culturally. In addition, QOL may change over time, and normative data may become outdated. For example, it is hoped that with the advent of targeted cancer therapies, cancer treatment will become increasingly less toxic[26]; thus, current norms for cancer-related QOL will become inappropriate comparisons in the future. Results from single studies should be replicated, and the sample sizes expanded. However, as more QOL questionnaires are validated for use in different cultures, normative data should become more stable, interpretation of the meaning of specific numerical scores for patient well-being clarified, and comparisons like the one in Table 1 increasingly informative.

COMPARATIVE STUDIES

As shown in Table 2,[23, 27-39] a number of studies have compared QOL in two or more different groups within a single study.[27] Fourteen studies were identified. Medline searches for the terms "cancer," "QOL," and "cultural or ethnic" were supplemented by searches with the names of specific ethnicities, races, and nationalities, and additional studies were identified through hand searches of relevant journals. Criteria for including studies in Table 2 were that more than one ethnic/cultural group was represented, that empirical patient-reported findings were presented and that at least one dimension of QOL was assessed. Studies that looked only at variables such as social support or coping were not included. Given the challenges of this kind of search, it is probable that we did not identify all studies in the published literature; however, Table 2 provides a representative listing.

All of these studies have used quantitative methods, although some sample sizes are so small that the data interpretation takes on a qualitative tone.[31] Two studies were from Europe,[32,33] one compared QOL in the United States with a Portuguese sample,[34] and the remainder compared subgroups within the United States. The most frequent comparisons were between African Americans and Whites (six studies), or African Americans, Whites, and Hispanics (two studies), or African Americans and Hispanics (one study). Two studies compared Whites and Asians, with the addition of Pacific Islanders in one study. Consistent with much of the psychosocial oncology literature, the majority of studies focused on or included breast cancer patients.[40] As shown in Table 2, every study except one[35] found ethnic or cultural differences, many of which persisted even after multivariate analyses that controlled for socioeconomic and other factors.

TABLE 2. Comparative Studies of QOL in Cancer Patients of Multiple Ethnicities

Study	No. of Patients	Patient Characteristics	Cancer Type	QOL Measures	Findings
Gotay et al.[23]	227	All American: Filipino (N = 30), Hawaiian (N = 25), Japanese (N = 73)	Diagnosed with breast or prostate cancer 4-6 months before	QLQ-C30	Filipinos reported worse QOL re: emotional functioning, nausea and symptoms (breast) and fatigue, nausea, symptoms, coping (prostate); differences maintained in multivariate analyses for breast but not prostate patients
Wan et al.[27]	761	African American (N = 320), Hispanic (N = 441)	Breast, lung, colon, head, and neck cancers	FACT	Hispanics had lower satisfaction with treatment in multivariate analysis
Moadel et al.[28]	248	African American (N = 62), Hispanic (N = 48), White (N = 118)	Oncology outpatients	New existential/spiritual scale	Hispanics highest, then African Americans, then Whites on both univariate and multivariate analyses
Eton.[29]	256	African American (N = 27), White (N = 229)	Localized prostate cancer within 7 weeks of treatment	SF-36 Prostate-specific QOL	Whites had better urinary, bowel, and physical functioning (co-morbidity, treatment, age controlled)
Lubeck et al.[30]	1178	African American (N = 161), White (N = 958)	Newly diagnosed prostate caner	SF-36, Prostate specific QOL	Blacks had lower QOL at baseline, but higher sexual function. Over time, all improved but Blacks more slowly
Kagawa-Singer et al.[31]	34	Anglo (N = 12), Chinese American (N = 11), Japanese American (N = 11)	Breast cancer 6 months 3 years post-treatment	CARES Social Support CES-D	Chinese had most problems with care providers, older Anglos most depressed
Bernhard et al.[32]	2220	Patients from 9 national/language groups: Slovenia, Sweden, Switzerland (German-speaking)/Germany, Spain, Italy, Switzerland (French-speaking), Australia/New Zealand, South Africa, Switzerland (Italian-speaking)	Stage II breast cancer patients on randomized treatment trial	5 Linear analogue scales (LASA)	Significant differences found on all 5 measures: highest, Italian, Swiss, lowest, Slovenians; clinical and sociodemographic factors also affected QOL
de Haes et al.[33]	689	Patients from 6 national/language groups: Eastern Europe, English-speaking, Finnish, French speaking, German, Latin countries	Stage 1 node positive breast cancer patients in randomized treatment trial	Rotterdam Symptom Checklist	Psychometric analysis confirmed RSCL stable across groups. Consistent differences across groups, French worst, Finnish best

Continued

TABLE 2. *Continued*

Study	No. of Patients	Patient Characteristics	Cancer Type	QOL Measures	Findings
Forjaz and Guarnaccia.[34]	207	American (N = 109), Portuguese (N = 98)	Outpatients with hematologic malignancy	Functional Living Index-Cancer (FLIC)	Portuguese had better physical and social functioning, less pain, more vitality, better overall (demographics controlled)
Rodrigue.[35]	98	African American (N = 42), White (N = 56)	Mixed cancers and stages	SCL-90, coping, family relationships, social support, satisfaction with health care	No differences in adjustment, depression, anxiety. African Americans used avoidance coping more, had more family disruption, had smaller social networks
Spencer et al.[36]	223	African American (N = 24), Hispanic (N = 48), White (N = 151)	Early stage breast cancer	New concerns about breast cancer scale, POMS, CES-D, Global QOL, social activities disruption, psychosexual well-being	Hispanics had most distress, social and psychosexual disruption, African Americans had least distress
Bourjolly et al.[37]	102	African American (N = 41), White (N = 61)	Breast cancer treated with breast conservation surgery and radiation	Social functioning	African Americans had lower social functioning and household activities (both bivariate and multivariate analyses)
Ashing-Giwa et al.[38]	278	African American (N = 117), White (N = 161)	Breast cancer, 7 years post-diagnosis	CARES SF-36 Ladder of life, Life stress, Quality of care	Univariate ethnic differences were explained by other factors (particularly life stress) in multivariate analyses
Deimling et al.[39]	180	African American (N = 90), White (N = 90)	Breast, colorectal, prostate cancer, 5+ years post-diagnosis	Functional limitations (IADL), self-rated health	African Americans had more functional limitations (both bivariate and multivariate analyses) and worse self-rated health (bivariate only)

The breast cancer studies, or studies of more than one site that presented results separately for breast cancer, are discussed in more detail in order to give a sense of the research that has been conducted to date. Two studies in breast cancer patients assessed QOL in largely European samples (although both studies[32,33] included patients from Australia, and Bernhard et al.[32] also from New Zealand and South Africa). Both studies were in the context clinical trials of cancer treatment. Such trials offer methodological advantages including the ability to specify tumor and treatment, large sample size, and attention to quality control of the data. In one study, Bernhard et al.[32] assessed QOL in a large sample of women from various countries who had received initial surgery for Stage II breast cancer. The report found significant differences between ethnic groups in all five QOL dimensions measured. For example, regarding mood, the Slovenian-speaking patients reported the lowest mood, while the Italian-speaking Swiss reported the highest. De Haes and colleagues[33] assessed QOL in Stage I breast cancer patients. Their national/language groups were largely nonoverlapping with the groups of Bernhard et al.,[32] and the QOL measure was different. Nonetheless, ethnic differences were found with consistent and large differences between the group with the lowest (French) and the highest scores (Finnish).[33]

The study of Kagawa-Singer et al.[31] of White ($N = 12$), Chinese American ($N = 11$), and Japanese American ($N = 11$) breast cancer survivors found that both age and acculturation affected communication of distress. Older women, particularly older Asian women, were less likely to report depression. Less acculturated women reported fewer psychosocial problems and more medical problems than more acculturated Asian women, whose responses were similar to those of the White women. In addition, the White women were three times more likely to request help than Japanese Americans, and two times more likely than Chinese Americans to do so.

Gotay et al.[23] assessed breast cancer patients from four ethnic groups (Filipino, Native Hawaiian, Japanese, White) within 5 months of diagnosis using the QLQ-C30. Scores for emotional functioning, nausea and vomiting, and symptom count varied significantly according to ethnicity. In all instances, the Filipino women reported worse outcomes than the other groups, which did not differ. In almost every other subscale, Filipinos were the population experiencing the lowest level of functioning among the four groups and the highest symptom levels, even though the differences were not statistically significant. In multiple regression analyses, ethnicity explained additional variance in all three outcomes (emotional functioning, nausea/vomiting, and symptom count) even after clinical and demographic variables were entered.

Spencer et al.[36] investigated psychosocial issues in White, Hispanic, and African American breast cancer patients who had been diagnosed during the past year. They found that, controlling for age and clinical variables, Hispanic women reported the highest levels of distress, while African American women reported the lowest levels. This pattern of results held across both the concerns reported by the women (including "life and pain," a factor derived from data reduction in this study, sexuality, work concerns, partner concerns, and concerns about seeing one's children grow up) and subjective well-being (including emotional distress, social disruption, sexual disruption, and femininity).

Bourjolly et al.[37] studied African American and White women who had received breast conserving surgery and radiation therapy for early stage breast cancer. They assessed social functioning as well as a number of predictive factors, including social support network, coping style, health locus of control, religiosity, and appraisal of cancer's impact. Results indicated that African American women had worse social functioning, even controlling for a number of other medical and social variables. The same relationships were found for household activities.

The study of Ashing-Giwa et al.[38] on African American and White long-term breast cancer survivors found univariate differences between the groups on several standardized measures of QOL, with African Americans expressing poorer QOL, general self-rated health, and stress. However, in multivariate analyses controlling for demographic variables and life stress, no ethnic differences were found. The authors suggest that socioeconomic, life stress, co-morbidity, and living situation were important predictors of QOL in breast cancer patients. This study points out the importance of considering additional variables that may be correlated with ethnicity, rather than concluding that differences among ethnic groups in a particular study are due to ethnicity per se.

Advantages and Disadvantages of Comparative Studies

Advantages to including multiple groups in the same study include a standard approach to recruiting and enrolling study participants, collection of data at the same time, use of common metrics, and the ability to put the findings for any one group into context. One challenge is identifying common metrics that are equally applicable for all groups in the study, as will be discussed in more detail below. It is a common temptation in comparative studies for investigators to choose QOL measures that have been used by other researchers in the target ethnic groups and have demonstrated reasonable psychometric properties, without really examining the questionnaires in terms of their items and match to study purposes. Careful selection of questionnaires is important, since content varies, as well as additional psychometric development that may sometimes be required.

It is difficult to draw conclusions about trends in these studies, given that there is so much variability in cultural groups, types of cancer and other clinical characteristics, and QOL measures used. However, it is clear that sometimes, apparent ethnic or cultural differences may be due to other factors. For example, the univariate or bivariate ethnic differences found in Ashing-Giwa et al.,[38] Deimling et al.[39] and the Gotay et al.[23] prostate cancer analysis were not maintained in multivariate analyses that controlled for other variables such as age, life stress, co-morbidity, and other factors. However, the univariate and bivariate analyses are still important and may be especially useful for clinicians, as they are likely to see patients as whole individuals, not in terms of multiple predictors. Thus, an oncologist may find it useful to know that QOL may be lower in Filipino prostate cancer patients, who may also be younger, recent immigrants, and less likely to have received radiation therapy (data from Gotay et al.[23]). In a number of studies, as shown in Table 2, ethnic differences remained after many other variables were controlled for,[23,27,28,34,37,39] indicating that ethnic group membership per se can be an important correlate of cultural differences in QOL.

MEASUREMENT OF QOL

Given the centrality of patients' evaluations of their own well-being to QOL, self-reports obtained from the individuals themselves are the primary way such information is collected. In cancer research, self-reports are most commonly gathered using standardized questionnaires and interviews. This methodology stems to some degree from the prevalence of QOL assessment in clinical trials of cancer therapy. In the setting of clinical trials, measures that are minimally intrusive in the busy clinic environment and that can be readily replicated over multiple sites of data collection are required. It is clear that the questions included in such surveys must be easily understood and language-appropriate. We will discuss briefly equivalence across cultures, and some QOL instruments that have been useful in cross-cultural cancer patient studies to date. The reader is referred to publications that provide detailed discussions of how to develop and ensure cross-cultural validity of QOL instruments.[38-44]

Assessment tools used in cross-cultural comparisons need to be examined to ensure that they are equivalent across groups. Several types of equivalence are desirable[45]: semantic equivalence (do the words and phrases have similar meaning?); idiomatic equivalence (do any idioms or colloquialisms have the same meaning?); experiential equivalence (are illustrative situations comparable: eg, asking if a patient can drive as an indication of access to transportation may not be meaningful in a culture where personal automobiles are rarely used); and conceptual equivalence (is the concept being measured equally meaningful in across cultures?). Stewart and Napoles-Springer[47] include three additional aspects of equivalence: operational equivalence (is the mode of administration, survey format, respondent burden, patient recruitment consistent across groups?), psychometric equivalence (are the standard psychometric properties, such as factor structure, internal consistency, and test-retest reliability comparable?), and criterion equivalence (eg, is interpretation of scores and cut-offs the same?). Clearly, developing instruments that meet standards for cultural equivalence of QOL instruments is a rigorous process.

Several comprehensive reports analyzing the performance of QOL questionnaires across cultures have been reported[45,46] Although these reviews did not examine every aspect of equivalence listed above, they provide a useful evaluation of current QOL questionnaires used in cancer patient populations. Aaronson[49] focused on five leading QOL questionnaires that had been applied cross-culturally: the Functional Living Index-Cancer (FLIC),[50] the Cancer Rehabilitation Evaluation System (CARES),[51] the Rotterdam Symptom Checklist (RSCL),[33] the EORTC QLQ-C30,[21] and the FACT.[19] All of these questionnaires were developed for cancer patient populations, to assess multiple aspects of patient functioning, and are designed to be self-administered questionnaires. They are currently available in multiple languages: FLIC—19; CARES—4; RSCL—at least 7; QLQ-C30—37; and the FACT—more than 40, and the EORTC and FACT teams have established standardized translation and review guidelines.[49] According to Aaronson,[49] considerable information on the psychometric properties of the QLQ-C30 and FACT are available, and less on the other three questionnaires. Aaronson[49] found that the psychometric performance of all five scales has been very good, and the weaknesses of the questionnaires that were apparent from the original validation tests of the different tools were confirmed in studies based in other cultures. For example, the cognitive functioning and emesis subscales of the QLQ-C30 consistently demonstrate lower consistency than the other subscales, as do the social and emotional subscales of the FACT. Aaronson[49] recommends that any of the questionnaires may be reasonable choices to assess QOL in a given study; however, because the specific content of the scales varies, the investigator needs to review the items and wording to determine which is the best choice for use in a given study.

DISCUSSION

Much of the literature discussed in this chapter is recent, having been published in just the past few years. Thus, it is apparent that more interest is being directed at understanding how cultural factors affect QOL and other outcomes in cancer patients and survivors.[52,53] There is considerably more work that needs to be done. We will focus on three areas that deserve special attention.

The Need to Include Members of the Target Cultural Groups in Study Design and Implementation

Researchers need to consider what is important to members of a particular culture to develop a meaningful QOL instrument. In addition, it is also important to consider the cultural appropriateness of the research methods themselves. For example, in many cultures, such as Native Hawaiians, face-to-face communication is very important. For this reason, techniques such as telephone interviews or mailed surveys may be seen as culturally inappropriate, irrelevant, or insulting. While many North American patients are quite experienced in completing survey forms and answering questions using scaled responses, linear scales, or computer scannable "bubble forms," other groups without these experiences may find such approaches impossible to understand. The cultural implications of the gender, age, and ethnicity of the interviewer, or person who administers an outcome assessment, may have a considerable influence on the data obtained, as suggested in the discussion of the Moore[13] study. For instance, a female might be very unlikely to discuss certain topics with a male, an older person to self-disclose to a younger interviewer, an African American with a White, and so forth. The importance of input and involvement of informants and/or collaborators who are knowledgeable about the target culture cannot be overestimated.

The Need to Recognize that Cultural Considerations are Important for all Patients

A considerably larger body of literature could have been used to inform this chapter if the emphasis had been on "American perspectives on QOL" since much of the literature to date has been based on studies in White, non-Hispanic cancer patients in the United States. However, cultural variables within the American experience are seldom pulled out for intensive examination; the Freedman[12] study illustrates an exception. However, it is worth reiterating that all patients are part of a culture, not only individuals who belong to minority groups, people who live in other countries, or those who are immigrants. Cultural aspects of values and appropriate behaviors are often invisible to members of "majority" groups, or when all individuals share the same values; however, it is through comparison with other groups that implicit cultural assumptions often become apparent. These cultural factors are key variables, along with life experiences, SES, and personality differences that affect the meaning of cancer for individuals and families, as well as its impact on QOL. As Burkett[54] points out, "culture ... is not an optional factor that only sometimes influences health and illness; it is a prerequisite for all meaningful human experiences, including being ill ... among all people, not just members of 'exotic' cultures" (p. 287).

The Need for Theory in Studies of Cultural and Ethnic Differences in QOL

The majority of the studies in this nascent literature attempted to see if there were, in fact, ethnic, cultural, or national differences in QOL outcomes. This is a reasonable start to understanding group differences. For instance, considerable effort goes into activities such as documenting differences in cancer incidence and survival in various groups across the US and internationally to understand patterns of cancer. Yet, the documentation of such differences is only the first step in understanding why such variation occurs and how negative outcomes can be modified. Some of the studies described herein were remarkably devoid of explanatory mechanisms for the ethnic differences detected. For example, the studies by Bernhard et al.[32] and de Haes et al.[33] uncovered major group differences within a largely Western European sample that might have been expected to be homogenous. Some findings seem contradictory: for example, in the Bernhard[32] study, Swedes had among the lowest scores, while in the de Haes[33] study, Finnish had among the highest scores. Still, because no additional information was collected beyond national origin and language group, it was impossible to know why such profound and perplexing differences emerged, and no explanations were offered.

More work is needed to understand the interplay of different QOL assessment tools in various population groups, as well as the effects of response styles, which have been shown to differ from one culture to the other. For example, Asians have been shown to avoid extreme responses on scales of emotion (eg, Lee[55]), and respondents of different ethnicity have been shown to be more likely to give socially desirable responses.[56] It may be that comfort in disclosing emotions varies cross-culturally. In an upcoming study, we are planning to explore this hypothesis by including a measure of emotional expressiveness to try to understand if the consistently higher distress reported by Filipinos in our studies reflects greater emotional expressiveness in Filipino culture. Such studies are needed to move this field beyond a study of ethnic differences to a study of cultural differences. Ethnicity can serve as a "shorthand" for shared cultural values, beliefs, and behaviors; however, to truly understand culture, values, beliefs, and behaviors need to be assessed directly. In fact, as underlying principles are elucidated, the distinctions among "ethnicity," "race," and "culture" become less relevant. In the future, we may not need to ask cancer patients to choose ethnic labels to describe themselves, but instead ask them questions such as how comfortable they feel discussing their feelings, the significance of independence in their lives, and the differential importance of group versus individual achievement—all areas that are thought to underlie cultural variations.[57]

In addition, the important role of traditional medical care needs to be considered in understanding QOL in diverse populations. Patients often turn to complementary and alternative (CAM) medicine to treat their cancer, many of which are based in their cultural beliefs about causes of cancer and appropriate remedies to treat the disease (see also chapter 10 by Ernst, this volume). Current uses of CAM treatments, generally, are widespread among the United States population. Eisenberg et al.[58] in a United States nationally representative study found that 42% of adults used some CAM during the previous year for various illnesses. Within the United States, there is evidence that CAM use in cancer varies according to ethnicity. Lee and colleagues[59] studied CAM use in newly diagnosed breast cancer patients of multiple ethnicities ($N = 373$). Differences were found among ethnic groups, as African Americans were most likely to use spiritual healing, Chinese women were most likely to choose herbal remedies and dietary therapies, Whites were most likely to choose psychological therapies such as counseling, meditation or imagery, and dietary therapies, and Hispanics were most likely to use dietary methods and spiritual healing. Maskarinec et al.[60] included 1 168 patients with invasive cancer and found that CAM use was highest among Filipino and Caucasian patients, intermediate for Native Hawaiians and Chinese, and significantly lower among Japanese. Some ethnic preferences for CAM followed ethnic folk medicine traditions, for example, herbal medicines by Chinese, Hawaiian healing by Native Hawaiians, and religious healing or prayer by Filipinos. Further research is needed to understand and how it is linked to cultural beliefs and values and how CAM use affects QOL.[61]

CONCLUSION

Research on QOL in cancer patients from different cultures offers the potential for fascinating insights that will guide the development of culturally appropriate cancer treatment and supportive care to improve patient well-being. Such studies will help to explain which impacts of cancer and cancer treatments are invariant across groups, and which aspects are culture-specific. With increased cultural mixing—both internationally and interpersonally, as a result of increased numbers of inter-ethnic marriages—the situation becomes even more interesting and challenging. The literature to date has documented that there are ethnic and cultural differences in cancer-related QOL, and there are validated approaches to measure QOL across cancer patients from different cultural groups. Further development of this field will depend on complementary information from both qualitative and quantitative methods. Such research has the potential to further our understanding of the impact of cancer on QOL in the international arena, as well as closer to home.

REFERENCES

1. WHOQOL Group. Study protocol for the World Health Organisation project to develop a Quality of Life assessment instrument (the WHOQOL). *Qual Life Res.* 1993;2:153-159.
2. WHOQOL Group. The World Health Organization Quality of Life assessment (WHOQOL): position paper from the World Health Organization. *Social Sci Med.* 1995;41:1403-1409.
3. Stjernsward J, Teoh N. Current status of the global cancer control program of the World Health Organization. *J Pain Symptom Manage.* 1993;8:340-347.
4. Mark N, Roberts L. Ethnosensitive techniques in the treatment of Hasidic patients with cancer. *Cancer Pract.* 1994;2:202-208.
5. Peretz T, Baider L, Ever-Hadani P, De-Nour AK. Psychological distress in female cancer patients with Holocaust experience. *Gen Hosp Psychiatr.* 1994;16:413-418.
6. Baider L, Peretz T, Hadani PE, Perry S, Avramov R, Kaplan De-Nour A. Transmission of response to trauma? Second-generation Holocaust survivors' reaction to cancer. *Am J Psychiatr.* 2000;157:904-910.
7. McDermott JF, Tseng W, Maretzki TW. *People and Cultures of Hawaii.* Honolulu, HI: University of Hawai'i Press; 1980.
8. Tseng WS, Hsu J. *Culture and Family: Problems and Therapy.* New York, NY: Haworth; 1991.
9. Chaturvedi SK. What's important for quality of life to Indians-in relation to cancer. *Soc Sci Med.* 1991;33:91-94.
10. Donovan K, Sanson Fisher RW, Redman S. Measuring quality of life in cancer patients. *J Clin Oncol.* 1989;7:959-968.
11. Juarez G, Ferrell B, Borneman T. Perceptions of quality of life in Hispanic patients with cancer. *Cancer Pract.* 1998;6:318-324.
12. Freedman TG. Social and cultural dimensions of hair loss in women treated for breast cancer. *Cancer Nurs.* 1994;17:334-341.
13. Moore RJ. African American women and breast cancer. *Cancer Nurs.* 2001;24:35-42.
14. Northouse LL, Caffey M, Deichelbohrer L, et al. The quality of life of African American women with breast cancer. *Res Nurs Health.* 1999;22:449-460.
15. Wilmoth MC, Sanders LD. Accept me for myself: African American women's issues after breast cancer. *Oncol Nurs Forum.* 2001;28:875-879.
16. Molassiotis A, Chan CWH, Yam BMC, Chan ESJ, Lam CSW. Life after cancer: adaptation issues faced by Chinese gynaecological cancer survivors in Hong Kong. *Psychoncology.* 2002;11:114-1123.

17. Lam WWT, Fielding R. The evolving experience of illness for Chinese women with breast cancer: a qualitative study. *Psychooncology.* 2003;12:127-140.
18. Pandey M, Singh SP, Behere PB, Roy SK, Singh S, Shukla VK. Quality of life in patients with early and advanced carcinoma of the breast. *Eur J Surg Oncol.* 2000;26:20-24.
19. Cella DF, Tulsky DS, Gray G, et al. The functional assessment of cancer therapy scale: development and validation of the general measure. *J Clin Oncol.* 1993;11:570-579.
20. Navon L. Cultural views of cancer around the world. *Cancer Nurs.* 1999;22:39-45.
21. Aaronson NK, Ahmedzai S, Bergman B, et al. The European organization for research and treatment of cancer QLQ-C30: a quality of life instrument for use in clinical trials in oncology. *J Natl Cancer Inst.* 1993;85:365-376.
22. Gotay CC, Blaine D, Haynes SN, Holup J, Pagano I. Assessment of quality of life in a multicultural cancer patient population. *Psychol Assess.* 2002;14:439-450.
23. Gotay CC, Holup JL, Pagano I. Ethnic differences in quality of life among early breast and prostate cancer survivors. *Psychooncology.* 2002;11:103-113.
24. Carlsson M, Hamrin E. Measurement of quality of life in women with breast cancer: development of a Life Satisfaction Questionnaire (LSQ-32) and a comparison with the EORTC QLQ-30. *Qual Life Res.* 1996;5:265-274.
25. Hjermstad MJ, Fayers PM, Bjordal K, Kaasa S. Using reference data on quality of life: the importance of adjusting for age and gender, exemplified by the EORTC QLQ-C30 (+3). *Eur J Cancer.* 1998;3:1381-1387.
26. Atkins JH, Gershall LJ. Selective anticancer drugs. *Nat Rev: Drugs Discovery.* 2002;1:491-492.
27. Wan GJ, Counte MA, Cella DF, et al. The impact of socio-cultural and clinical factors in health-related quality of life reports among Hispanic and African American cancer patients. *J Outcomes Meas.* 1999;3:200-215.
28. Moadel A, Morgan C, Fatone A, et al. Seeking meaning and hope: self-reported spiritual and existential needs among an ethnically-diverse cancer patient population. *Psychooncology.* 1999;8:378-385.
29. Eton DT, Lepore SJ, Helgeson VS. Early quality of life in patients with localized prostate carcinoma: an examination of treatment-related, demographic, and psychosocial factors. *Cancer.* 2001;92:1451-1459.
30. Lubeck DP, Kim H, Grossfeld G, et al. Health related quality of life differences between black and white men with prostate cancer: data from the cancer of the prostate strategic urologic research endeavor. *J Urol.* 2001;166:2281-2285.
31. Kagawa-Singer M, Wellisch DK, Durvasula R. Impact of breast cancer on Asian American and Anglo American women. *Cult Med Psychiatr.* 1997;21:449-480.
32. Bernhard J, Hurny C, Coates AS, et al. Factors affecting baseline quality of life in two international adjuvant breast cancer trials. *Br J Cancer.* 1998;78:686-693.
33. de Haes JC, Olschewski M. Quality of life assessment in a cross-cultural context: use of the Rotterdam symptom checklist in a multinational randomized trial comparing CMF and Zoladex (Goserlin) treatment in early breast cancer. *Ann Oncol.* 1998;9:745-750.
34. Forjaz MJ, Guarnaccia CA. A comparison of Portuguese and American patients with hematological malignancies: a cross-cultural survey of health-related quality of life. *Psychooncology.* 2001;10:251-258.
35. Rodrigue JR. An examination of race differences in patients' psychological adjustment to cancer. *J Clin Psychol.* 1997;4:271-280.
36. Spencer SM, Lehman JM, Wynings C, et al. Concerns about breast cancer and relations to psychosocial well-being in a multiethnic sample of early-stage patients. *Health Psychol.* 1999;18:159-168.
37. Bourjolly JN, Kerson TS, Nuamah IF. A comparison of social functioning among black and white women with breast cancer. *Soc Work Health Care.* 1999;28:1-20.

38. Ashing-Giwa K, Ganz PA, Petersen L. Quality of life of African American and white long term breast carcinoma survivors. *Cancer.* 1999;85:418-426.

39. Deimling GT, Schaefer ML, Kahana B, Bowman KF, Reardon J. Racial differences in health of older-adult long-term cancer survivors. *J of Psychosocial Oncol.* 2002;20:71-94.

40. Gotay, CC, Muraoka, MY. Quality of life in long-term survivors of adult-onset cancers. *J Natl Cancer Inst.* 1998;90:656-667.

41. Acquadro C, Jambon B, Ellis D, Marquis P. Language and translation issues. In: Spilker B, ed. *Quality of Life and Pharmacoeconomics in Clinical Trials.* 2nd ed. Philadelphia, PA: Lippincott-Raven Publishers; 1996:575-585.

42. Anderson RT, McFarlene M, Naughhton MJ, Shumaker SA. Conceptual issues and considerations in cross-cultural validation of generic health-related quality of life instruments. In: Spilker B, ed. *Quality of Life and Pharmacoeconomics in Clinical Trials.* 2nd ed. Philadelphia, PA: Lippincott-Raven Publishers; 1996:605-612.

43. Bullinger M, Power MJ, Aaronson NK, Cella DF, Anderson RT. Creating and evaluating cross-cultural instruments. In: Spilker B, ed. *Quality of Life and Pharmacoeconomics in Clinical Trials.* 2nd ed. Philadelphia, PA: Lippincott-Raven Publishers; 1996:659-668.

44. Cella DF, Lloyd SR, Wright B. Cross-cultural instrument equating: current research and future directions. In: Spilker B, ed. *Quality of Life and Pharmacoeconomics in Clinical Trials.* 2nd ed. Philadelphia, PA: Lippincott-Raven Publishers; 1996:707-715.

45. Guillemin F, Bombardier C, Beaton D. Cross-cultural adaptation of health-related quality of life measures: literature review and proposed guidelines. *J Clin Epidemiol.* 1993; 46:1417-1432.

46. Hilton A, Skrutkowski M. Translating instruments into other languages: development and testing processes. *Cancer Nurs.* 2002;25:1-7.

47. Stewart AL, Napoles-Springer A. Health related quality of life assessment in diverse population groups in the United States. *Med Care.* 2000;38:II-102-II-124.

48. Anderson, RT, Aaronson NK, Leplege AP, Wildin D. International use and application of generic health-related quality of life instruments. In: Spilker B, ed. *Quality of Life and Pharmacoeconomics in Clinical Trials.* 2nd ed. Philadelphia, PA: Lippincott-Raven Publishers; 1996:613-632.

49. Aaronson NK. Cross-cultural use of health-related quality of life assessments in clinical oncology. In: Lipscomb J, Gotay CC, Snyder C, eds. *Outcomes Assessment in Cancer.* Cambridge, MA: Cambridge University Press; in press.

50. Schipper H, Clinch J, McMurray A, Levitt M. Measuring the quality of life of cancer patients: the functional living index-cancer: development and validation. *J Clin Oncol.* 1984;2:472-483.

51. Ganz PA, Schag CA, Lee JJ, Sim HS. The CARES: a generic measure of health-related quality of life in patients with cancer. *Qual Life Res,* 1992;1:19-29.

52. Aziz NM, Rowland JH. Cancer survivorship research among ethnic minority and medically underserved groups. *Oncol Nurs Forum.* 2002;29:789-801.

52. Meyerowitz BE, Richardson J, Hudson S, Leedham B. Ethnicity and cancer outcomes: behavioral and psychosocial considerations. *Psychol Bull.* 1998;123:47-70.

54. Burkett GL. Culture, illness, and the biopsychosocial model. *Fam Med.* 1991;23:2867-2891.

55. Lee JW, Jones PS, Mineyama Y, Zhang XE. Cultural differences in responses to a Likert scale. *Res Nurs Health.* 2002;25:295-306.

56. Warnecke RB, Johnson TP, Chavez N, et al. Improving question wording in surveys of culturally diverse populations. *Ann Epidemiol.* 1997;7:334-342.

57. Gotay CC. Cultural variations in family adjustment to cancer. In: Baider L, Cooper GL, Kaplan De-Nour A, eds. *Cancer and the Family.* New York, NY Wiley; 1996:31-52.

58. Eisenberg DM, Davis RB, Ettner SL, et al. Trends in alternative medicine use in the United States, 1990-1997: results of a follow-up national survey. *JAMA.* 1998;280:1569-1575.

59. Lee MM, Lin SS, Wrensch MR, Adler SR, Eisenberg DM. Alternative therapies used by women with breast cancer in four ethnic populations. *J Natl Cancer Inst.* 2000;92:42-47.
60. Maskarinec G, Shumay DM, Kakai H, Gotay CC. Ethnic differences in complementary and alternative medicine use among cancer patients. *J Altern Complement Med.* 2000;6:531-538.
61. Maskarinec G, Gotay CC, Tatsumura Y, Shumay DM, Kakai H. Perceived cancer causes: use of complementary and alternative therapy. *Cancer Pract.* 2001;9:183-190.

CHAPTER 4

Cancer and Aging

A Biological, Clinical, and Cultural Analysis

Lodovico Balducci, Darlene Johnson, and Claudia Beghe

INTRODUCTION

By and large, cancer is a disease of old age. In the Western world, more than 50% of all cancers occur in the 12% of the population aged 65 to 95.[1,2] Due to the extended life expectancy of certain populations in the Western context, this percentage is expected to increase with the aging of the global population.[1,2] As such, strategies for effectively preventing, managing, and controlling cancer hinge on the successful communication between clinicians and aged individuals. Clinicians should be able to illustrate preventative and treatment options available to the older person, patients should be able to state their desire and priorities for the conduction of their own lives; clinicians and patients together should reach a consensus for the most suitable choices in individual situations. Additionally, to be effective, these messages need be congruent with the special needs and aspirations of increasingly culturally diverse patients with cancer.[3] In this chapter, we establish a conceptual frame of reference where different experiences of aging may be accommodated, and different strategies for care may be explored. We specifically seek to address the following concerns: What is aging? We will first define aging. Then we illustrate the biological, functional, medical, social, and emotional changes associated with aging. We further propose an assessment of physiologic rather than chronological age. We then proceed to investigate the influence of life expectancy, age-related changes in function, co-morbidity, social and emotional support on cancer prevention and treatment. What are the age-related barriers to cancer prevention and treatment, with special focus on agism? Finally, what are the ways in which we can effectively communicate with the older person across culturally diverse contexts? In particular, we will examine the effects of social and cultural contexts and of personal belief on communication.

DEFINITION OF AGING: BIOLOGICAL, PHYSIOLOGICAL, FUNCTIONAL, MEDICAL, AND SOCIAL PARAMETERS

Aging may be thought of as a progressive reduction in tolerance of stress due to a progressive declining functional reserve of multiple organs and systems.[4] As a consequence of this decline, susceptibility to disease is increased and ultimately the life expectancy is shortened. The causes of aging are multiple and seemingly include an exhaustible functional reserve, whose exhaustion is hastened by traumatic life events, such as diseases, accidents, and financial and emotional stress. A number of biological events are recognizable with aging which include:

1. Molecular abnormalities of cellular aging, such as an increase in the formation of DNA adducts, DNA hypermethylation, point mutation, expression of genes such as P16, that inhibit the cell cycle. Some of these mutations mimic early carcinogenesis and enhance the vulnerability of older individuals to environmental carcinogens. All of these events may compromise cell function and viability.[5-7]
2. Synthesis of abnormal proteins also may compromise cell function and metabolism.[5-7] These changes may result in abnormal metabolism of cytotoxic drug and decreased sensitivity to these agents.
3. Decreased cell proliferation. Evolutionary pressures have selected this for successful reproduction, making it likely that the aging of an organism is an epigenetic and pleiotropic manifestation of the optimization for early fitness. Indeed, antagonistic pleiotropy, wherein genes that enhance early survival and function but are disadvantageous later in life, may play an overriding role in aging.[8] This phenomenon, also known as proliferative senescence, may paradoxically enhance the risk of cancer.[9-10] Senescent cells have lost the ability to undergo apoptosis and produce a number of

growth factors and proteolytic enzymes that may promote genomic instability in terms of carcinogenesis and metastases.

4. Changes in body environment, including immune-senescence,[12] may increase the risk of infections and neoplastic diseases, endocrine senescence, which may lead to osteoporosis, genito-urinary atrophy, dementia, and a generalized catabolic status.[13] Of special interest, aging has been associated with increased concentration in the circulation of catabolic cytokines, such as Interleukins (Il),[1,2,6,10] tumor necrosis factor (TNF), tissue growth factor-β (TGF-β), which may be responsible for reduced anabolic activity and dysfunction of the central nervous system,[12] bones,[13] muscles,[14] and may inhibit hemopoiesis.[15] These findings underlie the hypothesis of aging as a chronic inflammation, and further propose that signs of chronic inflammation, such as increased concentrations of D-Dimer and C-reactive protein in the circulation may reflect loss of functional reserve, that is, the ability to cope with stress.[16-18]

5. Reduced function of different organs and systems: for example, a decline in glomerular filtration rates, maximal respiratory capacity, and splanchnic circulation is almost universal, whereas nerve conduction is remarkably preserved.[4]

In addition, personal and environmental resources, including formal and informal support networks, may also decline with aging. Moreover, as cognition declines so does the ability to process new information and to adapt to new situations. Decline in taste, social and emotional isolation, and depression may lead to malnutrition. For instance, reduced eyesight may compromise access to transportation and performance of simple activities, and these problems are generally worsened by social isolation.[19,20]

Clearly, aging involves the interaction of different domains and is highly individualized. Thus, the clinical evaluation of the older person needs to account for individual changes in each of these domains. For these reasons, a multidimensional assessment of the older person may provide necessary clues to individual life expectancy, functional reserve, emotional and social needs, and allows the formulation of individual management plans.

THE ASSESSMENT OF AGING

The Comprehensive Geriatric Assessment (CGA)

A CGA (Table 1) has been used for a long time as the standard form of assessment of older individuals.

TABLE 1. The Comprehensive Geriatric Assessment (CGA)

Parameter	Assessment
Function	*Activities of Daily Living (ADL)* Eating, dressing, continence, grooming, transferring, going to the bathroom *Instrumental Activities of Daily Living (IADL)* Use of transportation, management of money and medications, shopping, ability to provide own meals, ability to perform laundry, house management, and use of telephone Performance status
Co-morbidity	Number of co-morbid conditions *Seriousness of co-morbid conditions (co-morbidity index)*
Socioeconomic issues	Living conditions *Presence and adequacy of caregiver* *Income* *Access to transportation*
Geriatric Syndromes	Dementia Minimental status (MMS), other Depression Geriatric depression scale (GDS) Delirium For minimal infection or medication Falls ($\geq$1/month) Osteoporosis (spontaneous fractures) Neglect and abuse *Failure to thrive* *Dizziness*
Polypharmacy	Number of medication *Drug-drug interaction*
Nutrition	Nutritional risk Mini nutritional assessment (MNA)

Function

Function is assessed as performance status (PS), Activities of Daily Living (ADLs), and Instrumental Activities of Daily Living (IADLs). Function is predictive of mortality, which at 2 years is less that 10% for individuals aged 70 and older who are fully independent, increases to around 15% for those dependent in one or more of the IADLs, and is higher than 20% for those dependent in one or more ADLs.[21-23] Dependence in IADLs is also associated with increased risk of dementia at 2 years and has been associated with increased risk of chemotherapy-induced neutropenia in two prospective studies. IADL, ADL, and PS appeared poorly correlated with each other in two perspective studies and it is recommended that they be independently evaluated.[24,25]

Co-morbidity

Co-morbidity is also associated with increased mortality,[21,26,27] increased risk of functional dependence,[27] and reduced tolerance of cytotoxic treatment.[28-30] The assessment of co-morbidity remains controversial for a variety of reasons.[31] Satariano and Ragland demonstrated that the risk of mortality in older women with breast cancer was correlated to the number of co-morbid conditions, chosen among seven conditions.[26] This simple approach fails to account for the severity of each condition that is instead reflected in the co-morbidity scales, devised by several authors. Of these, the Cumulative Index of Related Symptoms-Geriatrics (CIRS-G) is the most manageable in our opinion, because it proved more sensitive than other scales[31] and its final score may be translated into the score of another scale of common use in epidemiological studies, the Charlson's scale.

Among co-morbid conditions, anemia is of special interest.[31] The incidence and prevalence of anemia that increase with age is an independent risk factor for death,[32-34] myelosuppression from cytotoxic chemotherapy,[31,35] fatigue and functional dependence.[34] In studies involving patients with chronic renal failure, anemia was associated with increased risk with congestive heart failure and dementia, which were averted by correcting anemia with erythropoietin.[36-38] In cancer patients, anemia was associated with reduced survival, while correction of anemia with erythropoietin may improve survival.[34]

Geriatric Syndromes

These are conditions typical, if not specific, to aging and are associated with decreased life expectancy.[39,40] Geriatric syndromes are associated with reduced life expectancy and are considered a hallmark of frailty,[39,40] a condition with negligible functional reserve. Only when these conditions interfere with a person's daily life are they considered the *Geriatric Syndrome*. For instance, delirium must be unexpected and occurs in association with medications or mild infections that do not cause delirium in a healthy elderly. Incontinence must be complete and irreversible. Falls must occur at least three times a month or the fear of falling prevents regular activities, such as walking, and vertigo must be continuous and must interfere with a person's movements. As a characteristic of *geriatric syndromes*, depression deserves special attention. The scope of this condition is broad and its consequences on survival and quality of life are far-reaching. While only severe depression is generally considered a geriatric syndrome, the clinician should be aware that even subclinical forms of depression are associated with increased risk of mortality.[41] For this reason, older individuals should be considered at high risk for depression and should undergo screening for this condition, which may be reversible, particularly in the early stages of cancer.[42,43] The high prevalence of depression may derive in part from the social changes of aging including isolation from dissolution of nuclear family and waning of social relationship due to disease, disability, and death. Depression may also underlie the high rate of suicide among elderly individuals. For example, they are both also particularly high among certain ethnic groups such as the Chinese.[44-46] In addition, several simple instruments, including the Geriatric Depression Scale may be used to screen cancer patients for depression.[43]

Social Resources

The issue of social resources is of particular relevance in the Western context, where the dissolution of the nuclear family has coincided with the dissolution of the informal support network, while the formal network may be expensive and cumbersome.[19,20] Of these social resources, of central importance is the home caregiver who should be able to recognize and manage emergencies, to provide physical and emotional support to the patient, to mediate conflicts within the family and between the family and clinicians.[47] Caregiving for an ill elderly person may be very stressful and could be a cause of morbidity and mortality to the caregiver. For instance, recent studies suggest that many caregivers consider their health to be poorer than that of age-matched peers and approximately 80% of caregivers suffer from depression. The stressful situation of caregivers makes their job more difficult because the carereceiver's symptoms and emotional state[48] influence it. As the caregiver may turn into the most effective ally of the clinician, it behooves the clinician to provide adequate training and support to the caregiver, and to maintain this uniquely precious resource.

Nutrition

The prevalence of protein/calorie malnutrition increases with age. Malnutrition is a risk factor for functional dependency,[49,50] mortality,[51,52] and chemotherapy-associated complications.[53] In the majority of cases, malnutrition of older individuals is preventable or reversible. A simple screening test of international use, the Mini Nutritional Assessment (MNA) identifies patients who are malnourished and those at risk of becoming malnourished.[54]

Polypharmacy

Polypharmacy is the assumption of multiple drugs, some of which are redundant or unnecessary.[55] The prevalence of polypharmacy increases with age. Among cancer patients aged 70 and older, polypharmacy was present in 41% of cases.[24,25] Polypharmacy reflects a common problem of elderly patients in developed country: the absence of a primary care clinician.[56] This problem is further compounded by the availability of alternative medicine products. Although polypharmacy may be appropriate in few cases, it may increase the risk of drug interactions and iatrogenic diseases as well as the cost of care.

The benefits of the CGA in the general geriatric population include reduction in the number of hospitalizations, maintenance of functional independence, and the potential improvement of survival and related outcomes.[57-59] In the management of the older cancer patients, the CGA has succeeded in the following.

1. Preparing the patient for cancer treatment by discovering unsuspected conditions that may interfere with the treatment.[24,25,60,61] For example, the application of the CGA to 15 women aged 70 and over has resulted in 17.2 new intervention for patients that would have been omitted without the CGA.[62] Three studies explored prospectively the CGA in cancer patients aged 70 and above. Dependence in IADL was present in approximately 70% of these subjects, some degree of co-morbidity in more than 70%, and dementia, malnutrition, and depression in approximately 20% each.[24,25,61]
2. Estimation of life expectancy and treatment tolerance. The risk of mortality increases with the risk of functional dependence, the severity of co-morbidity, the degree of dementia and depression, malnutrition, failure to thrive, falls and neglect and abuse (Table 2).[21-25,63-65] Two recent studies demonstrated that IADL dependence was an independent risk factor in chemotherapy complications.[28,30] In addition, the discovery of certain co-morbid conditions, such as history of heart disease, diabetes, or peripheral neuropathy may exclude medications that are toxic to certain organs.
3. The assessment of the social situation, living conditions, economic resources, and caregiving opportunities.

TABLE 2. The Vulnerable Elderly Survey 13 (VES-13)

Element of Assessment	Score
A. Scoring system	
Age	
• 75-84	1
• ≥85	3
Self-reported health	
• Good or excellent	0
• Fair or poor	1
ADL/IADL. Needs helps in	
• Shopping	1
• Money management	1
• Light housework	1
• Transferring	1
• Bathing	1
Activities. Needs help in	
• Stooping, crouching or kneeling	1
• Lifting or carrying 10 lbs	1
• Writing or handling small objects	1
• Reaching or extending arm above shoulder	1
• Walking 1/4 mile	1
• Heavy housework	1

B. Vulnerability scores, functional decline, and survival

Score	Risk of functional decline or death (%)
1-2	11.8
3+	49.8
1-3	14.8
4+	54.9

4. The institution of a common language in the description of older individuals. This common language may facilitate the interpretation of clinical data and clinical trials, which are often marred by the diversity of the older population. Hamerman in important research has recognized four states[39] and has proposed a conceptual framework for the nosology of aging. These include a primary state of full independence, an intermediate state in which persons start developing dependence, a secondary state or "frailty" in which patients have exhausted every functional reserve, and a fourth state, or near death.

However, the application of this model to clinical practice is hindered by two problems: lack of a common definition of frailty and the wide gamut of conditions encompassed by the intermediate state. Most definitions of frailty include dependence in one or more ADLs, the presence of one or more geriatric syndromes, and serious co-morbidity, which interferes with the person's daily life. Still, it is not farfetched that in a near future we will be able to reach a clinical consensus about this condition and study its clinical implications in the clinical arena. Rather, the boundaries of the intermediate state represent a more serious problem and more precise clinical criteria to subclassify this state appear desirable. Despite these limitations, the CGA is the basis of an algorithm for cancer treatment in the older person and is of common use in our institution for management of patients aged 70 and older with chemotherapy (Figure 1). In this algorithm it should be noticed that symptom management may include low doses of chemotherapy, such as capecitabine, low doses of taxanes, navelbine, and gemcitabine, that in some frail patients may be more effective and better tolerated than opioids.[40] This algorithm may be used as frame of reference in clinical practice and fine-tuned as our understanding of aging improves.

Limits and Evolution of the CGA

Undoubtedly, the CGA has given an important contribution to the understanding of aging and to the management of older individuals. However, the CGA in its present form has two major limitations:

- It is time- and resources consuming.
- The wealth of information of the CGA needs to be integrated into simple index predicting life expectancy, risk of chemotherapy-related toxicity, and more in general of the risk of functional decline.

As a consequence, a number of simple and timesaving screening tests have been proposed "in lieu" of a comprehensive assessment. Elderly who screen positive are considered at increased risk of death and functional decline and need a more comprehensive assessment to establish whether their condition is reversible with appropriate medical and social care. Of these screening tests, two deserve special attention. The Vulnerable Elderly Survey 13 (VES-13) is a 13-item questionnaire that may be self-administered in the clinic waiting room and requires only few minutes (Table 3).[66] This instrument is appealing, because it has been tested in home dwelling elderly, that reflect the majority of older cancer patients. And it has been well validated as a score of 4 or higher indicates an almost fourfold increase in

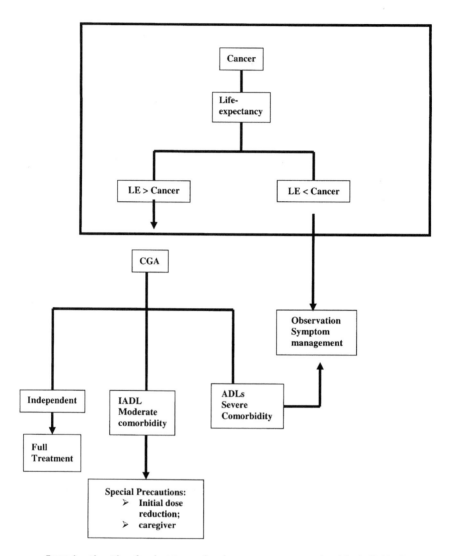

FIGURE 1   Algorithm for decisions related to cancer treatment in older individuals.

risk of death and functional decline. In addition, the VES-13 score may also reflect the influence of co-morbidity on survival and functional decline, because the addition of a co-morbidity score did not change the predictive value of the VES-13. Of concern is the fact that the VES-13 is heavily weighted by age. Thus, it may tend to overestimate the risk of death and

TABLE 3. Pharmacologic Changes of Age That May Influence Cancer Chemotherapy

Pharmacokinetic changes		
Absorption	Reduced	Does not seem to affect bioavailability of oral agents
Renal excretion	Reduced	May increase toxicity of agents whose parent compounds are excreted from the kidneys; and of active metabolites of other agents
Hepatic metabolism	Reduced activity of phase I reaction, the effects of phase II reactions not clear	Unknown consequences
Biliary excretion	Probably unchanged	Irrelevant
Volume of distribution (Vd) for hydrosoluble drugs	Reduced due to decreased total body water and serum albumin concentration. May be worsened by anemia, as many agents are bound to red blood cells	May be associated with increased toxicity; correction of anemia is recommended
Pharmacodinamic changes		
Increased prevalence of multidrug resistance	• Increased prevalence of MDR1 expression in AML • Decreased tumor growth fraction • Increased tumor anoxia • Abnormalities of enzymes that are the target of chemotherapy	Decreased treatment effectiveness
Decreased intracellular drug metabolism	Decreased intracellular concentration and activity of drug metabolizing enzymes	Enhanced risk of toxicity
Reduced ability to repair DNA damage	Longer persistence of cellular damage in normal cells	Enhanced risk of toxicity
Susceptibility of special organ-systems		
Hemopoiesis	• Reduced reserve of hemopoietic stem cells • Reduced production of growth factors • Malnutrition	Increased risk of neutropenia and thrombocytopenia for moderately toxic chemotherapy (CHOP and regimens of similar dose-intensity)

continued

TABLE 3. *(continued)*

	• Increased concentration of circulating cytokines that inhibit hemopoiesis	
Gastrointestinal mucosas	• Reduced stem cell concentration • Enhanced proliferation of cryptal cells	Increased risk and severity of mucositis from fluorinated pyrimidines
Myocardium	Reduced concentration of sarcomeres	Increased risk of cardiotoxicity
Central and peripheral nervous system	Reduced number of neurons	Increased risk of neurotoxicity

functional decline for the oldest individuals. Also of concern is the lack of questions related to nutrition, pharmacy, social support, cognitive, and emotional status.

The other screening test is a test of physical performance (get up and go) that consists in asking a person to get up from an armchair, walk ten feet and back, and sit again. A score of 1 is given for each one of these points: requiring more than 10 s to complete the movement, uncertain gait, and the need to use the elbow to get up. The higher the score, the higher the risk of functional dependence in the next two years.[67] It appears reasonable to perform an "in depth" CGA in all patients with a score of 1 and higher. No information exists about the sensitivity of this test for co-morbidity, depression, memory disorders, and the need for social support. Prior to being used "in lieu" of the complete CGA, this test needs validation in clinical trials.

A clear interrelation exists between function, co-morbidity, cognition, depression, and nutrition.[49,50,67-70] Two possible models of interaction are considered (Figure 2). In Model A, function recapitulates all other parameters in the assessment of life expectancy, functional decline, and risk of chemotherapy-related toxicity. The independence of the VES-13 score from co-morbidity supports this approach. In Model B, a combined index is required to integrate the various assessment parameters. This approach is also supported by other studies, which indicate that life expectancy and functional decline are complex functions.[21,63]

It should be noticed that the clinical impression is quite accurate in the diagnosis of frailty.[71] The real and yet unsolved problem is to establish how many assessment parameters one needs to correctly classify that elusive intermediate state to which the majority of older cancer patients belong.

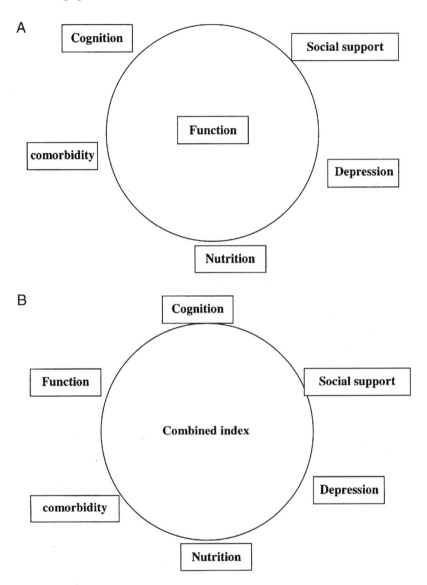

FIGURE 2 Interrelations of comorbidity and other age-related changes.

For what concerns prediction of chemotherapy-related toxicity, an index integrating the different risk of toxicity of different chemotherapy regimens and the characteristics of individual patients is being studied in our institution. This index is called Chemotherapy Related Assessment High age patients (CRASH).

Other Forms of Aging Assessment

The increased concentration of catabolic cytokines in the blood of older individuals may aid in predicting which individuals may be at greater risk of dying and functional decline. For sometime now it has been known that the concentrations of IL-6 were increased in the circulation of patients with different geriatric syndromes, and that these concentrations may predict functional decline. Recently, Cohen et al. demonstrated that increased concentrations of both IL-6 and D-dimer in home-dwelling independent elderly are associated with an almost threefold increased risk of functional decline over 2 years.[72] These data suggest for the first time the ability to assess aging with laboratory tests. Other substances that may be helpful for this purpose include C-reactive protein[73] and TNF.[14]

Geriatric Assessment in a Culturally Diverse Society

The construct of aging as a progressive loss of functional reserve is universal, but the effective assessment and management of aging may vary in different cultural and ethnic contexts. For example, some of the IADLs may be sex-specific in some cultures. Older men from Southern Europe or from Southeast Asia may be uncapable of activities as housekeeping and laundering, because these are considered mainly as womanly activities, whereas in the same society, older women seldom are responsible for financial management. Likewise, in the Mediterranean and Latin world, as well as in Southeast Asia, the main source of support may be represented by the informal network (extended family) and in North America and Northern Europe by the formal network (home care, government agencies, etc.), and the evaluation of the social support may have a different focus. Especially in the developing world, older individuals that grew up in a tribal context may find themselves disoriented in an urban environment. More in general, rapid developments in science and technology have produced substantial societal changes that may affect the availability and the effectiveness of cancer care in older individuals.

Few examples may illustrate the impact of these changes:

1. Medicine has become more and more specialized and primary care providers as well as coordinators of care are becoming progressively scarcer,[56] with a progressive loss of care coordination. Older individuals with multiple co-morbidity may then require multiple visits to different medical offices and receive redundant and interactive prescription, which may hinder treatment compliance,

increase the confusion about management, and enhance the risk of treatment. In addition, with the fading of home care, elderly individuals need to negotiate complex drives as well as complex health structure to be able to receive outpatient care.[74-78]

2. The society has become increasingly mobile, which has contributed to the dissolution of the nuclear family resulting in the loneliness and paucity of social resources of older individuals.

3. Communication technology has changed dramatically over the last decade with the pervasiveness of electronic communication. The web has become a household tool probably of more common use that the telephone was only 20 years ago. Older individuals may feel intimidated by these new forms of communication that may cause progressive social estrangement. It is important to note, however, that the new technology may also represent an opportunity of better care for the elderly. In general, individuals over 65 appear very receptive to learn computer technology and to benefit from it in terms of quality of life.[79] Additionally, telecommunication can be of special help to the caregiver[80] and may reduce the need of difficult clinic visits for the disabled elderly.[81] Provision of this tool may be highly beneficial to the older cancer patient.

4. Ethnic differences may be accentuated with aging. The Nobel laureate (1990), Octavio Paz, has described in very convincing terms how expression of one's feeling is perceived as a form of self-destruction in the Mexican American culture.[82] While one must be careful of such generalizations, certain cultural characteristics may be particularly rooted in older individuals and may prevent the adequate disclosure of medical problems.

Clearly, cultural competence does influence the way a person ages and highlights the need for effective individualized communication.

In summary, aging is associated with a progressive reduction in the functional reserve of different organ systems and in personal and social resources. Some of these changes are universal, while others are culture sensitive, may be complicated by rapid societal evolution and may influence effective communication with the clinician.

These age-related changes that tend to reduce life expectancy and tolerance of stress occur at a different rate in different persons and are poorly reflected in chronological age. The CGA may provide a number of important insight on the life expectancy, tolerance of stress, medical, and social needs of the older person, but it is time consuming. Furthermore, the CGA is inadequate in to classifying the largest group of elderly individuals, those who are neither completely independent nor obviously frail.

The ongoing challenges of aging research include:

1. validation of a screening test, capable of identifying those individuals in need of an "in depth" CGA. The VES-13 and the get-up-and-go test appear promising for this purpose;
2. integration of the different elements of the CGA in a single reproducible index capable of estimating life expectancy, risk of functional dependence, and stress tolerance. The VES-13 and other index seem useful for this purpose, while the CRASH index may identify individual risks of chemotherapy-related toxicity;
3. integration of laboratory and of physical performance tests in the geriatric assessment.

After reviewing universal characteristics of aging, we will explore the practical implication of aging for the management of cancer, in the American Society and around the world.

UNIQUE AGE-RELATED QUESTIONS IN THE PREVENTION AND TREATMENT OF CANCER

Four age-related questions have been noted in the literature and have been shown to impact the effective treatment and care of elderly patients with cancer[83]:

- Is the patient going to die of cancer or with cancer?
- Is the cancer going to influence a person's function and quality of life?
- Is the patient able to tolerate cancer treatment?
- What role can effective communication play facilitating better care in these culturally diverse elderly patients?

Considerations of life expectancy mainly impact cancer treatment and prevention efforts, including the management of slowly growing tumors (localized prostate cancer, chronic lymphocytic leukemia, low grade lymphomas), or adjuvant treatments for cancer, whose benefits are expected years after treatment administration.[84] The average survival rate of metastatic cancer, or of some hematological malignancies such as intermediate grade lymphomas or acute leukemia, is usually shorter than the life expectancy of most elderly persons.[21] While few clinicians would recommend radical prostatectomy in a 90-year-old man, or adjuvant chemotherapy of breast cancer in a 90-year-old woman, the majority would recommend chemotherapy for advanced large cell lymphoma in either person, because the benefits in terms of life expectancy and quality of life in general overwhelm the risk of treatment complications.[85]

Nevertheless, the issues related to cancer prevention and adjuvant management of cancer in culturally diverse and elderly patients remain less clear. Evidence from randomized controlled clinical trials demonstrates that serial mammography reduces the mortality from breast cancer among women aged 50 to 70, and that serial examination of fecal occult blood reduces the mortality from cancer of the large bowel for persons aged 50 to 80.[86-88] The number of older individuals included in these trials is inadequate to reach any firm conclusions. Retrospective analyses of Surveillance, Epidemiology and End Result (SEER) data indicated that serial mammography reduces breast cancer related mortality at least up to age 85, in the absence of life-threatening co-morbidity.[89,90] Based on these findings it appears reasonable to recommend some form of screening for mammary and colorectal cancer for persons with a life expectancy of 5 years and longer, irrespective of age.[91] In the case of adjuvant treatment of cancer, the long-term benefits in reduction of cancer-related morbidity and mortality should be balanced by the immediate risk of treatment. Presumably, with age, the risk of dying of unrelated conditions increases and lessens the benefits of adjuvant chemotherapy. Extermann et al. provided a framework of reference for deciding when adjuvant chemotherapy is beneficial to older women with breast cancer.[84] Considering an absolute reduction of breast cancer-related mortality of 1% as a desirable outcome, the threshold for risk of recurrence above which chemotherapy appears beneficial increases with life expectancy, determined by age and co-morbidity. For healthy women, it is around 30% at age 70 and 40% at age 80; for women affected by severe co-morbidity, it is much higher. This approach could be adapted to other tumors, especially adjuvant chemotherapy of cancer of the large bowel and local treatment of adenocarcinoma of the prostate.

It is legitimate to separate questions of quality of life and survival for older individuals, as indolent cancers become more prevalent with age.[83] Breast or prostate cancer metastatic to the bones may not hasten the death but may certainly cause a progressive deterioration in the quality of life of the older person, with pain, disability, and deconditioning. As in the case of survival, the risk of recurrence and of cancer-related complications is determined by the patient's life expectancy and by the aggressiveness of the tumor.

The effectiveness of cancer chemotherapy may decline with age due to lessened benefits and enhanced risk of complications. Though surgical-related mortality increases with age, the increase concerns mainly emergency surgery: elective surgery appears reasonably safe up to age 100 in the absence of other risk factors.[92,93] Data for patients over 100 are scanty. The need for emergency abdominal surgery, the most lethal for older individuals, may be minimized by early detection of colorectal cancer through screening.[92]

Several patient series support the safety of radiation therapy in standard doses in older individuals.[94-96] This form of treatment is particularly helpful in soothing the symptoms of cancer in older individuals, including pain, visceral and vascular obstruction, and bleeding. In combination with cytotoxic chemotherapy, radiation therapy may allow the preservation of larynx, esophagus, bladder, and rectum in the management of tumors of these organs, and may improve the survival of patients with stage 3 lung cancer or early rectal cancer.[97] Though the information is limited, this form of treatment appears reasonable in older individuals. Besides preventing disfiguration, organ preservation may be beneficial in that it avoids the need to negotiate an ostomy, which may be particularly hard for older individuals with limited vision and fine movements. Nutritional counseling seems to reduce the risk of malnutrition from esophagitis, to which older individuals are particularly subjected during radiation of the chest.[97]

Aging is associated with a number of pharmacological changes that may influence effectiveness and tolerance of cytotoxic chemotherapy (Table 3).[98] Fortunately, the bioavailability of oral medications does not appear compromised despite reduced intestinal absorption. A new spate of oral medication, including oral etoposide, capecitabine, and other oral forms of fluoro-uracil, temozolamide, oral forms of platinum, idarubicin, and navelbine are rapidly becoming available. The oral formulation allows home administration and increased dose flexibility and is thus more convenient for older individuals.[99] The decline in glomerular filtration rate is almost universal and causes a reduction in the excretion of carboplatin, bleomicine, and methotrexate, and of the active metabolites of anthracyclines, especially idarubicinol and daunorubicinol. A special case is that of cytarabin in high doses that results in the generation of ara-uridine, a neurotoxic metabolites, excreted from the kidney. Age-related decline in renal function may account for enhanced risk of cerebellar toxicity in older individuals.

Hepatic uptake of drugs and their metabolism through phase I reaction decrease with age, due to reduced splanchnic circulation and enzymatic activity, but does not seem to affect the effectiveness and toxicity of cytotoxic chemotherapy. A number of studies have demonstrated that anemia is associated with increased risk of chemotherapy-related toxicity, as the percentage of free drugs in the circulation may increase in the presence of anemia.[32,35]

Pharmacodinamic changes are largely theoretical, with exception for the well-demonstrated increase in the prevalence of MDR-1 in the myeloblasts of elderly acute leukemics, which may account in part for the worst prognosis of acute myeloid leukemia in elderly individuals.[100] Rudd et al. reported that cisplatin-induced DNA adducts persisted more that 70 h in the monocytes of individuals over 70 and less that 20 h in those under 50. Reduced ability of DNA repair by normal cells may account for enhanced toxicity.[101]

For example, a number of studies in patients with large cell non-Hodgkin's lymphoma, indicated that the risk of neutropenia, neutropenic infections, and infectious deaths was increased among individuals aged 70 and older treated with CHOP and CHOP-like regimens,[102-111] and that prophylactic use of filgrastim prevented such complication in 50% to 75% of cases.[102,110,111] Increased risk of myelotoxicity with age was also reported in patients treated with other regimens.[112-114] It is important to notice that in a number of retrospective studies involving patients treated for different malignancies, age over 70 did not seem associated with increased risk of myelodepression.[115-120] The patients in these studies were highly selected and only a negligible portion was aged 80 and older.

The risk of mucositis, and related death appears also to increase with age and is particularly true for persons treated with fluorinated pyrimidines.[121,122] Unfortunately no antidote for mucositis is available, but studies with keratinocyte growth factors are encouraging.[123] The substitution of intravenous fluorinated pyrimidines with capecitabine may in part obviate this complication as capecitabine is a prodrug activated in the tumor cell itself, so that the exposure of normal tissues to the active principle is minimized.[99] Timely intravenous fluid resuscitation may prevent death from dehydration in patients with diarrhea or severe esophagitis. And no prophylactic measures are indicated at present for the prevention of cardiomyopathy and neurotoxicity. Ongoing studies may establish whether liposomal anthracyclines are preferable in older individuals.

In lieu of an awareness of the increased risk of some forms of chemotherapy-related toxicity among older individuals, the National Cancer Center Network (NCCN) has recently issued a number of guidelines for the management of older individuals with cytotoxic chemotherapy.[60,124] These include:

- Adjust the dose of chemotherapy to maximize renal function. Dose escalation is highly recommended if toxicity is not observed after the first dose, to avoid the risk of undertreatment.
- Prophylactic use of filgrastim or pegfilgrastim in patients aged 70 and older treated with a form of chemotherapy with dose intensity comparable to CHOP. Dose reduction may be considered instead of growth factors when the goal of treatment is palliative.

- Maintenance of hemoglobin levels $\geq 12\,\mathrm{gm/dl}$. In addition to preventing myelotoxicity, these levels of hemoglobin may prevent fatigue and functional dependence.
- Substitution of intravenous fluorinated pyrimidines with capecitabine.
- Aggressive management of mucositis involving fluid resuscitation and hospitalization.
- All patients aged 70 and older should undergo some form of geriatric assessment, to assess life expectancy, treatment tolerance, and presence of conditions that may influence the treatment of cancer.

The last recommendation, related to geriatric assessment stems from the need of assessing physiological rather than chronological age, at the time of treatment-related decisions.

AGING IN THE COUNTRY AND IN THE WORLD

The aging of the population is a worldwide phenomenon. In addition, the diversity in the cultural, demographic and biomedical environment may complicate the effective management of oncology care in the older population. Indeed, central to effective oncology care is the clinician-patient relationship. A recent study revealed that smiling, nodding, and frowning were associated with improvements in physical, cognitive, and psychological functioning in elderly patients.[125] This is merely one example of the importance of effective communication to oncology outcomes in older patients with cancer.

Agism

Before discussing ethnical, cultural, and geographic differences of aging, we need to address this universal prejudice. Agism is a ubiquitous part of everyday life, occurring in every ethnic group, in every country. Thus, it needs to be addressed and assessed in the specific cultural context and environment in which each person ages.[126] Agism in the West, in the broadest sense, involves discrimination of older individuals based on their age, which adversely affects their care.[127] Such discrimination may vary from open disrespect to assumption of frailty and disability, to restricted access to any form of social activity, including health care. In its subtlest form, agism may take the form of special care: "let's not compromise the dear one's quality of life with useless aggressive treatment."[128,129] These attitudes, which are common among family members as well as clinician, may effectively shut older individuals out from decisions related to their own health care.[130,131] Even in the United States, older individuals are less likely to have their pain effectively managed[132] and to have less input regarding the place of their death.[133] They are also less likely to be offered screening for cancer,[134] and participation in clinical trials of cancer treatment,[135,136] or simply to receive standard treatment for their cancer.[129,130,136,137] This also occurs in other instances; for example, in the United Kingdom, despite socialized medicine, older lung cancer patients are less likely to be offered surgery and more likely to die prematurely compared to younger patients.[137] The absurdity of such attitudes is highlighted by the fact that older individuals are just as likely as younger individuals to participate in clinical trials when these are offered to them[138] and to participate in cancer screening programs, when these are made available and the information is properly provided.[134,139,140] Not unexpectedly, older individuals from minority groups suffer the most from the effects of agism,[139] due to a combination of factors including socioeconomic, inadequate and inappropriate information, racial and ethnic discrimination, and even lack of interest and professional preparation of their clinicians.[139,140] For instance, other North American research suggests that both older patients and African American patients with breast carcinoma are more likely to present with distant disease and are less likely to receive appropriate diagnostic evaluation and therapeutic intervention compared with younger patients.[139-141] Nonetheless, as the aging population expands, agism may prevent adequate care of the majority of the population and may eventually unleash a generational conflict. Agism may also become an important barrier in the clinician-patient communication, should the patient perceive condescension and the lack of interest by the clinician and biomedical team.

While there is not an universal recipe against agism, some important factors should be clearly remembered by the clinicians and highlighted to the public as necessary:

- Aging is not equivalent to frailty: many older individuals are still independent and able to tolerate aggressive medical treatment under proper circumstances.[83] Failure to offer effective treatment on account of a person's age may result in shortening that person's survival and compromise of that person's quality of life.
- Aging is not equivalent to lack of understanding or a lack of comprehension. One of the most offensive and common attitudes of clinicians, nurses, social workers, and other health care professionals is to address the younger children of the older person rather than the patient himself/herself. Even in the presence of serious dementia, the patient appreciates being addressed in a form that is appropriate in his/her culture. In North America this may include frequent touch and eye contact.
- Aging does not imply impaired decisional ability. The majority of older individuals can decide their preferred course of treatment, and

even the most demented person may decide what he/she wishes to eat at lunch. It behooves the health care professional to allow enough space to the older person to make all decisions related to their care that they are able to make.

- Aging does not justify inferior care as a form of resources management. Our medical ethics hinges on the principle of justice, which implies that the medical care customary in their community should be offered to all persons independent of individual characteristics, as long as the expected benefits overcome the potential risks. In other words, the provision of inferior care to an older person because the person has a reduced life expectancy is equivalent to a value judgment that the duration of life is more valuable that its personal implication; it is equivalent to say that an older life has less value that a younger one.
- The study of aging is an evolving field. More importantly, each generation reaches old age with different physical and cultural characteristics.

Therefore, to attend to this pervasive prejudice across cultural contexts, clinicians must foster a more accommodating medical environment for older individuals. This includes more cultural sensitivity to patient in culturally diverse elderly patient populations. Major threats in the present system include:

- Hospital and clinical structures that are difficult to negotiate and have difficult access, as they are located in high traffic downtown areas.
- The progressive shortening of time allocated by health maintenance organizations to individual clinic visits, affects the oncology care that elderly patients receive. Older individuals need more time on account of slow movements, reduced hearing and eyesight, and difficulties comprehending current medical concepts and increasingly complex clinical protocols.
- Lack of economic incentive for a CGA that is currently not reimbursed by Medicare.
- Poor communication between oncology clinicians and culturally diverse elderly patients.

Accounting for Cultural, Ethnic, and Geographical Differences in the Management of Older Individuals

As we have previously stated, aging is a universal phenomenon. At the same time, the average life expectancy and the prevalence of older individuals are quite diverse in different parts of the world. In North America and Western Europe, the aging of the population resulted from a combination of more prolonged life expectancy and reduced natality rate, whereas persistently high natality and mortality rate during infancy, together with infectious epidemics, inadequate nutrition, and local warfare are responsible for lower life expectancy in the developing world. Even in North America, life expectancy varies between different ethnic groups. Life expectancy in, for example, African Americans and Hispanics is shorter than among Caucasians, due at least in part to persistently high natality and reduced access to health care.[142-145] Thus, the demographics of aging is quite different for one part of the world from the other and for an ethnic group from the other within the same country, and so are the resources available for the management of older individuals.

Within the Western world different attitudes toward aging may be encountered among different populations and ethnic groups. Discussing agism, for example, we emphasized how the utilization of screening asymptomatic persons for cancer is lower among older minority patients[134,146] and how misbelieve or lack of information and of clinician support may be as much responsible for this deficiency as economic and social restrictions. While the presence of cultural differences among different ethnic groups is well recognized,[3,147] it is important that clinicians do not assume that all persons belonging to the same ethnic group will behave the same way. For example, while it is more common for Hispanic American than for Anglo American to conceal the diagnosis of terminal disease, a clinician should not automatically assume that every older Hispanic American does not want to deal with the diagnosis and every Anglo does. Rather, awareness of cultural competence should make one cautious in the way that serious information is conveyed and wait for each patient to manifest how much he/she wishes to know. Though it is not always possible to conciliate the clinician ethical and legal imperatives with the patient's desire and expectations, in most cases a satisfactory compromise may be reached. For example, lying to a patient is seldom acceptable, but it is legitimate to answer "I do not know" to a person asking how long he/she has to live, if the clinician feels that that person cannot handle the information, as the survival statistics do not necessarily comprehend the individual cases.

General rules for communicating with older individuals include speaking slowly and clearly with a heightened voice timber, to overcome hearing impairment, allowing extra time for questions, without showing impatience, using touch as an important medium of communication, as touch is the best preserved of all senses, trying to establish eye contact, and including the designed caregiver in the discussion.

A common approach to the older cancer patient in different cultures and different societies is desirable. An understanding of a number of central issues may also facilitate this task. These include:

1. *Family composition.* Hispanic Americans, and to some extent Asian Americans, or some of the new migrants, especially from Northern Africa or China, are more likely to have an extended family and to take care of their elders at home. In these situations, the training of the family caregiver is essential to assure that all problems emerging during cancer treatment are timely addressed. Obviously this situation is not unique to some ethnic groups and the training to the caregiver may apply to all extended families willing to care for their own elders at home.

2. *The decision maker.* The physician can never renounce her/his responsibility toward the patient, but she/he may accept that the patient depends on somebody else's decisions for his/her care. In this situation, once the wish of the patient is confirmed and documented in the chart, the clinician may refer to the "decision maker" for further treatment plans. It is therefore desirable that the patients be kept informed as he/she may decide at anytime to revoke that decision to him/herself.

3. *Patient beliefs.* Essentially three types of beliefs may be identified that influence the management of cancer and medicine in general: medical scientific, naturalistic, and magical religious.[140] Attempts to situate the medical message concordant with an understanding of the patient's belief systems is generally more productive than to try to fight the beliefs themselves. Actually the clinician can use the patient's beliefs as a context effect to enhance the care of patients in this population.

4. *Economical and social situation.* It behooves any health care operator to assure that the patient is not undergoing any form of direct or subtle abuse, and when this is present, it should be immediately reported to the proper authority. It is possible however that even within the caring family the ideal medical care cannot be administered due to economic or time restrictions. In this condition, the most productive attitude is probably to negotiate with the patient family the most effective care that can be delivered under the circumstances.

CONCLUSIONS

Cancer will become the leading cause of morbidity and death as the global population ages. While health and health care disparities have been well documented in culturally and linguistically diverse patients with cancer, aging involves unique biological, medical, and social considerations that must be further explored as it also influences cancer prevention and cancer treatment in these populations. Further, even though aging is common to all cultures and latitudes, the cultural context in which the experience occurs varies even within the Western context. As such, cancer specialists must learn to not only account for the functional but also for the cultural diversity of the older population in medical decisions related to cancer prevention and cancer treatment. In addition, use of screening instruments such the CGA also represent a milestone in the management of older individuals. It is also currently being modified to become more cost effective and to provide more precise information related to life expectancy and tolerance of cancer treatment. The increase in cultural diversity in the oncology setting also influences cancer treatment. A clinician must be able to act within the boundaries of cultural competence when ministering to older cancer patients. Cultural specific instruments to assess older individuals are particularly desirable in a multicultural society, but also strive to effectively communicate with these individuals in these populations, their families and significant others. With proper patient selection and information, older individuals may obtain the same degree of benefits from cancer prevention and cancer treatment as younger individuals, and age should never be a criteria for health care discrimination.

REFERENCES

1. Yancik R, Ries LAG. Aging and cancer in America: Demographic and epidemiologic perspectives. *Hematol/Oncol Clin N Am.* 2000;14:17-24.
2. Yancik RM, Ries L. Cancer and age: Magnitude of the problem. In: Balducci L, Lyman GH, Ershler WB eds. *Comprehensive Geriatric Oncology.* London: Harwood Academic Publishers, 1998; 95-104.
3. Butow PN, Tattersall MH, Goldstein D. Communication with cancer patients in a culturally diverse society. *Ann N Y Acad Sci.* 1997;809:317-329.
4. Duthie E, Anisimov VN. Physiology of aging: Relevance to symptom perceptions: Age as a risk factor in multistage carcinogenesis. In: Balducci L, Lyman GH, Ershler WB eds. *Comprehensive Geriatric Oncology,* 2nd ed. Amsterdam: Harwood Academic Publishers; 2003; in press.
5. Collins K. Mammalian telomeres and telomerase. *Curr Opin Cell Biol.* 2000;12:378-383.
6. Liggett WH, Sidransky D. Role of the P16 tumor suppressor gene in cancer. *J Clin Oncol.* 1998;16:1197-1206.
7. Anisimov VN. Age as a risk factor in multistage carcinogenesis. In: Balducci L, Lyman GH, Ershler WB eds. *Comprehensive Geriatric Oncology,* 2nd ed. Amsterdam: Harwood Academic Publishers; 2003; in press.
8. Troen BR. The biology of aging. *Mt Sinai J Med.* 2003;70(1):3-22.
9. Campisi J. Cancer and age: The double-edged sword of proliferative senescence. *J Am Ger Soc.* 1997;43:482–490.
10. Warner HR. Aging and regulation of apoptosis. *Curr Top Cell Regul.* 1997;35:107-121.

11. Eskandari F, Sternberg EM. Neural-immune interactions in health and disease. *Ann N Y Acad Sci.* 2002;966:20-27.
12. Webster JI, Tonelli L, Sternberg EM. Neuroendocrine regulation of immunity. *Annu Rev Immunol.* 2002;20:125-163.
13. Wilson CJ, Finch CE, Cohen HJ. Cytokines and Cognition—The case for a Head to Toe Inflammatory paradigm. *J Am Ger Soc.* 2002;50:2041-2056.
14. Hamerman D, Berman JV, Albers W, et al. Emerging evidence of inflammation in conditions frequently affecting older adults: Reports of a symposium. *J Am Ger Soc.* 1999;47:1016-1102.
15. Ferrucci L, Penninx BWJH, Volpato S, et al. Change in muscle strength explains accelerated decline of physical function in older women with high interleukin 6 serum levels. *J Am Ger Soc.* 2002;50:1947-1954.
16. Leng S, Chaves P, Koenig K, et al. Serum interleukin 6 and hemoglobin as physiological correlates in the geriatric syndrome of frailty: A pilot study. *J Am Ger Soc.* 2002;50:1268-1271.
17. Chaves PH, Volpato S, Fried L. Challenging the world health organization criteria for anemia in the older woman. *J Am Ger Soc.* 2001;49:S3, A10.
18. Reuben DR, Cheh AI, Harris TB, et al. Peripheral blood markers of inflammation predict mortality and functional decline in high functioning community dwelling older persons. *J Am Ger Soc.* 2002;50:638-644.
19. Fees BS, Martin P, Poon LW. A model of loneliness in older adults. *J Gerontol B Psychol Sci Soc Sci.* 1999;54:231-239.
20. Steverink N, Westerhof GJ, Bode C, et al. The personal experience of aging, individual resources, and subjective well being. *J Gerontol B Psychol Sci Soc Sci.* 2001;56:P364-P373.
21. Walter LC, Brand RJ, Counsell SR, et al. Development and validation of a prognostic index for 1-year mortality in older adults after hospitalization. *JAMA.* 2001;285:2987-2994.
22. Inouye SK, Peduzzi PN, Robison JT, et al. Importance of functional measures in predicting mortality among older hospitalized patients. *JAMA.* 1998;279:1187-1193.
23. Ramos LR, Simoes EJ, Albert MS. Dependence in activities of daily living and cognitiver impairment strongly predict mortality in older urban residents in Brazil. *J Am Ger Soc.* 2001;49:1168-1175.
24. Extermann M, Overcash J, Lyman GH, et al. Comorbidity and functional status are independent in older cancer patients. *J Clin Oncol.* 1998;16:1582-1587.
25. Repetto L, Fratino L, Audisio RA, et al. Comprehensive geriatric assessment adds information to the Eastern Cooperative group Performance Status in elderly cancer patients. An Italian Group for Geriatric Oncology Study. *J Clin Oncol.* 2002;20:494-502.
26. Satariano WA, Ragland DR. The effect of comorbidity on 3-year survival of women with primary breast cancer. *Ann Int Med.* 1994;120:104-110.
27. Yancik R, Ganz PA, Varricchio CG, et al. Perspectives on comorbidity and cancer in the older patient: approach to expand the knowledge base. *J Clin Oncol.* 2001;19:1147-1151.
28. Zagonel V, Fratino L, Piselli P, et al. The comprehensive geriatric assessment predicts mortality among elderly cancer patients. *Proc Am Soc Clin Oncol.* 2002;21:365 a (abstract 1458).
29. Chen H, Cantor A, Meyer J, et al. Can older cancer patients tolerate chemotherapy? A prospective pilot study. *Cancer.* 2003;15:1107-1114.
30. Extermann M, Chan H, Cantor AB. Predictors of tolerance to chemotherapy in older cancer patients: a prospective pilot study. *Eur J Cancer.* 2002;38:1466-1473.
31. Extermann M. Measuring comorbidity in older cancer patients. *Eur J Cancer.* 2000;36:453-471.
32. Balducci L. Epidemiologi of anemia in the elderly: information on diagnostic evaluation. *J Am Ger Soc.* 2003;51(3 Suppl):S2-S9.

33. Chaves PH, Volpato S, Fried L. Challenging the world health organization criteria for anemia in the older woman. *J Am Ger Soc.* 2001;49:S3, A10.
34. Littlewood TJ, Bajetta E, Nortier JW, et al. Effects of epoetin alfa on hematologic parameters and quality of life in cancer patients receiving nonplatinum chemotherapy: results of a randomized, double-blind, placebo-controlled trial. *J Clin Oncol.* 2001;19(11):2865-2874.
35. Schijvers D, Highley M, DeBruyn E, et al. Role of red blood cell in pharmakinetics of chemotherapeutic agents. *Anticancer Drugs.* 1999;10:147-153.
36. Metivier F, Marchais SJ, Guerin AP, Pannier B, London GM. Pathophysiology of anaemia: focus on the heart and blood vessels. *Nephrol Dial Transplant.* 2000;15(3):14-18.
37. Wu Wc, Rathore SS, Wang Y, et al. Blood transfusions in elderly patients with acute myocardial infarction. *N Eng J Med.* 2001;345:1230-1236.
38. Pickett JL, Theberge DC, Brown WS, Schweitzer SU, Nissenson AR. Normalizing hematocrit in dialysis patients improves brain function. *Am J Kidney Dis.* 1999;33(6):1122-1130.
39. Hamerman D: Toward an understanding of frailty. *Ann Intern Med.* 1999;130:945-950.
40. Balducci L, Stanta G. Cancer in the frail patient: a coming epidemic. *Hematol Oncol Clin N Am.* 2000;14:235-250.
41. Lyness JM, Ling DA, Cox C, et al. The importance of subsyndromal depression in older primary care patients. Prevalence and associated functional disability. *J Am Ger Soc.* 1999;47:647-652.
42. Wholey MA, Simon GE. Managing depression in medical outpatient. *N Engl J Med.* 2000;343:1942-1950.
43. Valenstein M, Vijan S, Zeber JE, et al. The cost-utility of screening for depression in primary care. *Ann Intern Med.* 2001;134:345-360.
44. Draper B. Attempted suicide in old age. *Int J Geriatr Psychiatr.* 1996;11:577-587.
45. Frierson RL. Suicide attempts by the old and the very old. *Arch Intern Med.* 1991;151:141-144.
46. Yang CH, Tsai SJ, Chang JW, Hwang JP. Characteristics of Chinese suicide attempters admitted to a geropsychiatric unit. *Int J Geriatr Psychiatr.* 2001;16(11):1033-1036.
47. Weitzner MA, Haley WE, Chen H. The family caregiver of the older cancer patient. *Hematol Oncol Clin.* 2000;14:269-282.
48. Hosaka T, Sugiyama Y. Structured intervention in family caregivers of the demented elderly and changes in their immune function. *Psychiatr Clin Neurosci.* 2003;57(2):147-151
49. Jannsen I, Heymsfield SB, Ross R. Low relative skeletal mass (sarcopenia) in older persons is associated with functional impairment and physical disability. *J Am Ger Soc.* 2002;50:889-896.
50. Visser M, Kitchevsky SB, Goodpaster BH, et al. Leg muscle mass in relation to lower extremity performance in men and women aged 70-79: the health, aging, and body composition study. *J Am Ger Soc.* 2002;50:897-904.
51. Hu Peifeng, Seeman TE, Harris TB, et al. Does inflammation or undernutrition explain the low cholesterol-mortality association in high-functioning older persons? MacArthur Study of successful Aging. *J Am Ger Soc.* 2003;51:80-84.
52. Wedick NE, Barrett-Connor E, Knoke JD. The relationship between weight loss and all-cause mortality in older men and women with and without diabetes mellitus: the Rancho Bernardo Study. *J Am Ger Soc.* 2002;50:1810-1815.
53. Astani A, Smith RC, Allen BJ. The predictive value of body proteins for chemotherapy induced toxicity. *Cancer.* 2000;88:796-903.
54. Guigoz Y, Vellas B, Garry PJ. Mininutritional assessment: a practical assessment tool for grading the nutritional state of elderly patients. In: *Facts, Research, Interventions in Geriatrics.* New York, Serdi Publishing Company, 1997;15-60.
55. Corcoran ME. Polypharmacy in the older patient. In: Balducci L, Lyman GH, Ershler WB eds. *Comprehensive Geriatric Oncology.* Amsterdam: Harwood Academic Publishers; 2003, in press

56. Clarfield AM, Bergman H, Kane R. Fragmentation of care for frail older people-an international problem. Experience from three countries: Israel, Canada, and the United States. *J Am Ger Soc.* 2001;49:1714-1721.

57. Cohen HJ, Feussner JR, Weinberger M, et al. A controlled trial of inpatient and outpatient geriatric assessment. *N Engl J Med.* 2002;346:905-912.

58. Reuben DB, Franck J, Hirsch S, et al. A randomized clinical trial of outpatient geriatric assessment (CGA), coupled with an intervention, to increase adherence to recommendations. *J Am Ger Soc.* 1999;47:269-276.

59. Bula CJ, Berod AC, Stuck AE, et al. Effectiveness of preventive in-home geriatric assessment in well functioning, community dwelling older people: secondary analysis of a randomized trial. *J Am Ger Soc.* 1999;47:389-395.

60. Balducci L, Yates G. General guidelines for the management of older patients with cancer. *Oncology, NCCN Proc.* November 14:2000;221–227.

61. Ingram SS, Seo PH, Martell RE, et al. Comprehensive assessment of the elderly cancer patient: The feasibility of self-report methodology. *J Clin Oncol.* 2002;20:770-775.

62. Balducci L, Extermann M, Meyer J, et al. Comprehensive geriatric intervention in older breast cancer patients. A pilot. *Proc Am Soc Clin Oncol.* 2001;20:314b (abstract 3008).

63. Hirdes JP, Frijters DH, Teare GF, et al. The MDS-CHESS Scale: a new measure to predict mortality in institutionalized older people. *J Am Ger Soc.* 2003;51:96-100.

64. Stump TE, Callahan CM, Hendrie HC, et al. Cognitive impairment and mortality in older primary care patients. *J Am Ger Soc.* 2001;49:934-940.

65. Blazer DG, Hybels CF, Pieper CF. The association of depression and mortality in elderly persons: a case for multiple independent pathways. *J Gerontol Med Sci.* 2001;56: M505-M509.

66. Saliba D, Elliott M, Rubenstein LZ, et al. The vulnerable elders survey: a tool for identifying vulnerable older people in the community. *J Am Ger Soc.* 2001;49:1691-1699.

67. Gill TM, Baker DI. Gottschalk M, et al. A program to prevent functional decline in physically frail elderly persons who live at home. *N Engl J Med.* 2002;347:1068-1074.

68. Nourhashemi F, Andrieu S, Gillette-Guyonnet S, et al. Instrumental activities of daily living as a potential marker of frailty: a study of 7364 community-dwelling elderly women (the EPIDOS study). *J Gerontol Med Sci.* 2001;56:M448-M453.

69. Njergovan V, man-Son-Hing M, Mitchell SL, et al. The hierarchy of functional loss associated with cognitive decline in older persons. *J Gerontol.* 2001;56 A:M638-M643.

70. Kivela S-L, Pahakala K. Depressive disorders as predictors of physical disability in old age. *J Am Ger Soc.* 2001;49:290-296.

71. Brody KK, Johnson RE, Ried LD, et al. A comparison of two methods for identifying frail medicare aged persons. *J Am Ger Soc.* 2002;50:562-569.

72. Cohen HJ, Pieper CF, Harris T. Markers of inflammation and coagulation predict decline in function and mortality in community-dwelling elderly. *J Am Ger Soc.* 2001;49:S1, A3.

73. Taaffe DR, Harris TB, Ferrucci L, et al. Cross-sectional and prospective relationships of interleukin-6 and C-reactive protein with physical performance in elderly persons: MacArthur Studies of successful aging. *J Gerontol Med Sci.* 2000;55A:M709-M715.

74. Knickman JR, Snell EK. The 2030m problem: caring for aging baby boomers. *Health Serv Res.* 2002;37:849-884.

75. Nolan M. Successful ageing: keeping the person in person centred care. *Br J Nurs.* 2001;10:450-454.

76. Dossey L. Longevity. *Altern Ther Health Med.* 2002;8:12-16.

77. Tinker A. The social implications of an aging population. *Mech Ageing Dev.* 2002;123: 729-735.

78. Karner TX. Caring for an aging society. *J Aging Social Policy.* 2001;13:15-36.

79. White H, Mcconnell E, Clipp E, et al. A randomized controlled trial of the psychosocial impact of providing internet training and access to older adults. *Aging Mental Health.* 2002;6:213-221.
80. Czaja SJ, Rubert MP. Telecommunications technology as an aid to family caregivers of persons with dementia. *Psychosom Med.* 2002;64:469-476.
81. Wilson LS, Gill RW, Sharp IF, et al. Building the hospital without walls: a CSIRO home telecare initiative. *Telemed J.* 2000;6:275-281.
82. Octavio Paz: *el labirinto de la soledad*
83. Repetto L, Balducci L. A case for geriatric oncology. *Lancet Oncol.* 2002;3:289-297.
84. Extermann M, Balducci L, Lyman GH. What threshold for adjuvant therapy in older breast cancer patients? *J Clin Oncol.* 2000;18:1709-1717.
85. Monfardini S, Carbone A. Non-Hodgkin's lymphomas. In: Balducci L, Lyman GH, Ershler WB, eds. *Comprehensive Geriatric Oncology.* London: Harwood Academic Publishers, 1998;577-595.
86. Balducci L, Beche C. Prevention of cancer in the older person. *Clin Ger Med.* 2002; 18:723-738.
87. Kerlikowske K, Grady D, Rubin SM, et al. Efficacy of screening mammography. A meta-analysis. *JAMA.* 1995;273:149-154.
88. Walsh JME, Terdiman JI. Colorectal cancer screening: scientific evidence. *J Am Med Ass.* 2003;281:1288-1296.
89. Mccarthy EP, Burns RB, Freund KM, et al. Mammography use, breast cancer stage at diagnosis, and survival among older women. *J Am Ger Soc.* 2000;48:1226-1233.
90. McPherson CP, Swenson KK, Lee MW. The effects of mammographic detection and comorbidity on the survival of older women with breast cancer. *J Am Ger Soc.* 2002;50:1061-1068.
91. Walter LC, Covinsky CE. Cancer screening in elderly patients. *J Am Med Ass.* 2001;285:2750-2756.
92. Kemeny MM, Bush-Devereaux E, Merriam LT, et al. Cancer surgery in the elderly. *Hematol/Oncol Clin N Am.* 2000;14:169-192.
93. Davila Miguel. Anesthesia in older cancer patients. In: Balducci L, Lyman GH, Ershler WB eds. *Comprehensive Geriatric Oncology* 2nd ed. Amsterdam: Harwood Academic Publishers; 2003, in press.
94. Olmi P, Ausili Cefaro GP, Balzi M, et al. radiotherapy in the aged. *Clin Ger Med.* 1997;13:143-168.
95. Scalliet P, Pignon T. Radiotherapy in the elderly. In: Balducci L, Lyman GH, Ershler WB eds. *Comprehensive Geriatric Oncology,* London: Harwood Academic Publishers; 1998; 421-428.
96. Zachariah B, Balducci L. Radiation therapy of the older patient. *Hematol Oncol Clin N Am.,* 2000;14:131-167.
97. Balducci L and Trotti A. Organ preservation: an effective and safe form of cancer treatment. *Clin Ger Med.* 1997;13:185-202.
98. Cova D, Balducci L. Cytotoxic chemotherapy in the older patient. In: Balducci L, Lyman GH, Ershler WB, eds. *Comprehensive Geriatric Oncology.* 2nd ed. Amsterdam: Harwood Academic Publishers; 2003; in press.
99. Balducci L, Carreca I. Oral chemotherapy of cancer in the elderly. *Am J Cancer* 2002;1:101-108.
100. Lancet JE, Willman CL, Bennett JM. Acute myelogenous leukemia and aging: clinical interactions. *Hematol/Oncol Clinics N Am.* 2000;16:251-268.
101. Rudd GN, Hartley GA, Souhani RL. Persistence of cisplatin-induced interstrand crosslinking in peripheral blood mononuclear cells from elderly and younger individuals. *Cancer Chemother Pharmacol.* 1995;35:323-326.

102. Zinzani PG, Storti S, Zaccaria A, et al. Elderly aggressive histology non-Hodgkin's lymphoma: First line VNCOP-B regimen: expereince on 350 patients. *Blood*. 1999;94:33-38.
103. Sonneveld P, de Ridder M, van der Lelie H, et al. Comparison of doxorubicin and mitoxantrone in the treatment of elderly patients with advanced diffuse non-Hodgkin's lymphoma using CHOP vs CNOP chemotherapy. *J Clin Oncol*. 1995;13:2530-2539.
104. Gomez H, Mas L, Casanova L, et al. Elderly patients with aggressive non-Hodgkin's lymphoma treated with CHOP chemotherapy plus granulocyte-macrophage colony-stimulating factor: identification of two age subgroups with differing hematologic toxicity. *J Clin Oncol*. 1998;16:2352-2358.
105. Tirelli U, Errante D, Van Glabbeke M, et al. CHOP is the standard regimen in patients ≥ 70 years of age with intermediate and high grade non-Hodgkin's lymphoma: results of a randomized study of the European organization for the research and treatment of cancer lymphoma cooperative study. *J Clin Oncol*. 1998;16:27-34.
106. Bastion Y, Blay J-Y, Divine M, et al. Elderly patients with aggressive non-Hodgkin's lymphoma: disease presentation, response to treatment and survival. A Groupe d'Etude des Lymphomes de l'Adulte Study on 453 patients older than 69 years. *J Clin Oncol*. 1997;15:2945-2953.
107. Bertini M, Freilone R, Vitolo U, et al. The treatment of elderly patients with aggressive non-Hodgkin's lymphomas: feasiblity and efficacy of an intensive multidrug regimen. *Leukemia Lymphoma*. 1996;22:483-493.
108. Reilly SE, Connors JM, Howdle S, et al. In search of an optimal regimen for elderly patients with advanced-stage diffuse large-cell lymphoma: results of a phase II study of P/DOCE chemotherapy. *J Clin Oncol*. 1993;2250-2257.
109. Armitage JO, Potter JF. Aggressive chemotherapy for diffuse histiocytic lymphoma in the elderly. *J Am Ger Soc*. 1984;32:269-273.
110. Bjorkholm M, Osby E, Hagberg H, et al. Randomized trial of R-methu granulocyte colony stimulating factors as adjunto to CHOP or CNOP treatment of elderly patients with aggressive non-Hodgkin's lymphoma. Proc ASH, *Blood* (suppl). 1999;94:599a (abstract 2665).
111. Balducci L, Lyman GH, Ozer H. Patients aged ≥ 70 are at high risk for neutropenic infection and should receive hemopoietic growth factors when treated with moderately toxic chemotherapy. *J Clin Oncol*. 2001;19:1583-1585.
112. Balducci L, Hardy CH, Lyman GH. Hematopoietic growth factors in the older cancer patient. *Curr Opin in Hematol*. 2001;8:170-187.
113. Dees EC, O'Reilly S, Goodman SN, et al. A prospective pharmacologic evaluation of age-related toxicity chemotherapy in women with breast cancer. *Cancer Invest*. 2000; 18:521-529.
114. Kim YJ, Rubenstein EB, Rolston KV, et al. Colony-stimulating factors (CSFs) may reduce complications and death in solid tumor patients with fever and neutropenia. *Proc ASCO*. 2000;19:612a (abstract 2411).
115. Begg C, Carbone P. Experience of the Eastern Cooperative Oncology Group. *Cancer*. 1983;52:1986-1992.
116. Christman K, Muss HB, Case D, et al. Chemotherapy of metastatic breast cancer in the elderly. *JAMA*. 1992;268:57-62.
117. Giovannozzi-Bannon S, Rademaker A, Lai G, et al. Treatment tolerance of elderly cancer patients entered onto phase II clinical trials. An Illinois Cancer Center study. *J Clin Oncol*. 1994;12:2447-2452.
118. Ibrahim N, Frye DK, Buzdar AU, et al. Doxorubicin based combination chemotherapy in elderly patients with metastatic breast cancer. Tolerance and outcome. *Arch Intern Med*. 1996;156:882-888.

119. Ibrahim NK, Buzdar AU, Asmar l, et al. Doxorubicin based adjuvant chemotherapy in elderly breast cancer patients: the M D Anderson experience with long term follow-up. *Ann Oncol.* 2000;11:1-5.

120. Gelman RS, Taylor SG. Cyclophosphamide, methotrexate and 5 fluorouracil chemotherapy in women more than 65 year old with advanced breast cancer. The elimination of age trends in toxicity by using doses based on creatinine clearance. *J Clin Oncol.* 1984;2:1406-1414.

121. Stein BN, Petrelli NJ, Douglass HO, et al. Age and sex are independent predictors of 5-fluorouracil toxicity. *Cancer.* 1995;75:11-17.

122. Jacobson SD, Cha S, Sargent DJ, et al. Tolerability, dose intensity and benefit of 5FU based chemotherapy for advanced colorectal cancer (CRC) in the elderly. A North Central Cancer Treatment Group Study. *Proc Am Soc Clin Oncol.* 2001;20:384a (abstract 1534).

123. Spielberger RT, Stiff P, Emmanouilides C, et al. Efficacy of recombinant human keratinocyte growth factor (rHuKGF) in reducing mucositis in patients with hematologic malignancies undergoing autologous peripheral blood progenito cell transplantation after radiation-based conditioning. Results of a phase 2 trial. *Proc Am Soc Clin Oncol.* 2001;20:7a (abstract 25).

124. Repetto L, Carreca I, Maraninchi D, et al. Use of growth factors in elderly patients with cancer: a report from the second international Society of Geriatric Oncology (SIOG) meeting. *Crit Rev Hematol Oncol.* 2003;45:123-128.

125. Ambady N, Koo J, Rosenthal R, Winograd CH. Physical therapists' nonverbal communication predicts geriatric patients' health outcomes. *Psychol Aging.* 2002;17(3):443-445.

126. Nolan M. Ageism: what is in a word? *J Adv Nurs.* 2003;41:8-93.

127. Palmore E. The ageism survey: first findings. *Gerontologist.* 2001;41:572-575.

128. Dunlop DD, Manheim LM, Song J, et al. Gender and ethnic/racial disparities in health care utilization among older adults. *J Gerontol B Psychol Sci.* 2002;57:S221-S233.

129. Glanz K, Croyle RT, Chollett VY, et al. Cancer-related health disparity in women. *Am J Publ Health.* 2003;93:292-298.

130. Patriseck AC, Laliberte LL, Allen SM, et al. The treatment decision making process: age differences in a sample of women recently diagnosed with non-recurrent, early stage breast cancer. *Gerontologist.* 1997;37:598-608.

131. Kearney N, Miller M, Paul J, Smith K. Oncology healthcare professionals' attitudes toward elderly people. *Ann Oncol.* 2000;11(5):599-560.

132. Won A, Lapane K, Gambassi G, et al. Correlates and management of nonmalignant pain in the nursing home. SAGE study group. Systematic assessment of geriatric drug use via epidemiology. *J Am Ger Soc.* 1999;47:936-942.

133. Weitzen S, Teno JM, Fennell M, et al. Factors associated with site of death: a National study of where people die. *Med Care.* 2003;41:323-325.

134. Fox SA, Roetzheim RG, Kington RS. Barriers to cancer prevention in the older person. In: Balducci L, Lyman GH, Ershler WB eds. *Comprehensive geriatric Oncology.* Amsterdam; Harwood Academic Publishers, 1998;351-362.

135. Hutchins Hutchins LF, Unger JM, Crowley JJ, et al. Underepresentation of patients 65 years of age and older in cancer treatment. *N Engl J Med.* 1999;341:2061-2067.

136. Lewis JH, Kilgore ML, Goldman DP, et al. Participation of patients 65 years of age or older in cancer clinical trials. *J Clin Oncol.* 2003;21(7):1383-1389.

137. Peake MD, Thompson S, Lowe D, et al. Ageism in the management of lung cancer. *Age Ageing.* 2003;32:171-177.

138. Kemeny M, Muss HB, Kornblith AB, et al. Barriers to participation of older women with breast cancer in clinical trials. *Proc Am Soc Clin Oncol.* 2000;19:602a (abstract 2371).

139. Fox SA, Stein JA, Sockloskie RJ, et al. Targeted mailed materials and the medicare beneficiary: increasing mammogram screening among the elderly. *Am J Publ Health.* 2002;92:805-810.

140. Markens S, Fox SA, Taub B, et al. Role of black churches in health promotion programs: lessons from the Los Angeles mammography promotion in churches program. *Am J Publ Health.* 2002;92:805-810.

141. Maly RC, Leake B, Silliman RA. Health care disparities in older patients with breast carcinoma: informational support from physicians. *Cancer.* 2003;97(6):1517-1527.

142. Arias E. United States life tables 2000. *Natl Vital Stat Rep.* 2002;51:1-38.

143. Lillie-Blanton M, Brodie M, Rowland D, et al. Race, ethnicity, and the health care system: public perceptions and experiences. *Med Care Res Rev.* 2000;57(suppl 1):218-235.

144. Levine RS, Foster JE, Fullilove RE, et al. Black-white inequalities in mortality and life-expectancy, 1933-1999: implication for healthy people 2010. *Publ Health Rep.* 2001;116:474-483.

145. Bach PB, Schrag D, Brawley OW, et al. Survival of blacks and whites after a cancer diagnosis.

146. Levkoff S, Sanchez H. Lessons learned about minority recruitment and retention from the centers of minority aging and health promotion. *Gerontologist.* 2003;43:18-26.

147. Galambos CM, Moving cultural diversity toward cultural competence in health care. *Health Soc Work.* 2003;28:3-7.

CHAPTER 5

Children with Cancer

Cultural Differences in Communication between
the United States and the United Kingdom

Edward J. Estlin and Javier R. Kane

INTRODUCTION TO CHILDHOOD CANCER

Cancer in childhood is relatively rare, and the total incidence of childhood cancer (cancer in children less than 15 years of age) is about 1% of that of the adult population. In the United Kingdom, the risk of developing a malignancy in childhood has been estimated at 1 in 581.[1] In the United States, there has been no substantial change in incidence for the major pediatric cancers since the mid-1980s, when modest increases, which probably reflected diagnostic improvements or reporting changes, were reported for central nervous system (CNS) tumors, leukemia, and infant neuroblastoma.[2] In the pediatric setting, the most frequently encountered diagnostic tumor groups are acute leukemia, CNS tumors, lymphomas and soft tissue sarcomas (Table 1).

The relative incidence of overall and individual cancers can vary internationally, and according to racial origin within a single country. For example, the rate of childhood cancer in Ibadan, Nigeria is four times higher than that reported for the Indian population of Fiji.[3] For acute lymphoblastic leukemia, CNS tumors, and neuroblastoma, higher rates are found in Western Europe and the United States than in Africa and Asia. Within the

TABLE 1. Age-Standardized Incidence Rates of the Common Childhood Cancers[1]

Diagnostic group	Age-standardized incidence rates (per million/year)
Leukemia	
Acute lymphoblastic	32.3
Acute non-lymphocytic	5.9
Lymphomas	
Hodgkin's disease	4.6
Non-Hodgkin's lymphoma	6.2
Central nervous system	
Astrocytoma	10.0
Primitive neuroectodermal tumor	6.0
Ependymoma	3.1
Sympathetic nervous system	
Neuroblastoma	8.1
Renal	
Wilms' tumor	7.6
Bone	
Osteogenic sarcoma	2.5
Ewing's tumor	2.3
Soft-tissue sarcoma	
Rhabdomyosarcoma	5.2
Fibrosarcoma	1.0
Other tumors	
Retinoblastoma	3.7
Germ-cell tumors	3.6
Epithelial	3.0

United States, acute leukemia and Ewing's tumor are found more commonly in the White compared with the African American childhood population. Overall, childhood cancer is more common in boys than girls.[3]

Unlike cancer in adults, where the overwhelming majority of cancers are carcinomas that originate in epithelial surfaces, most of the common forms of childhood non-hematological cancer mimic developing or embryonal tissue development. For example, rhabdomyosarcoma and Wilms' tumor resemble developing myogenic mesenchyme and renal tissue respectively.[4] Moreover, certain childhood tumors, such as neuroblastoma and Wilms' tumor are more common in the first 5 years of life,[1] suggesting that many cases of childhood cancer represent gestation-related defects in tissue growth and differentiation. However, whereas CNS tumors and acute lymphoblastic leukemia also have a higher incidence in early childhood, the peak incidence of Ewing's tumor, Hodgkin's disease, and osteogenic sarcoma is found in early adolescence.[5]

Despite the histological features and age of onset of many childhood cancers, less than 5% of cases are associated with a known genetic or cancer-predisposition syndrome.[6] However, certain conditions are associated with an inherited predisposition to cancer.[5] For instance, children with the constitutional chromosomal abnormality of Down syndrome (trisomy 21) have a 20-fold increased risk of developing acute leukemia during the first 10 years of life.[5] The study of the genetic abnormalities found in childhood malignancies and the identification of certain cancer-predisposition genes provide invaluable information for the understanding of the pathogenesis of childhood cancer. For example, the inappropriate activation of normal growth promoting genes, or cellular proto-oncogenes, as seen with the t(8,14) translocation found with Burkitt's lymphoma, are increasingly recognized as playing a role in the pathogenesis of childhood cancers.[7] Alternatively, the functional inactivation of tumor suppressor genes can cause a cancer predisposition phenotype with autosomal recessive characteristics, and the example of the retinoblastoma tumor suppressor gene (RB-1) on chromosome 13q14 has become a paradigm for the analysis of the inherited cancer predisposition syndromes.[7] Other syndromes or conditions that predispose to cancer in children[5,6,8-10] are listed in Table 2.

In summary, epidemiological studies have played an important role in the clinical characterization of individual childhood cancers. Although the vast majority of childhood cancer occurs in children who do not have a predisposing factor, and the importance of environmental factors are largely uncertain, the identification of cancer predisposition syndromes has allowed the evolution of the molecular genetic characterization of diseases such as Wilms' tumor. Such information is providing an invaluable insight into the pathogenesis of childhood cancer.

TREATMENT OF CHILDHOOD CANCER

The standard approach in the treatment of childhood cancer consists of integrating multiple therapeutic modalities to the treatment regimen. This multimodality approach incorporates chemotherapy to eradicate systemic metastatic disease and surgery and/or radiation to provide local disease control. Although the philosophies or the treatment of diseases such as Wilms' tumor (immediate vs delayed, post-chemotherapy nephrectomy) and rhabdomyosarcoma (earlier and more widespread use of radiotherapy for local control) are sometimes different between the United Kingdom/Europe and United States, the conduct of trials is usually along similar lines internationally.

TABLE 2. Predisposition to Childhood Cancer (Malignant Peripheral Nerve Sheath Tumor, MPNST)

Predisposing factor	Genetic abnormality	Associated cancer
Loss of tumor suppressor gene		
Wilms-anhiridia-genitourinary abnormalities-retardation (WAGR)	Loss of tumor suppressor gene at 11p13	Wilms' tumor
Beckwith-Wiedeman syndrome	Loss of tumor suppressor gene at 11p15	
Li-Fraumeni syndrome	Germ line mutation of p53 tumor suppressor gene	Sarcoma Leukemia CNS tumors
Other genetic abnormalities		
Multiple endocrine neoplasia (MEN 2A and 2B)	10q11.2 mutation activating RET oncogene	Medullary thyroid carcinoma
Von Hippel-Lindau disease		Renal cell carcinoma Phaemchromocytoma
Phakomatoses		
Neurofibromatosis type 1	17q11.2	Low-grade glioma Soft-tissue sarcoma MPNST AML
Tuberose sclerosis	9q34 and 16p13	Giant cell astrocytoma
DNA repair defects and hereditary immunodeficiency disorders		
Ataxia-telangiectasia		Acute leukemia
Fanconi's anemia		Lymphoma
Immunodeficiency		
Exogenous factors		
Ultraviolet irradiation	Xeroderma pigmentosum/albinism	Malignant melanoma
Ionizing irradiation		Acute leukemia Thyroid cancer

The prognosis for childhood cancer has improved dramatically since the introduction of chemotherapy. The 5-year survival rate for all forms of childhood cancer at the end of the 20th century was 75%, compared to the dismal outcomes seen in the pre-chemotherapy era.[11] Most types of childhood cancers are treated using conventional frontline treatment regimens designed to eradicate all cancer cells. The efficacy of these drug regimens appears to correlate with low tumor burden.[12] Multidrug combination regimens are used to overcome drug resistance or provide a synergistic cytotoxic effect. Adjuvant chemotherapy is used to eliminate micro-metastatic tumor deposits before the development of clinically evident metastatic disease or for patients without residual tumor after local control has been achieved with surgery or radiation.[13] In general, chemotherapy is used at maximum dose intensity as this correlates with efficacy and improved clinical outcomes, particularly for certain types of tumors.[14-16] Myeloablative chemotherapy is also a key component of stem cell transplantation in which high doses of chemotherapy agents are given as part of the preparative regimen with or without total body irradiation. Stem cell transplantation is a therapeutic intervention for a variety of leukemias, lymphomas, and some solid tumors.[17-19]

Surgery is an important component of the multi-modal treatment of cancer.[20] Surgical intervention is required to establish an accurate diagnosis for most childhood tumors. The use of a correct biopsy technique is essential to avoid contamination of uninvolved body cavities or lymphatic drainage. More recently, fine needle aspirate biopsies and other minimally invasive surgical techniques such as thoracoscopy or laparoscopy have become common practice. Expert surgical approach is important to establish an adequate staging of the tumor, which is disease specific and often used to dictate the intensity of chemotherapy.[21] Surgical intervention is also essential to achieve local control of the tumor by attaining a complete resection with negative microscopic margins, which often correlates with improved patient outcomes.[22-24] Surgery also plays a role in supportive care as in the implantation of gastrostomy feeding tubes for patients at risk of malnutrition or placement of central venous catheters to facilitate administration of chemotherapy and blood sampling. In some situations, surgery may even be used for the treatment of metastatic disease or as a component of supportive care.

Radiation has important antitumor activity for most childhood cancers but tumor cells vary considerably in their sensitivity to radiation. In general, radiation therapy is employed for primary tumor control, as part of a conditioning regimen for stem cell transplantation and in the palliation of cancer-related symptoms. The radiation dose usually depends on tumor size and tumor histology,[25] and modifications of total dose in children are usually justified by age-related toxicity.[26]

The majority of children diagnosed with cancer in the United States, and over 90% of those diagnosed in the United Kingdom are registered in clinical trials, which reflect the best that science and clinical practice have to offer.[27,28] In addition to its recognized therapeutic utility offering children the best possibility of cure, these trials aim to provide important and accurate information about the benefits of expensive and potentially toxic treatments, and are increasingly linked to studies of molecular, biological, and pharmacological factors. New therapeutic approaches are developed following a well-planned scientific approach, in which toxicity and efficacy of particular treatments are established and a determination is made on whether the treatment is better than what is currently available. According to the National Cancer Institute (NCI) drug development program, this scientific approach in cancer clinical trials is categorized into phase I, II, and III trials,[29] and the same approach has been made by the United Kingdom and European organizations.[28] Information regarding the maximum tolerated dose (MTD), dose limiting toxicities, and pharmacokinetics associated to a particular drug and schedule of administration are determined through a phase I study.[30] A phase II trial estimates the activity of the agent at the MTD against individual tumor types.[31] Active compounds are incorporated into phase III trials and compared in effectiveness and toxicity against standard therapy or the natural history of the disease.[32] A major challenge ahead for the development of new therapies for the treatment of children with cancer will be the evaluation of novel compounds that inhibit the processes of angiogenesis and cell cycle control.[33]

ORGANIZATION OF HEALTH CARE FOR CHILDREN WITH CANCER

Funding

In the United States, low-income and needy families receive medical care covered by Medicaid, a jointly funded Federal and State health insurance program. Medicaid covers approximately 36 million individuals including children. Each individual State administers its program and establishes its own eligibility standards, scope of services, and rate of payment for services. Other patients are medically insured by private commercial insurance companies that, like Medicaid, establish their own standards for eligibility and services. By the late 1990s, a significant reduction in the number of children with private insurance was reported, probably reflecting the increasing premium cost. In response to the growing number of uninsured children, the US government created the State run Children's Health Insurance Program (CHIP) which, despite delayed implementation and other problems, is estimated to eventually cover two thirds of the 11 million uninsured children.[34] Unfortunately, the number of uninsured children continues to grow even as the number of children covered by public insurance is increasing.[35] Recent data suggests that as many as 20% of all American children do not have health insurance. The majority of uninsured children diagnosed with cancer in the United States, however, will become eligible for public insurance at some point after diagnosis. Unfortunately, many adult long-term childhood cancer survivors will lose insurance coverage after their 21st birthday.

In the United Kingdom, children with suspected cancer will present to their regional specialist treatment center, having been referred by their family doctor or a district hospital pediatrician or surgeon. Some services, such as surgery for bone tumors or retinoblastoma, are now funded on a supra-regional basis by the national health service (NHS), with a concentration of expertise in a limited number of centers. The health care system with respect to pediatric cancer is almost entirely funded through the NHS, which is essentially a single payer system for health care. The NHS covers all aspects of diagnosis and treatment, although there is involvement of funding from the charitable sector in terms of the provision of a wider multidisciplinary team.

Over the last several years, strategies for cost containment and changes in the structure and organization of health care in the United States have succeeded in containing the burden of explosive medical costs. These changes in managed care have threatened to constrain the integrity of the medical profession by directly interfering with the communication that must exist between physicians, patients, and their caregivers. There is a growing sense that the current model threatens to preempt the personal, the professional and, more fundamentally still, the moral dimension of the patient-physician relationship.[36] A further important barrier to effective communication in the American health care system is the fact that practitioners often do not recover reimbursement for time spent communicating with their patients suggesting that open communication as a medical intervention is not good business practice.[37] Physician reimbursement for services in the United States follows a complex system of billing codes defined by the Current Procedural Terminology (CPT) that has been criticized for discouraging patient-physician interaction by selectively reimbursing for brief procedure-related visits.[38] A "Prolonged Physician Service" code exists to obtain reimbursement for conversations with children and their families regarding diagnosis, relapse, complications of therapy, issues related to death and dying, and advanced care planning. There are, however, many practical problems with the current system and lengthy counseling time is not being reimbursed at all. Lack of reimbursement or poor reimbursement for prolonged service codes is a serious problem that affects the quality of medical care for American children with cancer in a significant way. For example, parents must often be counseled without the child patient present in the conversation but charges to Medicaid using codes for non face-to-face interaction are often rejected.

National Organization of Children's Cancer Services

Clinical trials in the United States are developed and coordinated by a national cooperative formed by 4500 members and 238 member institutions, the Children's Oncology Group (COG), an organization devoted exclusively to research in childhood and adolescent cancer. The COG is funded by the NCI and is supported by the National Childhood Cancer Foundation (NCCF), which serves as the grantee and manager of the COG grant.[39] Patients entering COG studies do so at member institutions throughout the country via a web-based remote data entry system, and approximately 80% of all children with cancer in the United States are now entered into clinical trials. Patients receive treatment under the care of pediatric hematology oncology specialists who are COG members and work for one of its member institutions. All COG studies are reviewed rigorously for scientific merit and patient safety by a multidisciplinary team of cancer specialists, by the NCI and by the local review boards of each COG institution.

The United Kingdom Children's Cancer Study Group (UKCCSG) was founded in 1977. The activities of the group include the registration of all cases of childhood cancer (in collaboration with the National Registry of Childhood Tumors), the organization and running of national treatment programs, collaborating with similar international organizations, facilitating basic scientific research and investigating the late effects of treatment. It is responsible for a range of phase I, II, and III studies in all areas of childhood cancer, except for childhood leukemia, which is administered through the auspices of the Medical Research Council. The UKCCSG Data Center in Leicester is the coordinating center for the Group in terms of registrations, clinical trials, and administration. The Group now has over 300 members, working in 22 Regional pediatric oncology treatment centers throughout the country. Membership of the UKCCSG is multidisciplinary and includes clinicians, pathologists, epidemiologists, and basic scientists,[40] and the activities of the Group are divided amongst various Working Groups in the areas of specific tumors, late effects, modalities of therapy, biological studies, and new agents/pharmacology.

Interdisciplinary Care and Fragmentation of Care

Care of pediatric oncology patients routinely involves multiple professionals from various disciplines including oncology, surgery, radiotherapy and other specialties, nursing, psychology, social work, child life, and pastoral care among others. It also requires the coordination of multiple services within hospitals and in the community, such as school, church, home health agency, and hospice. Ideally, the services should be coordinated and seamless. In the United States, care coordination and supportive services are usually readily available when treatment is delivered with a curative intent while the oncology program serves as a medical home. Clinical experience, however, demonstrates that for patients with advanced disease, when life prolongation or comfort care is the primary goal of care, pediatric oncology programs have difficulty in providing proper coordination of care leading to fragmentation and poorly timed delivery of palliative care services.[41] This fragmentation is of greater significance for patients with advanced disease and results primarily from the lack of a coordination entity required for an increasingly complex care and the separation that exists between tertiary care children's hospitals, home health agencies, and hospice care organizations. Indeed, there are many problems in the delivery of pediatric palliative medicine and end-of-life care in the United States. Hospice care continues to be the main source of care of American patients at the end of their lives.[42] Unfortunately, current hospice admission guidelines and reimbursement practices in the United States are not consistent with optimal palliative care of seriously ill children.[43,44] For example, hospice rules and payments are influenced strongly by the Medicare Hospice Benefit, which requires relinquishing reimbursement for potentially life-prolonging treatment in favor of just palliative care at home.[45] It is well known that these and other barriers make timely admission of pediatric oncology patients into hospice an impossible task. It is estimated that only 5000 children of the 53000 who die from all causes in the United States every year receive hospice care and over half of the pediatric deaths occur in the hospital.[46,47]

In the United Kingdom, the care of children with cancer is also multidisciplinary. Each Regional treatment center will have a core of NHS-funded pediatric hematologists and oncologists, nursing staff to cover inpatient and outpatient therapy, social workers, teachers, and input from dieticians, teachers, physiotherapists, occupational therapists, and pharmacists. Historically, the MacMillan Cancer Relief and Cancer and Leukaemia in Childhood charities have also played a very important role in establishing a network of Outreach Nurses in the United Kingdom, with many of the nurses being funded directly by the NHS. The role of the Oncology Outreach Nurse Specialist is developing as a major influence for the communication between the specialist units and primary care teams and schools. In addition, these nurse specialists provide an educational role for the families of children with cancer, and also play a major role in the provision of care for children in the terminal phase of their illness. In the United Kingdom, the Outreach Nurses will coordinate the care of the child receiving palliative care with the pediatric Hospice, or as is the case for the vast majority of children, at home in conjunction with primary care and district teams.[48] Each Regional pediatric cancer center in the United Kingdom will have access to at least one hospice, that are generally funded by charity, that is dedicated to the care of children. The link between hospital- and community-based services has allowed individual districts (in terms of administration) to establish multidisciplinary teams dedicated to pediatric palliative care.[49] This is perhaps one of the strengths of the health service in the United Kingdom.

COMMUNICATION AND STAGES OF CARE

General Issues in Communication

Children with cancer and their families experience a great deal of suffering.[50] The medical care of these children demands effective communication with children and their parents or guardians in order to avoid unnecessary suffering. Caregivers, as surrogate decision-makers, need to be well informed and empowered to make decisions in the best interest of the child.[51] There are several situations when good communication is essential for effective medical care: at the time of diagnosis, complications or relapse, during hospitalizations or other crisis, at disease progression, death, and bereavement. Communication regarding prognosis for life expectancy and quality of life, treatment alternatives, goals of care, and advance care planning is also necessary at different stages of the disease trajectory. Earlier recognition of poor prognosis by both parents and physicians is important and correlates with having earlier discussions of hospice care, better quality of home care, less cancer-directed therapy, and earlier institution of orders to withhold artificial life sustaining therapies.[52]

Communication about difficult issues, however, varies across geographical regions and factors such as physician and family values influence the process. Physicians in Western countries, for example, are less likely to withhold unfavorable information, use euphemisms, and give treatments known not to be effective so as not to destroy hope.[53]

Maintaining adequate communication with both patients and their caregivers is also of utmost importance in end-of-life care when compassionate decisions to withhold or withdraw curative and/or other life prolonging therapies must be made. For the most part pediatric oncologists in the United States are not well trained in end-of-life care.[54] A recent report suggests that these physicians have learned to care for dying children and their families by trial and error.[55] Treatment of pediatric oncology patients demands greater communication regarding issues related to coping, self-efficacy, family cohesion, parental self-care, and similar issues which, in general, are briefly discussed by physicians and often assigned to psychologists, counselors, or other supportive staff. There is no standardized approach for health care professionals to communicate with patients and their parents regarding their medical care in these circumstances. Health care organizations and individual institutions promote ethical standards of practice; whether conversations with patients and their families in the process of medical decision-making occur in a way that is goal directed, culturally sensitive, and compassionate depends primarily on the personal attributes of the individual professionals providing the care. Standardization of the communication process utilizing tools such as the Final Stage Conference, although helpful to facilitate discussion of difficult issues with patients and families, are not widely implemented.[56]

Diagnosis and Treatment: Issues of Consent, Assent, and Dissent

In the United States, participation of children in research trials requires parental or legal guardian consent after they have been fully informed through a process that intends to honor the ethical principles of respect for human dignity and individual autonomy.[57] Except for emancipated minors, American children under the age of 18 are not considered adults and can only legally assent or dissent to participate. It is usually their parents or other authorized surrogate decision-maker who must go through the process of consent. This process involves a parent-friendly disclosure of the purpose and nature of the study, risks, benefits, and treatment. In recognition of this challenge, the International Society of Paediatric Oncology (SIOP) has issued guidelines for communication, which include recommendations for planning discussions well, involving other members of staff and provision for follow up meetings.[58] Similarly, the Institutional Review Board Guidebook published by the National Institutes of Health Office for Human Research Protection suggests that "the child should be given an explanation of the proposed research procedures in a language that is appropriate to the child's age, experience, maturity, and condition".[59] Many ethicists, institutional review boards, and researchers in the United States believe that too much information is provided to obtain participation consent, but accept the process of obtaining permission from parents and having the child agree to participate if he or she is over the age of 7 years.[60] There is no national agreement, however, on whether a child's decision to dissent should be honored. This is broadly similar to the guidelines adhered to in the United Kingdom, where children and parents are involved in discussions about diagnosis, treatment, and permission for tumor, and data storage.

The area of diagnosis and informed consent has been the subject of study within pediatric oncology. In a study of families with children entering Children's Cancer Group clinical trials, parents described that discussions of diagnosis and treatment options occurred amidst tremendous stress. In addition, a sense of constraint and lack of control was common, and parents experienced variable degrees of choice regarding their child's participation in a clinical trial.[61] In a survey of principal investigators and parents, satisfaction with informed consent in relation to Children's Cancer Group trials was not related to ethnicity or educational level. Parents generally found the discussions to be more helpful than consent documents, and were less likely to feel that too much information had been imparted in comparison to the pediatric oncologist.[62] In contrast, in the United Kingdom, this area has not been the subject of widespread study. However, one study warned of the potential social positioning of young people in relation to adults, which may lead to the executive role of parents leading to the marginalization of children in the discussion process.[63] The practice of directing information toward the parents or carers, and not necessarily the child or young person with cancer, perhaps reflects a more widespread culture within pediatrics. Children's cancer specialists may therefore need to acquire the communication skills necessary to discuss medical-technical issues with their patients themselves.[64]

Issues relating to culture and ethnicity may be particularly important in relation to children's cancer therapy. The relative under-representation of ethnic minorities in the ranks of health professionals, the under-funding of hospice care in the United States, and cultural differences in relation to the discussion of issues relating to terminal care pose enormous challenges.[65] Fundamental philosophical differences exist between "Western" thinking and that of terminally ill adults who are of African American, Hispanic Latino, and native American origin, where terminal care focuses on living and prolonging life and less on coping with eventual death. It is not known if these influences relate to the terminal care of children from different ethnic origins in the United States. However, more is known about the influence of racial and ethnic differences in survival for children with acute lymphoblastic leukemia. For children in the United States, a poorer outcome has been described for children with standard risk (African American children) and higher risk (Hispanic children) acute lymphoblastic leukemia, than for Caucasian children or those from an Asian origin. These differences in survival did not relate to socioeconomic status (SES), and whether ethnic differences in compliance or pharmacogenetics are important in this setting is unknown.[66] In the United Kingdom, although there are many similarities in the use of cancer services between ethnic minority groups and individuals with lower SES[67] in the adult setting, no difference has been found for childhood cancer survival between Caucasian and non-Caucasian children with cancer.[68] This may indicate that the care afforded by the multidisciplinary team and the willingness of parents to comply with their children's treatment is able to overcome difficulties in communication and cultural differences.

End-of-Life Care: Issues of Communication

Advance Care Planning includes specific conversations regarding resuscitation orders, advanced directives, and medical power of attorney.[69] In the United States, most States require completion of a "Do Not Resuscitate" (D.N.R.) form signed by both parents and doctors, and used to instruct health care providers to withhold some forms of artificial life sustaining therapies. Adult patients may use the "Advanced Directives" document to inform family members and doctors about their wishes regarding artificial life sustaining therapies and other treatments in case they become unable to communicate these wishes personally. In the case of minors who are not legally required to make their own medical decisions, some institutions advocate the use of a "Directive to Physicians" where parents may alert their doctors regarding their health care wishes for their child. This document is not legally binding and serves more as a communication tool for health care providers rather than an Advanced Directive. The Medical Power of Attorney is a document used to assign a surrogate decision-maker in case the patient becomes unable to make decisions on his own. Except in cases of emancipated minors, this form is rarely needed for pediatric patients. In the United Kingdom, the system is less formal. Where death is foreseen and agreed as inevitable by both parents/carers and health professionals, a handwritten annotation is made to the hospital record to prevent full resuscitation in the event of collapse. However, the vast majority of children die at their homes or in hospice, where intensive care measures would not be undertaken anyway with full counseling of the parents.

In end-of-life care, when quality of life is the main focus of care, most palliative care physicians in the United States believe that children's dissent, adolescents in particular, to participate in clinical trials deserves special attention. Here, the Institute of Medicine report on Improving Palliative Care for Cancer recommends that children's decision should be respected if they have reached the age of assent, understand their condition and treatment alternatives, and the consequences of their choices.[70] Having the child and his or her parents participate in the medical decision-making process is certainly a goal of treatment and a priority of the COG.[71] Indeed, in a survey of pediatric hematologists/oncologists from the UKCCSG and Pediatric Oncology Group in North America, the consent of parents and children was raised as an ethical consideration by many respondents.[72] Nevertheless, whether a different consent process is needed for enrollment of children with advanced disease in phase I clinical trials has not yet been the subject of formal study.

CONCLUSIONS

As discussed in the preceding sections, health care professionals are faced with many important challenges when caring for children with cancer. The visible improvements made in survival for children with cancer over the last 30 years owes perhaps as much to the development of national organizations such as the COG and the UKCCSG, as to the inherent sensitivity to treatment of these cancers. In addition, the intensification of multi-modality therapy, and the inclusion of biological and pharmacological studies into frontline treatment protocols are causing tremendous challenges in terms of the informed consent of children and parents at a very difficult time.

In relation to issues of communication in general, the lack of effective reimbursement of physicians for parental counseling, especially if the consultation does not directly involve the child may be an important barrier to effective communication in the United States. For the provision of health care beyond the boundaries of the pediatric oncology unit, the link between community-based health care teams and the specialist unit that exist under the auspices of the NHS in the United Kingdom seem to facilitate a more even and home-centered approach to palliative care. The diverse ethnic mix of cultures in the United States, and to a lesser extent the United Kingdom, pose unique challenges to effective communication. This may be one variable that influences the outcome of childhood ALL, and therefore perhaps other forms of cancer in the United States and formal studies are needed to investigate the importance of communication for potentially important issues such as compliance.

Considering the importance of communication within the area of childhood cancer, there has been a paucity of formal studies in this area. From their review of the subject, Scott et al.[73] concluded that interventions to enhance communication involving children and adolescents with cancer have not been widely or rigorously assessed. The weak evidence that exists suggests that some children and adolescents with cancer derive some benefit from specific information-giving programs and from interventions that aim to facilitate their reintegration into school and social activities. Also gained from studies performed in the United States and United Kingdom are the findings of parental executive action, potential marginalization of children, parental senses of constraint and lack of control, and an appreciation of discussions over consent forms. There is an increasing volume of information faced by the parents of newly diagnosed children with cancer. Further studies of communication are required at all stages of care, from diagnosis through to end-of-life issues. Such studies could investigate the importance of the environment of the discussion, the length of time pediatricians are able to spend with families to discuss important issues such as diagnosis, randomization, and relapse and end-of-life care. The cooperation of national groups such as the COG and the UKCCSG would provide for an excellent and informative study of the influence of cultural variables, health system funding, and community provision for care on this process.

REFERENCES

1. Stiller CA, Allen MB, Eatock EM. Childhood cancer in Britain: the national registry of childhood tumours and incidence rates 1978–1987. *Eur J Cancer.* 1995;31A:2028-2034.
2. Linet MS, Ries LA, Smith MA, Tarone RE, Devesa SS. 1999. Cancer surveillance series: recent trends in childhood cancer incidence and mortality in the United States. *J Natl Cancer Inst.* 1999;91:1051-1058.
3. Robison LL. General principles of the epidemiology of childhood cancer. In: Pizzo PA, Poplack DG, ed. *Principles and Practice of Pediatric Oncology.* Philadelphia, PA: Lippincottt-Raven Publishers; 1997:1-10.
4. Triche TJ. Tumour pathology section 1: Methodology and specific applications. In: Pinkerton CR, Plowman PN, eds. *Paediatric Oncology: Clinical Practice and Controversies.* 2nd ed. London: Chapman & Hall Medical; 1997:67-92.
5. Plon SE, Peterson LE. Childhood cancer, hereditary and the environment. In: Pizzo PA, Poplack DG, ed. *Principles and Practice of Pediatric Oncology.* Philadelphia, PA: Lippincott-Raven Publishers; 1997:11-36.
6. Narod SA. Genetic epidemiology of childhood cancer. *Biochim Biophys Acta.* 1996;1288: F141-F150.
7. Pritchard-Jones K. Genetics of childhood cancer. *Br Med Bull.* 1996;52:704-723.
8. Matsui I, Tanimura M, Kobayashi N, Sawada T, Nagahara N, Akatsuka J. Neurofibromatosis type 1 and childhood cancer. *Cancer.* 1993;72:2746.
9. Eisenbarth I, Vogel G, Krone W, Vogel W, Assum G. An isochore transition in the NF1 gene region coincides with a switch in the extent of linkage disequilibrium. *Am J Hum Genet.* 2000;67:873-880.
10. Langkau N, Martin N, Brandt R, et al. TSC1 and TSC2 mutations in tuberous sclerosis, the associated phenotypes and a model to explain observed TSC1/TSC2 frequency ratios. *Eur J Pediatr.* 2002;161:393-402.
11. Greenlee RT, Murray T, Bolden S, Wingo PA. Cancer statistics, 2000. *CA Cancer J Clin.* 2000;50:7-33.
12. Goldie JH, Coldman AJ. Theoretical considerations regarding the early use of adjuvant chemotherapy. *Recent Results Cancer Res.* 1986;103:30-35.
13. Dawson JW, Taylor I. Principles of adjuvant therapy. *Br J Hosp Med.* 1995;54:249-254.
14. Gaynon P, Steinherz P, Bleyer WA, et al. Association of delivered drug dose and outcome for children with acute lymphoblastic leukemia and unfavorable presenting features. *Med Pediatr Oncol.* 1991;19:221-227.
15. Bacci G, Picci P, Avella M, et al. The importance of dose-intensity in neoadjuvant chemotherapy of osteosarcoma: a retrospective analysis of high-dose methotrexate, cis-platinum and adriamycin used preoperatively. *J Chemother.* 1990;2:127-135.
16. Cheung N-KV, Heller G. Chemotherapy dose-intensity correlates strongly with response, median survival, and median progression-free survival in metastatic neuroblastoma. *J Clin Oncol.* 1991;9:1050-1058.
17. Kobrinsky NL, Sposto R, Shah NR, et al. Outcomes of treatment of children and adolescents with recurrent non-Hodgkin's lymphoma and Hodgkin's disease with dexamethasone,

etoposide, cisplatin, cytarabine, and l-asparaginase, maintenance chemotherapy, and transplantation: Children's Cancer Group Study CCG-5912. *J Clin Oncol.* 2001;19:2390-2396.

18. Feig SA, Harris RE, Sather HN. Bone marrow transplantation versus chemotherapy for maintenance of second remission of childhood acute lymphoblastic leukemia: a study of the Children's Cancer Group (CCG-1884). *Med Ped Oncol.* 1997;29:534-540.

19. Sands SA, van Gorp WG, Finlay JL. Pilot neuropsychological findings from a treatment regimen consisting of intensive chemotherapy and bone marrow rescue for young children with newly diagnosed malignant brain tumors. *Childs Nerv Syst.* 1998;14:587-589.

20. Zimmermann T, Blutters-Sawatzki R, Flechsenhar K, Padberg WM. Peripheral primitive neuroectodermal tumor: challenge for multimodal treatment. *World J Surg.* 2001;25: 1367-1372.

21. Katzenstein HM, London WB, Douglass EC, et al. Treatment of unresectable and metastatic hepatoblastoma: a pediatric oncology group phase II study. *J Clin Oncol.* 2002;20: 3438-3444.

22. Schnater JM, Aronson DC, Plaschkes J, et al. Surgical view of the treatment of patients with hepatoblastoma: results from the first prospective trial of the International society of pediatric oncology liver tumor study group. *Cancer.* 2002;94:1111-1120.

23. Katzenstein HM, London WB, Douglass EC, et al. Treatment of unresectable and metastatic hepatoblastoma: a pediatric oncology group phase II study. *J Clin Oncol.* 2002;20: 3438-3444.

24. Sirvent N, Kanold J, Levy C, et al. Non-metastatic Ewing's sarcoma of the ribs: the French society of pediatric oncology experience. *Eur J Cancer.* 2002;38:561-567.

25. Laver JH, Mahmoud H, Pick TE, et al. Results of a randomized phase III trial in children and adolescents with advanced stage diffuse large cell non-Hodgkin's lymphoma: a pediatric oncology group study. *Leuk Lymphoma.* 2002;43:105-109.

26. Merchant TE. Conformal therapy for pediatric sarcomas. *Semin Radiat Oncol.* 1997;7: 236-245.

27. Benowitz S. Children's oncology group looks to increase efficiency, numbers in clinical trials. *J Natl Cancer Inst.* 2000;92:1876-1878.

28. Estlin EJ, Ablett S. Practicalities and ethics of running clinical trials in paediatric oncology—the UK experience. *Eur J Cancer.* 2001;37:1399-1401.

29. Muggia FM, Carter SK, Macdonald JS. The cancer therapy evaluation program of the National Cancer Institute. *Semin Oncol.* 1981;8:394-402.

30. Shah S, Weitman S, Langevin AM, Bernstein M, Furman W, Pratt C. Phase I therapy trials in children with cancer. *J Pediatr Hematol Oncol.* 1998;20:431-438.

31. Weitman S, Ochoa S, Sullivan J, et al. Pediatric phase II cancer chemotherapy trials: a pediatric oncology group study. *J Pediatr Hematol Oncol.* 1997;19:187-191.

32. Bleyer A. Older adolescents with cancer in North America deficits in outcome and research. *Pediatr Clin North Am.* 2002;49:1027-1042.

33. Estlin EJ. Novel targets for therapy in paediatric oncology. *Curr Drug Targets Immune Endocr Metabol Disord.* 2002;2:141-150.

34. Kaiser Family Foundation and Health Research Educational Trust. *Employer Health Benefits: 1999 Annual Survey.* Menlo Park, CA, and Chicago, IL, 1999.

35. Cunningham PJ. Recent trends in children's health insurance coverage: no gains for low-income children. *HSC.* 2000:1-6.

36. Baker R, Emanuel L. The efficacy of professional ethics: the AMA code of ethics in historical and current perspective. *Hastings Cent Rep.* 2000;30(4 suppl):S13-S17.

37. Emanuel L. Structured advance planning. Is it finally time for physician action and reimbursement? *JAMA.* 1995;274:501-503.

38. Storey P, Knight C. UNIPAC six: ethical and legal decision making when caring for the terminally ill. Gainesville, FL: AAHPM; 1996.

39. Children's Oncology Group. Available at: www.childrensoncologygroup.org

40. Estlin EJ, Ablett S, Newell DR, Lewis IJ, Lashford L, Pearson AD. Phase I trials in paediatric oncology—the European perspective. The new agents group of the United Kingdom children's cancer study group. *Invest New Drugs.* 1996;14:432-435.

41. Wolfe J, Friebert S, Hilden J. Caring for children with advanced cancer integrating palliative care. *Pediatr Clin North Am.* 2002;49:1043-1062.

42. Miller PJ, Mike PB. The Medicare hospice benefit: ten years of federal policy for the terminally ill. *Death Stud.* 1995;19:531-542.

43. von Gunten CF, Ferris FD, D'Antuono R, Emanuel LL. Recommendations to improve end-of-life care through regulatory change in U.S. health care financing. *J Palliative Med.* 2002;5:35-41.

44. Field MJ, Cassel CK, eds. *Approaching Death. Improving Care at the End of Life.* Washington, DC: National Academy Press; 1997.

45. Kinzbrunner BM. Hospice: 15 years and beyond in the care of the dying. *J Palliat Med.* 1998;1:127-137.

46. Feudtner C, Silveira MJ, Christakis DA. Where do children with complex chronic conditions die? Patterns in Washington State, 1980-1998. *Pediatr.* 2002;109:656-660.

47. A call for change. Improving the lives of children living with life limiting illnesses. Report of the Children's International Project on Palliative Services of the National Hospice Organization. NHPCO Website at: http://www.nhpco.org/public/articles/Callfor Change.pdf

48. Goldman A. ABC of palliative care. Special problems of children. *Br Med J.* 1998;316:49-52.

49. Wallace AC, Jackson S. Establishing a district palliative care team for children. *Child Care Health Dev.* 1995;21:383-385.

50. Wolfe J, Grier HE, Klar N, et al. Symptoms and suffering at the end of life in children with cancer. *New Eng J Med.* 2000;342:326-333.

51. Wharton RH, Levine KR, Buka S, Emanuel L. Advance care planning for children with special health care needs: a survey of parental attitudes. *Pediatr.* 1996;97:682-687.

52. Wolfe J, Klar N, Grier HE, et al. Understanding of prognosis among parents of children who died of cancer: impact on treatment goals and integration of palliative care. *JAMA.* 2000;284:2469-2475.

53. Baile WF, Lenzi R, Parker PA, Buckman R, Cohen L. Oncologists' attitudes toward and practices in giving bad news: an exploratory study. *J Clin Oncol.* 2002;20:2189-2196.

54. Sahler OJZ, Frager G, Levetown M, Cohn FG, Lipson MA. Medical education about end-of-life care in the pediatric setting: principles, challenges and opportunities. *Pediatr.* 2000;105:575-584.

55. Hilden JM, Emanuel EJ, Fairclough DL, et al. Attitudes and practices among pediatric oncologists regarding end-of-life care: results of the 1998 American Society of Clinical Oncology survey. *J Clin Oncol.* 2001;19:205-212.

56. Nitschke R, Meyer WH, Sexauer CL, Parkhurst JB, Foster P, Huszti H. Care of terminally ill children with cancer. *Med Pediatr Oncol.* 2000;34:268-270.

57. The National Commission for the Protection of Human Subjects of Biomedical and Behavioral Research. *The Belmont Report.* Washington, DC: Government Printing Office (FR Doc 79-12065);1988.

58. Masera G, Chesler MA, Jankovic M, et al. SIOP Working Committee on psychosocial issues in pediatric oncology: guidelines for communication of the diagnosis. *Med Pediatr Oncol.* 1997;28:382-385.

59. Institutional Review Guidebook, Website.

60. American Academy of Pediatrics, Committee on Bioethics. Informed consent, parental permission, and assent in pediatric practice. *Pediatr.* 1995;95:314-317.

61. Levi RB, Marsick R, Drotar D, Kodish ED. Diagnosis, disclosure, and informed consent: learning from parents of children with cancer. *J Pediatr Hematol Oncol.* 2000;22:3-12.

62. Kodish ED, Pentz RD, Noll RB, Ruccione K, Buckley J, Lange BJ. Informed consent in the children's cancer group: results of preliminary research. *Cancer.* 1998;82:2467-2481.
63. Young B, Dixon-Woods M, Windridge KC, et al. Managing communication with young people who have a potentially life threatening chronic illness: qualitative study of patients and parents. *Br Med J.* 2003;326:305-306.
64. van Dulmen AM. Children's contributions to pediatric outpatient encounters. *Pediatr.* 1998;102:563-568.
65. Thomas ND. The importance of culture throughout all of life and beyond. *Holist Nurs Pract.* 2001;15:40-46.
66. Bhatia S, Sather HN, Heerema NA, et al. Racial and ethnic differences in survival of children with acute lymphoblastic leukaemia. *Blood.* 2002;100:1957-1964.
67. Lodge N. The identified needs of ethnic minority groups with cancer within the community: a review of the literature. *Eur J Cancer Care.* 2001;10:234-244.
68. Stiller CA, Bunch KJ, Lewis IJ. Ethnic group and survival from childhood cancer: a report from the UK children's cancer study group. *Br J Cancer.* 2000;82:1339-1343.
69. Choi YS, Billings JA. Changing perspectives on palliative care. *Oncology.* 2002;16:515-522.
70. Hilden J, Himelstein BP, Freyer DR, Friebert S, Kane JR. End-of-life care: special issues in pediatric oncology. In: Foley K, Gelband H, eds. *Improving Palliative Care for Cancer.* Washington, D.C.: Institute of Medicine. National Academy Press; 2001.
71. Spinetta JJ, Masera G, Jankovic M, et al. Valid informed consent and participative decision-making in children with cancer and their parents: a report of the SIOP working committee on psychosocial issues in pediatric oncology. *Med Pediatr Oncol.* 2003;40:244-246.
72. Estlin EJ, Cotterrill S, Pratt CB, Pearson AD, Bernstein M. Phase I trials in pediatric oncology: perceptions of pediatricians from the United Kingdom children's cancer study group and the pediatric oncology group. *J Clin Oncol.* 2000;18:1900-1905.
73. Scott JT, Entwhistle VA, Sowden AJ, et al. Communicating with children and adolescents about their cancer (Cochrane Review). In: *The Cochrane Library,* Issue 3, 2001. Oxford: Update Software.

CHAPTER 6

Cancer Risk Assessment

Clinically Relevant Information Is Key

Patricia T. Kelly

INTRODUCTION

Cancer Risk Assessment services are becoming more widely available as genetic testing for hereditary susceptibility to cancer gains acceptance. These services typically provide risk assessment and genetic testing for individuals with concerns about their family history of cancer. Many Cancer Risk Assessment services also help individuals to understand and make use of information about nonhereditary risks and assist them in making informed decisions about medical care and follow-up options. This chapter discusses some of the types of information that are most useful in discussing hereditary and nonhereditary breast and ovarian cancer risks with concerned individuals, specifically:

- risk over time
- absolute risk
- specificity about what a risk refers to

When these three elements are included in the Cancer Risk Assessment discussion process, individuals are more likely to understand their risks and are better prepared to participate in an informed health and medical care decision process.

Risk Over Time

Individuals who have a genetic change (mutation) in the *BRCA1* gene on chromosome 17 or the *BRCA2* gene on chromosome 13 have an increased risk of breast cancer, ovarian cancer, and to a far lesser extent, several other cancers as well. Initial studies on the risk of breast and ovarian cancer to BRCA mutation carriers were based on small groups of specially selected families.[1-3] Cancer risks in these studies are higher than those obtained in more recent studies in which families were ascertained by testing unselected individuals with breast and ovarian cancer.

In one recent study of 280 families with a BRCA1 mutation, carriers had a breast cancer risk of 65% to age 70.[4] Risk of ovarian cancer to age 70 was 39%. The age-specific risks are shown in Table 1. Age-specific risks provide information about both immediate and future risks and so are generally more useful in a clinical setting than are lifetime risks.

In Table 1 it can be seen that this study found a breast cancer risk of 26% from age 40 to 50 (about 25% a year) and 15% or 1.5% a year for women aged 50 to 60. As a woman goes through each age without a breast cancer diagnosis, she leaves behind the risk associated with that age. Therefore, in this study a 50-year-old BRCA1 carrier without a breast cancer diagnosis had a 27% risk of breast cancer (15% plus 12%) to age 70. A 60-year-old had a 12% risk of breast cancer and a 17% risk of ovarian cancer to age 70. These risks are approximate, since they are based on all mutations in the BRCAI gene and are adapted from cumulative life table analysis figures.

An assessment of risk by age and over time helps women to make informed decisions about health behaviors now and over the next years. Perusal of Table 1 also shows that about 30% of the breast cancer risk and

TABLE 1. Breast and Ovarian Cancer Risks to Age 70 in *BRCA1* Carriers

Age	Breast (%)	Ovarian (%)
Up to 40	12	2
40-50	26	11
50-60	15	9
60-70	12	17
Total	65	39

Source: Adapted from Antoniou et al. 2003.[4]

TABLE 2. Breast and Ovarian Cancer Risks To Age 70 in BRCA21 Carriers

Age	Breast (%)	Ovarian (%)
Up to 40	6	1
40–50	10	1
50–60	15	6
60–70	14	4
Total	45	11

Source: Adapted from Antoniou et al. 2003.[4]

over 60% of the ovarian cancer risk occurs after age 50. In assessing risk due to strong hereditary factors, it is important to recognize that even women whose relatives were diagnosed with breast and/or ovarian cancer at older ages may have an increased hereditary cancer risk.

In this same study women in the 218 families who were BRCA2 carriers were found to have a breast cancer risk of 45% and an ovarian cancer risk of 11% to age 70.[4] As can be seen in Table 2, the breast cancer risk from age 40 on was 1–1.5% a year. Almost all of the ovarian cancer risk occurred after age 50. A 50-year-old woman had a 29% risk of breast cancer (about 1.4% a year) and a 10% risk of ovarian cancer (about 0.5% a year) to age 70.

The risks in Tables 1 and 2 are approximate and may well change as more individuals and families are studied and as BRCA carriers are ascertained in other ways.[5] Some studies find that the location of the mutation within the *BRCA1* or *BRCA2* gene influences the cancer risk.[6,7] In future it may therefore be possible to provide risk information based on a specific mutation within one of these genes instead of on all mutations in a gene as a group.

ABSOLUTE RISK

In a clinical setting absolute risks are generally less confusing than risks presented in comparison formats—that is, as relative risks, odds ratios, hazard ratios, or as percent increases or decreases.

Relative Risks, Odds Ratios, and Hazard Ratios

Studies on breast cancer risk associated with the use of hormone replacement therapy (HRT) are generally reported as relative risks, odds ratios, or hazard ratios. A number of studies find no statistically significant increase in breast cancer risk to HRT users, even with 15 to 20 years of use.[8-11] However, one often cited study, the Nurses Study, found that women who used HRT for five or more years had a 1.5-fold increase in breast cancer risk that was statistically significant.[12]

This 1.5-fold increase has caused great concern. And, because it was reported in a comparison format, the actual size of the increase is not clean. Subsequently an international group calculated that in 10 years a 1.5-fold increase in risk would result in an additional 0.3 breast cancer per 100 women.[13] In most instances hearing about a 1.5-fold increase in risk is likely to raise more concern than learning there is a risk of less than one breast cancer per 100 women in 10 years.

A similar misunderstanding about a risk's magnitude occurred when the results of the Women's Health Initiative (WHI) study were announced. In this large randomized prospective study of over 161 000 women, one group was assigned to take daily conjugated equine estrogen plus medroxy progesterone acetate (Prempro) and the other a placebo.[14] At the end of 5.2 years, the group taking Prempro and the group taking the placebo did not differ statistically in their breast cancer risk. However, the risk to the Prempro group was reported as a hazard rate of 1.26 and as such gave rise to much concern to women and their physicians.

Some of this concern might have been ameliorated and the results of the study better understood if more attention had been paid to what the hazard ratio of 1.26 meant in absolute terms. In this case the absolute difference between the group that did and did not take Prempro was 8 in 10 000 breast cancers a year or eight hundredths of one percent. This very small difference was largely overlooked. Instead, discussions focused on the 1.26-fold increase—the same finding as 8 in 10 000, but presented in a different format.

Also overlooked were aspects of the WHI study that make it unlikely that even this very small difference in breast cancer risk was due to Prempro use. These include:

1. An average follow-up of 5.2 years. Breast cancers are estimated to take an average of 8 years to reach 1 cm,[15] with cancers in older women growing more slowly than in those who are younger. Therefore all or most of the breast cancers detected in this study were likely to have been present in an undetected state before the study began.
2. A drop out rate of 42% among women assigned to take Prempro. Risks were calculated on the group to which a woman was assigned, not actual Prempro use.

As the information just presented suggests, the WHI study does not provide firm evidence that HRT use increases breast cancer risk. Not only was the difference in breast cancer rate between the placebo and Prempro group very small, it was not statistically significant. Furthermore, the small difference of 8 in 10000 is unlikely to be due to hormone use because of the short follow-up. Also, in this study the mean age of study participants was 63, with most not using HRT before the study began. The results therefore apply to women who start HRT use some 10 years after menopause and not to those whose HRT use starts at menopause. In addition, the women in this study used Prempro, so the results do not apply to other, newer approaches in which other hormones are used and a woman's natural cycle is more closely approximated.

Percent Increase or Decrease

The Tamoxifen prevention trial found that among high-risk women assigned to take tamoxifen, breast cancer risk was reduced by 49%.[16] In this study, women who were calculated to have an increased breast cancer risk were assigned to take either tamoxifen or a placebo for 5 years. At the end of 5.75 years, tamoxifen users were found to have 49% fewer breast cancers than women who took a placebo. To many, a 49% reduction was reason enough to suggest that women at increased breast cancer risk should consider taking tamoxifen for prevention.

Here also, the absolute risk provides a different perspective than that of the comparison risk. In the tamoxifen prevention trial, the 49% reduction in breast cancer risk was an absolute difference of 1.8 breast cancers in 100 women at 5.75 years, as shown in Table 3. This means that if 100 high-risk women took tamoxifen and 100 high-risk women did not, at the end of 5.75 years, only 1.8 more breast cancers would be found in the group that did not take tamoxifen. Obviously, a 49% reduction in risk

TABLE 3. Breast Cancer Rates in Tamoxifen Prevention Trial

Number/Rate	No Tamoxifen	Tamoxifen
Number of Women	6 599	6 576
Number of Breast Cancers	175	89
Cumulative Rate Per 100 Women	3.8	2.0

Adapted from Fisher et al. (1998).[16]

appears to be greater than does a reduction of 1.8 breast cancers per 100 women at the end of nearly six years.

Even the small reduction in breast cancer risk found in this study is unlikely to be due to tamoxifen use however, since the follow-up in the study was 5.75 years. This is less than the average 8 years needed for a breast cancer to reach 1 cm in size, as discussed previously. Therefore, all or most of the breast cancers detected during the tamoxifen prevention study were probably present in an undetected state before the study began.

RISK SPECIFICATION

Women who have concerns about breast cancer risk often experience difficulty hearing or absorbing information about risk.[17] It is not uncommon for these women to think that a risk of being diagnosed with breast cancer is actually the risk of dying of it. This distinction is particularly important because breast cancers are being detected at smaller sizes, when they are more curable. For example, women whose invasive ductal breast cancers measure up to 9 mm were found in one study to have a 20-year prognosis of better than 90%.[18] As Table 4 shows, with Grade 1 node negative invasive ductal breast cancers less than 1 cm, the survival was 92% and with Grade 3 it was 91%. Even with node negative invasive ductal breast cancers measuring up to 1.4 cm, the 20-year breast cancer specific survivals are above 90% for grades 1 and 2. Most of the women in this study had no chemotherapy or tamoxifen treatments.

Ovarian cancer, on the other hand, is difficult to detect before it has spread. Only about 30% of ovarian cancers detected in the United States are localized at the time of detection.[19] The 5-year 30% survival rate for all stages is 53%.

In making decisions about medical care and follow-up practices, information about risk of disease is an important component, but as the different survivals for breast and ovarian cancer demonstrate, it is not sufficient. In addition to risk of disease, individuals who seek Cancer Risk

TABLE 4. Twenty-Year Survival for Women with Node Negative Invasive Ductal Breast Cancers 1-9 mm

Grade	Survival (%)
1	92
2	91
3	91

Source: Adapted from Tabar et al. (2000).[18]

Assessment need information about prognosis and the likelihood that a cancer will be diagnosed when it is associated with a good prognosis. Individuals also need help in appreciating the difference between cancer risk and the risk of death due to that cancer.

CONCLUSION

In Cancer Risk Assessment, individuals benefit by having an opportunity to learn about their risks of developing cancer due to hereditary and non-hereditary risk factors. Risk of developing cancer, prognosis, and the likelihood that a cancer can be detected when the prognosis is good also need to be included. In addition, the format in which these risks are presented will often shape an individual's perspective of its magnitude. In a clinical setting, risk information is more likely to be useful when it is presented with a time frame and in an absolute format than when a comparison format is used. In addition, individuals need time to absorb and process the information to enable them to make use of it in a manner that is congruent with their lifestyles and value systems.

REFERENCES

1. Easton DF, Ford D, Bishop DT, et al. Breast and ovarian cancer incidence in BRCA1-mutation carriers. *Am J Hum Genet.* 1995;6:265-271.
2. Ford D, Easton DF, Bishop DT, et al. Risks of cancer in BRCA1-mutation carriers. *Lancet.* 1994;343:692-695.
3. Breast Cancer Linkage Consortium. Cancer risks in BRCA2 mutation carriers. *J Natl Cancer Inst.* 1999;91:1310-1316.
4. Antoniou A, Pharoah PDP, Narods, et al. Average risks of breast and ovarian cancer associated with BRCAI or BRAC2 mutations detected in case series unselected for family history. A combined analysis of 22 studies. *Am J Hum Genet.* 2003;72:1117–1130.
5. Burke W, Austin MA. Genetic risk in context: calculating the penetrance of BRCA1 and BRCA2 mutations. *J Nat Cancer Inst.* 2002;94:1185-1187.
6. Brose MS, Rebbeck TR, Calzone KA, et al. Cancer risk estimates for BRCA1 mutation carriers identified in a risk evaluation program. *J Nat Cancer Inst.* 2002;94:1365-1372.
7. Thompson D, Easton DF, The Breast Cancer Linkage Consortium. Cancer incidence in BRCA1 mutation carriers. *J Nat Cancer Inst.* 2002;94:1358-1365.
8. Newcomb PA, Longnecker MP, Storer BE, et al. Long-term hormone replacement therapy and risk of breast cancer in postmenopausal women. *Am J Epidemiol.* 1995;142:788-795.
9. Kaufman DW, Palmer JR, Mouzon J. de, et al. Estrogen replacement therapy and the risk of breast cancer: results from the case-control surveillance study. *Am J Epidemiol.* 1991;134:1375-1385.
10. Palmer JR, Rosenberg L, Miller DR, et al. Breast cancer risk after estrogen replacement therapy: results from the Toronto breast cancer study. *Am J Epidemiol.* 1991;134:1386-1395.

11. Stanford JL, Weiss NS, Voigt LF, et al. Combined estrogen and progestin hormone replacement therapy in relation to risk of breast cancer in middle-aged women. *JAMA.* 1995;274:137-142.

12. Colditz GA, Hankinson SE, Hunter DJ, et al. The use of estrogens and progestins and the risk of breast cancer in postmenopausal women. *N Engl J Med.* 1995;332:1589-1593.

13. Collaborative Group on Hormonal Factors in Breast Cancer. Breast cancer and hormone replacement therapy: collaborative reanalysis of data from 51 epidemiological studies of 52,705 women with breast cancer and 108,411 women without breast cancer. *Lancet.* 1997;350:1047-1059.

14. Writing Group for the Women's Health Initiative Investigators. Risks and benefits of estrogen plus progestin in healthy postmenopausal women. *JAMA.* 2002;288:321-333.

15. Harris JR, Hellman S. Natural history of breast cancer. In: Harris JR, Lipman ME, Morrow MM, et al., eds. *Diseases of the Breast.* Philadelphia, Lippincott-Raven; 1996:75-391.

16. Fisher B, Costantino JP, Wickerham DL, et al. Tamoxifen for prevention of breast cancer: Report of the National Surgical Adjuvant Breast and Bowel Project P-1 Study. *J Natl Cancer Inst.* 1998;90:1371-1388.

17. Kelly PT. *Assess Your True Risk of Breast Cancer.* NY: H Holt & Co, 2000.

18. Tabar L, Vitak B, Chen H-H, et al. The Swedish Two-County Trial twenty years later. *Radiol Clin North Am.* 2000;38:625-651.

19. Ries LAG, Eisner MP, Kosary CL, et al., eds. *SEER Cancer statistics Review, 1975-2003.* National Cancer Institute. Bethesda, MD. Available at: http://seer.cancer.gov/csr/1975_2003/. 2003.

PART II

Cancer Interventions across Cultures

CHAPTER 7

Cancer Prevention

Lifestyle as the Definitive Means of Cancer Control

John H. Weisburger

INTRODUCTION

International research using the techniques of geographic pathology has provided sound information on the causes of major chronic diseases, including coronary and vascular diseases and many types of diverse cancers.[1-3] It turns out that most of these chronic diseases relate to personal lifestyle and habits anywhere in the world[4] (Table 1). In the United States, for instance, it can be calculated, based on the annual publications of the American Cancer Society, that currently about 36% of cancers in the lung, urinary bladder, kidneys, renal pelvis, and also pancreas occur mostly in tobacco users[1] (Table 2). Fortunately, tobacco use and cigarette smoking is decreasing more in men than in women, and so are the diseases caused by tobacco. Yet, more women in the United States die annually due to lung cancer, than due to the much-feared breast cancer. Individuals who also use alcohol and smoke have a high risk of cancer in the oral cavity and the esophagus. Extensive alcohol use alone, especially hard liquor, is a risk factor for cancer of the esophagus,[5] and cancer of the rectum.[6] A large proportion of the cancers that occur in Western populations are related to nutritional traditions. For example, cancer of the large bowel (distal colon and rectum), postmenopausal breast, prostate, ovary, and pancreas are associated with a

137

TABLE 1. Risks for Cancer and other Chronic Diseases

Most types of cancer and cardiovascular disease relate to personal lifestyle, tobacco use, nutritional habits, and lack of physical exercise. Lifestyle is a function of locally prevailing traditions, worldwide. These can and should be changed based on current knowledge, derived from research on causation, and thus, effective prevention.

TABLE 2. Estimated Causes of Cancer Mortality

Lifestyle	% of total
Diet-related	
High fat, fried foods, low fiber, low vegetables, low fruits, low tea:	
colorectal, breast, pancreas, prostate, ovary, endometrium, kidney	38
High salt, pickled foods, low vegetables, low tea: stomach	5
Tobacco-related: lung, larynx, mouth, bladder, kidneys	36
Tobacco and alcohol-related: oral cavity, sophagus, pancreas	4
Alcohol: liver, esophagus	4
Sunlight and genetic factors: melanoma	2
Also: lack of exercise, sedentary habits, obesity	
Also: similar lifestyle factors are causes of cardiovascular disease	

Calculated from data.[1]

traditional nutritional habits involving carcinogens in well-done meats, and also an intake of high fat, low fiber, and low vegetables and fruits.[4] The underlying mechanisms will be discussed in this chapter.

ETIOLOGY

Genetic

Small proportions of cancers have a purely genetic basis.[7-11] These account for less than 1% of all cancers, such as retinoblastoma and soft tissue sarcomas. In the last few years, it was discovered that premenopausal breast cancer might have a genetic base. The relevant factors are BRCA1 and BRCA2, but health promoting nutritional habits can reduce the risk of this type of cancer to some extent.[4] In the other instance, a genetic condition called familial polyposis raises the risk of intestinal cancer in those carrying the associated family of genes, the APC genes.[12,13] Clearly, many types of cancer have a genetic base, in the sense that individuals exposed to carcinogens display differential sensitivity. Some people have a higher risk for a number of reasons. Carcinogens require activation to reactive metabolites, in contrast to detoxified metabolites (Table 3). Also, many individuals are efficient in repairing the

TABLE 3. Types of Carcinogens

Genotoxic carcinogens
Direct-acting alkylating agents; some chemotherapeutic drugs.
Procarcinogens are converted biochemically in vivo or in vitro to reactive metabolites that bind covalently with cellular macromolecules, DNA (mutagens), RNA, proteins, membranes. Active in the laboratory animals, virtually all human cancers involve genotoxic carcinogens. These need to be defined for each cancer. Genotoxic carcinogens can be detected and measured through their mutagenicity or induction of DNA repair systems, and also by a procedure named ^{32}P-postlabeling. The DNA carcinogen adducts can be repaired by complex repair enzymes systems.

Reactive oxygen species (ROS)
This type of chemical, or endogenous products generated in cell systems, is composed of peroxides, hydroxy radicals, and other active oxygen compounds that can attack cellular macromolecules, DNA, or proteins. They have typical markers such as 8-hydroxy deoxyguanylic acid, visualized in hydrolyzed DNA, or as oxidized cysteines in hydroxylated proteins.

Promoters
Classically, such chemicals failed to produce covalent products with DNA, were not mutagenic, but enhanced carcinogenesis in cells already transformed by activated procarcinogens. Thus, they interfered with cell-to-cell signaling through gap junctions, increasing cell duplication, inflammation, proliferation, and tissue hyperplasia. ROS contributes possibly to the promoting mechanism through cycloxygenase gene expressions and higher levels of cyclin kinases. One marker is increases in ornithine decarboxylase (ODC) forming polyamines.

damage to the genetic material and DNA. Others are less likely to have this beneficial biochemical asset, and such people are at greater risk.[14]

Differences in individual sensitivity based on genetics are found in all populations worldwide. Yet, effective chronic disease and especially the prevention of diverse cancers depend on the removal or lowering exposure levels of risk factors. We will emphasize those associated with lifestyle. Smoking relates to about 33% of all cancers, nutritional habits, and lack of exercise in approximately 60% of all cancers. These same lifestyle factors also play similar roles in cardiovascular diseases. Thus, adjustment of lifestyle to a lower risk situation can prevent premature deaths in the majority of the world's population. A health promoting lifestyle can also be the basis for reaching old age in good physical and mental health. This change would have enormous economic benefits in light of the high cost of medical care.

Lifestyle Traditions

Stomach cancer has declined sharply in the United States in the last 70 years and has begun to decrease elsewhere, where food preservation techniques have changed, as discussed below. Historically, it was a prevalent form of cancer.[15-17] We have learned that it was related to the tradition of food preservation by salting and pickling.[18] This custom was fortunately replaced by the spread of household and commercial refrigeration, permitting the storage of foods in the refrigerator or a freezer. In countries where commercial refrigeration is not available, or not used, the old methods of food preservation are needed and thus, stomach cancer and incidentally also, high blood pressure still occur. Foods containing vitamin C, such as vegetables and fruits lower the risk of consuming salted foods, to some extent. Old traditions of consuming salted foods are still apparent in African Americans, who still have higher levels of stomach cancer[1,19,20] compared with Whites (Table 4).

The lower socioeconomic groups tend to have more obese people (body mass index [BMI] higher than 26) with hypertension and adult-onset diabetes, or cancer of the uterine corpus (endometrium), in the United States. The increased occurrence of obesity-related diseases is also associated with the metabolic syndromes such as insulin resistance but not in all cases of obesity. Moreover, due to the globalization of the American high fat diet, an increase in obesity is prevalent in many areas of the world, across socioeconomic groupings, due to increasingly sedentary and lifestyle habits, such as hours of television watching while consuming snacks, and lack of physical exercise.

Many years ago, before harvesting techniques of foods, such as peanuts, were perfected, these foods contained a mold that, produced mycotoxins, in the family of aflatoxin compounds, which had been shown to be one cause of cancer of the liver.[21] The risk of this basically untreatable cancer is now much lower now in the Western world due to an improvement in agricultural techniques with virtually no mould contamination. Of additional benefit is the fact that peanuts and peanut butter contain healthy oil, the monounsaturated peanut oil, and essential minerals so that modern times permit consumption of the health promoting foods. In contrast, in parts of Africa, peanuts are still grown under poor agricultural conditions, yet they constitute a sizeable part of the food intake, leading to appreciable amounts of dietary aflatoxin. As a consequence, primary liver cancer remains a main cause of mortality, more so in individuals also being infected with the hepatitis antigens.

In a few individuals of Celtic descent, namely people from northern Europe, Ireland, Scotland, and Australian Whites, the skin is sensitive to sunlight and ultraviolet light in general. Exposure may lead to skin cancer and also to melanoma. Fortunately, most individuals have an excision enzyme system that can repair the damage to the skin, but a few individuals are more sensitive because of a genetically controlled deficiency of the repair enzymes performing nucleotide excision.[14]

TABLE 4. African American to White Mortality Rate Ratios for Select Cancers in the US, 1995–1999

	Men				Women		
Cancer type	African American rate	White rate	African American/White ratio	Cancer type	African American Rate	White Rate	African American/White Ratio
Larynx	5.8	2.4	2.4	Stomach	6.8	3.0	2.3
Prostate	72.8	31.2	2.3	Uterine cervix	6.2	2.8	2.2
Stomach	14.2	6.3	2.3	Esophagus	3.5	1.7	2.1
Oral cavity and pharynx	8.3	4.2	2.0	Uterine corpus	6.9	3.9	1.8
Esophagus	12.9	7.2	1.8	Larynx	0.9	0.5	1.8
Lung and bronchus	109.1	79.7	1.4	Colon and rectum	25.4	18.0	1.4
Pancreas	16.2	12.0	1.4	Pancreas	13.0	9.0	1.4
Colon and rectum	34.4	25.8	1.3	Breast	37.1	28.2	1.3
Urinary bladder	5.7	8.0	0.7	Urinary bladder	3.1	2.3	1.3
Brain	3.2	6.0	0.5	Lung and bronchus	40.2	41.7	1.0
				Brain	2.3	4.1	0.6

Source: Calculated from data.[40,41]

ENVIRONMENTAL RISK FACTORS

The field of cancer causation through the environment was discovered more than 150 years ago when individuals were observed to have specific types of cancer based on high-level occupational exposure to specific cancer-causing agents. Study of the etiological factors led to discovery that certain aromatic amines utilized in dye production could cause cancer of the urinary bladder.[22] The factories manufacturing these dyes have now eliminated or tightened the standards of their production facilities, minimizing exposure to the harmful components. Even today, asbestos has a bad name as a carcinogen for the lung. In fact, many years ago when asbestos was used in construction and in the insulation of pipes, many of the workmen were customary smokers.[23] It was then found that heavy exposure to asbestos, an irritant to the lung tissue, sharply enhanced the risk of lung cancer in smokers. The irritation caused an increase in cell cycling of the pulmonary cells. Damage from the carcinogens in tobacco smoke is poorly repaired in a tissue undergoing rapid cell cycling. Extensive asbestos contamination in nonsmokers has a slight effect on the lung, but leads to a small risk of cancer in the pleural lining of the lung, namely, mesothelioma.[24] The relevant mechanism is the generation of ROS that has adverse effects and that could be moderated by a diet high in vegetables and fruits, providing antioxidants to destroy the ROS.[4,25] In addition, soy foods and green, oolong, or black tea are excellent sources of antioxidants.[4]

There are some types of cancer that can be caused by radiation and drugs. High-level radiation can damage some tissues, which cannot be repaired through appropriate DNA repair enzymes, because of the high dosage.[14] Even x-rays, and radioactive substances such as those discovered by Madame Curie led to cancers at the point of exposure. This no longer occurs because of precautions taken to avoid extensive contamination. In fact, radiation for diagnostic purposes, such as chest x-rays and clinical use of radiation under controlled conditions is certainly beneficial.

TYPES OF CARCINOGENS

The causation of cancer by chemicals involves two distinct types of carcinogens: genotoxic and non-genotoxic.[26] The first class is genotoxic carcinogens, meaning that they covalently react with DNA, the genetic material. As a consequence, such carcinogens can be assessed qualitatively and quantitatively by measuring their mutagenicity in bacterial systems such as those developed by Ames.[27] In addition, they elicit DNA repair that can be evaluated by the procedure of Williams, specifically the induction of DNA repair in hepatocytes and also in other cell systems.[28] At the American Health Foundation, we have developed a systematic Decision Point approach to effectively outline the properties of genotoxic chemicals.[29] Additional procedures such as cell transformation and the development of mutagens in mammalian cells have been used, but these are more cumbersome and time consuming.[27] All human cancers involve the action of specific genotoxic carcinogens causing mutations in cellular oncogenes, or in p53 tumor suppressor genes.[9,10] Thus, an evaluation of the causes of human cancers is important to define the relevant genotoxic carcinogens.[24]

Non-genotoxic agents are also involved in cancer development.[28] These are classically called promoters and the underlying mechanism is an effect on cell duplication rates, growth, and differentiation, as well as signaling. The mechanisms with this type of compounds mean that there is a dose response, with a threshold that can be determined, and therefore, evaluate the lowest level of promoters that do not have a risk of cancer development. Even with genotoxic carcinogens, a specific low-level threshold has been detected.[30] Research in laboratory animals (mice, rats, or hamsters of various strains) assist in outlining mechanistic aspects and dose-response relationships useful in extrapolating to human disease risk. Often 2-year experiments are performed to evaluate possible cancer risks associated with exposure to chemicals. A research group in Nagoya has also provided a short-term model for testing chemicals.[31]

In recent years, another type of agent, the ROS has been discovered.[25] These also affect the DNA, but they could also act in the development of tumors, by virtue of their unique property of causing inflammatory reactions, with consequent raised cell duplication rates. In this instance, the mechanism of action needs to be defined as to whether ROS operate as genotoxicants or simply affect the growth and development of cells. ROS can be eliminated by antioxidants. This certainly highlights the need for foods rich in antioxidants, such as vegetables, fruits, soy products, and tea.[4,32,33]

SPECIFIC CHRONIC DISEASES

Coronary Heart Disease

In the Western world, heart disease accounts for greatest mortality in the public.[1] For example, in the United States, there is a somewhat higher risk among individuals of African American and Hispanic (eg, Puerto Rican or Mexican American) descent. The reason is that coronary heart disease is observed in individuals on a high saturated fat dietary regimen that does not contain adequate amounts of foods with antioxidants. The relevant mechanism is related to a traditional intake of meats and milk that raise the LDL-cholesterol, the atherogenic principle upon oxidation by ROS.[4,25] Intake of fried meat and milk shakes, which are sources of saturated fats, is particularly high in young people, mostly in the lower socioeconomic groups who have the custom of buying a quick, inexpensive meal in the so-called fast food outlets. The meat is consumed in a white bread bun, without real nutritional value, except for high calories and a high glycemic index. In other countries such as Finland, the meat is served between two pieces of whole grain, high-fiber rye bread, providing better nutritional value. Nonetheless, in fast food restaurants, there is a general lack of vegetables, foods that could aid in lowering the risk associated with ROS, through their dietary antioxidants, as discussed above.

Yet, not all fats raise LDL-cholesterol, for which the main fat responsible is saturated fat (Table 5). In contrast, monounsaturated oils such as olive oil and canola oil are beneficial and do not increase LDL-cholesterol.[4,31,34] In fact, the ω-3 polyunsaturated oils found in fish and in flaxseed decrease the total cholesterol and are, therefore, beneficial. It has been recommended that people should consume three to four servings of fish a week. The ω-6 polyunsaturated oils consumed mostly as part of the American diet do not increase LDL-cholesterol. Nor does it affect heart disease risk. Instead, it is an effective promoter of nutritionally linked cancers, such as cancer of the breast, prostate, pancreas, ovary, and endometrium, through very specific mechanisms. Optimally, the monounsaturated oils should be consumed to meet the needs for essential fats. One example of an area of the world where these oils are standard is Southern Italy and Greece, the so-called Mediterranean dietary custom, with a fairly low risk of heart disease and of many types of cancer.[32-35]

Yet another dietary factor elevates the risk of heart disease. This was discovered from studies of people in Finland who displayed a high incidence of mortality from heart disease, even though there was a relatively low incidence of breast and especially of colon cancer. It was found that the adults loved to consume milk, which accounted for the high risk of

TABLE 5. Fats and Oils

Hydrogenated oils and trans fats are undesirable. Best are monounsaturated oils, olive oil (Mediterranean tradition), and canola oil. The ω-3 oils from fish, flaxseed, and also some in canola oil, lower the risk of heart disease and the nutritionally linked cancers. The ω-6 oils lower the risk of heart disease, but increase the risk of the nutritionally linked cancers. Saturated fats increase the risk of heart disease. All fats and oils contribute more calories per gram than proteins or carbohydrate. Nonetheless, about 25% to 30% of daily calories might be as fat, particularly as mono- or ω-3 polyunsaturated oils.

heart disease.[4,35] In contrast, adults in France rarely drink milk. Thus, even though their normal dietary habits are Western, they use relatively small portions and consume vegetables and fruits and drink red wine (often thought to account for protection against oxidation of LDL-cholesterol since red wine is rich in the antioxidant resveratrol). Still, the overriding element is that the children drink milk, but not adults. The critical milk factor is lactose, absent in cheeses or yoghurt. The latter two foods are not atherogenic for that reason.

While this document deals mainly with nutrition, a major risk factor for heart disease is the use of tobacco products, especially the smoking of cigarettes. In this instance, there have been successes in the last 50 years, mainly in males in the United States. In 1950, almost 70% of males were smokers and very few women smoked. In sharp contrast, currently 28% of women are smokers and more women die of lung cancer and other tobacco-related cancers, than of breast cancer. Also, after menopause, women have the same risk of heart attacks then men, if they have the smoking addiction.[23] At this point in time, only 22% deaths in men are due to smoking.[1] Worldwide, cigarette smoking is increasing, from about 1 500 cigarettes in 1950 to over 5 000 units now.[36]

Populations in Asia serve as a contrast to these observations. In Japan, for instance, there are more smokers than in the United States, but the lung cancer rate is appreciably lower. An explanation for this contrast is the fact that the traditional Japanese diet is relatively low in total fat and rich in fish oils that are protective in heart disease and cancer (Table 5). The Japanese also consume considerable amounts of green tea with a demonstrated protective effect in heart disease and lung cancer.[34,35,37,38] Nonetheless, smoking is increasing in China and it is feared that people may be subject to an epidemic of lung cancer, as is probably true in parts of Africa, where smoking is on the rise.[36,39]

In the United States, Hispanics and African Americans tend to have higher lung cancer rates, even though for economic reasons, individuals in these populations tend to smoke less.[19,37,38,40,41] This anomaly is currently under investigation. One hypothesis is that the cigarettes are smoked

TABLE 6. Carbohydrates

Simple carbohydrates such as glucose or sucrose absorb quickly, have a high glycemic index, raise blood insulin, and should be avoided. Use synthetic sweeteners to provide desirable gustatory sensations. Complex carbohydrates, especially with soluble fiber from vegetables and fruits, and insoluble fibers as in bran, unrefined cereals or whole grain bread are health promoting, and lower the risk of heart disease and several of the nutritionally linked cancers.

differently in these populations, namely almost up to the filter, so that more harmful substances are inhaled. Also, it could be that the customary diets of individuals in these populations are low in defensive antioxidants.[4,35] We have suggested that protective foods such as vegetables receive price support by the federal government so that they can be made available to the public at a lower cost. An example of governmental intervention for agricultural products is price support for many grains.

Hypertension and Stroke, Gastric Cancer

Except for many types of cancer, chronic diseases, such as hypertension, stroke used to have a much higher incidence.[1] These stem from the traditional intake of foods that are highly salted and pickled,[4,18,19,40] given that these procedures were used classically before the introduction of food storage was made safe by refrigeration and freezing. Since that time, these diseases have decreased in the last 70 years, as has gastric cancer.[15,20] More recent studies, however, have observed that gastric cancer risk is higher with a concurrent infection with *Helicobacter pylori*.[40,41] Unfortunately, due to dietary patterns that have evolved over time, ethnic and minority populations, such as the lower socioeconomic classes including African American, or non-Hispanic Whites in the United States, still consume foods with high amounts of salt, accounting for the higher risk for hypertension.[40,41] In addition, obesity plays a role in the occurrence of hypertension and stroke, and there are more heavy people among such ethnic minorities, who also develop more cancer of the endometrium and kidneys, given that fat cells also generate estrogen, a risk factor for a variety of cancers. ROS may be also playing an additional cellular risk factor.

CANCERS

Head and Neck Cancers

These diseases are the results of smoking, together with excessive drinking of alcoholic beverages. Actually, alcohol by itself can lead to this set of diseases.[5] Here also, minorities seem to have a higher proportion of people with these habits, and since the diet does not include many protective foods, these populations display a higher incidence.[19,40,41] People in parts of France who are high consumers of specific alcoholic beverages such as Calvados liqueur also display the associated disease, cancer of the esophagus.[42,43] Also, in Japan, this cancer is found in men who smoke and drink alcohol, but not in women who tend not to have these habits.[5,23]

Cancers of the Lung, Pancreas, Kidney, and Urinary Bladder

These types of cancer are all associated with tobacco use, mainly through the smoking of cigarettes.[23] While these tobacco products contain specific genotoxic carcinogens, it would seem that their actions also involve ROS.[25,38] This accounts for the fact that individuals on a protective diet rich in antioxidants have a lower incidence, at equal smoking rates and duration. Thus, dietary habits impinge importantly on diseases associated with smoking.[35] This is especially true for pancreatic cancer. In men, for example, smoking- and obesity-related diabetes mellitus remain risk factors, more so in African American males in the United States. In women, high BMI and appreciable alcoholic beverage intake play a role, more so in African American than in non-Hispanic White women.[41]

The Western Nutritionally Linked Cancers, Cancers of the Postmenopausal Breast, Distal Colon, Pancreas, and Prostate

The associated genotoxic carcinogens appear to be a fairly new class of agents discovered about 25 years ago, the heterocyclic amines, formed during frying and broiling of meats.[44-48] These affect not only the tissues mentioned, but may also be involved in the occurrence of coronary heart disease. Observations in humans show that these cancers and also heart disease are higher in regular consumers of appreciable amounts of well-done red meat that contains such genotoxic agents. These chemicals were originally detected by measuring the mutagenicity of well-done fried meat.[46] Also, they invariably cause cancer in animal models as these target organs relatively quickly. Thus, there is excellent evidence for the role of heterocyclic amines as the relevant genotoxic carcinogens for these organs.

In terms of cancer prevention, it is important to apply available methods to lower the formation of heterocyclic amines. Our group at the Institute for Cancer Research has shown that mixing 10% to 15% soy protein with ground beef decreases sharply the content of heterocyclic amines in the resulting hamburger. We also discovered that application of the active components of green or black tea, namely the appropriate tea polyphenols to the surface of meats inhibits the formation of heterocyclic amines upon cooking.[32,35] Meat contains creatine, a chemical that is essential to the formation of heterocyclic amines. However, Felton and associates showed that brief cooking in a microwave oven on a tray permits the run off of juices, which serves to eliminate most of the creatine. Thus, subsequent frying or broiling through standard methods is effective in decreasing amounts of heterocyclic amines.[49]

These dietary interventions are important given that heterocyclic amines upon ingestion are metabolized. A major reaction performed mainly in the liver is N-hydroxylation, yielding the corresponding N-OH compounds. In select target organs, such as breast, distal colon, prostate, and pancreas, there are acetyltransferases of two types, NAT-1 and NAT-2, that can convert the N-OH heterocyclic amines to a reactive N-acetoxy chemical that attacks DNA and yields a mutated DNA in cells, precursor to other mutated cells, which upon duplication lead to clinical tumor formation.[46,50]

Role of Type and Amounts of Dietary Fat

Meat is an important source of saturated fats, which are associated with the elevated risk of heart disease. This risk in increased due the widespread practice of frying or broiling meat, which also leads to the formation of heterocyclic amines, thereby enhancing the risk.[45,46] As noted above, saturated fats also contribute to atherogenèsis by raising LDL-cholesterol. Yet saturated fats contribute relatively little to the risk of the nutritionally linked cancers (Table 5). For these diseases, the ω-6 polyunsaturated oils are important, as demonstrated by the induction of the nutritionally linked cancers in animal models, such as the rat,[51,52] and to some degree in humans (although this is a controversial area), due to an increase in the rate of duplication of cells carrying a mutation induced by an N-acetoxy heterocyclic amine. There has, for instance, been a slight but definite rise in the incidence of postmenopausal breast cancer in women in Western context in the last 40 years. This is possibly due to the fact that people switched from their use of saturated fats because of a fear of heart disease and the ω-6 polyunsaturated oils were substituted at this time. As previously noted, monounsaturated oils (olive or canola oil) have not been shown to increase the risk of the nutritionally linked cancers[34,53] because they are poor promoters in animal models and in humans. For example, Mediterranean countries have lower rates of coronary heart disease and of the nutritionally linked cancers. They are the preferred oils for people at home and should be used in restaurants.

PROTECTIVE ROLE OF INSOLUBLE BRAN CEREAL FIBER

Types of Fiber-Soluble versus Insoluble-Different Metabolic Effects

The importance of bran cereal fiber was discovered in the study of the lower risk of colon and breast cancer in people in Finland, in the face of a high incidence of heart disease.[51] It was established that the latter was due to the high intake of milk, in turn associated with lactose, the milk sugar.[35] As a parenthesis, the lower risk of heart disease in France is often explained by the fact that French often drink red wine with their meals. Another explanation for the French paradox, eating Western style but with a lower risk of heart disease, is the fact that by tradition adult French people rarely drink milk, and therefore, are not exposed to lactose, the atherogenic principle (absent in cheese and yogurt). Yogurt is an excellent food with calcium and other desirable minerals such as magnesium and zinc, and should be consumed by people, including children (however, children will benefit by the nutrients in milk, and there is less likelihood of an effect on the heart at a young age). Breast-feeding of babies and young children is beneficial to the baby. Breast milk is rich in excellent nutrients, including the antioxidant oil DHA, important in brain development. Moreover, a functional breast is much less likely to undergo neoplastic change. Thus, there are important health benefits to mother and child associated with breast-feeding.

The Finns, by tradition, consume daily appreciable amounts of rye bread, rich in insoluble fiber.[51] A specific marker for this consumption of rye bread was that the Finns have a high stool bulk, in contrast to New Yorkers who do not (Table 6). It turns out that the large stool served to eliminate bile acids, associated with colon cancer risk, and conjugated estrogen related to breast cancer risk.[51] Therefore, there is merit in recommending an increase in foods that contain insoluble fiber, such as whole grain bread and cereals, and also to avoid drinking milk as adults. Bread, buns, rolls, and cereals made with white flour are also an undesirable source of calories and should be avoided.

Soluble fibers are present in vegetables and in some fruits. These are tasty sources of valuable antioxidants. The soluble fiber in these foods has an effect on the intestinal tract in modifying the bacterial flora, favoring health promoting bacteria, such as lactobacilli and lowering the titers of less desirable bacteria.[51,52] The soluble fibers also lead to the presence in the intestine of gums that serve to eliminate undesirable chemicals in the gut stemming from secretion in the bile of metabolites formed in the liver.

Thus, foods rich in soluble and insoluble fibers, vegetables, fruits, whole grain bread, and bran cereals are beneficial in lowering the risk of chronic diseases, particularly cancers.[50]

IMPORTANT FUNCTION OF VEGETABLES, FRUITS, SOY PRODUCTS, AND TEA

In the past, many people in the United States were meat and potato eaters, accounting for the high risk of many chronic diseases, described above.

TABLE 7. Protective Foods

Virtually all vegetables and fruits are wholesome. Recommendations for prevention are 5 to 10 such foods a day, mainly because of their valuable content in antioxidants. In the Orient, soy foods play such a role, as does green tea (also 5 to 10 cups a day). Black and green tea are desirable, disease preventing beverages, with small amounts of 40 to 50 mg of caffeine per cup. Caffeine is a stimulant, without other adverse effects. Children up to age 12 should be offered decaffeinated tea, also rich in antioxidants.

An example of good nutrition was set by President Jefferson, who was reported to use vegetables as the main element on his dinner plate and used meat not as a center piece, as most American do, but had it as a side dish. We need to introduce similar schemes, and actually eat fish, a source of ω-3-polyunsaturated oils, three or four times a week preventing heart disease and many types of cancer. Vegetables are rich not only in essential vitamins, minerals, and similar micronutrients, but they are also a good source of antioxidants (Table 7). The importance of antioxidants is that cells in the body generate ROS, associated with heart disease and many types of cancer, together with the heterocyclic amines in cooked meats.[21,22,46] In addition, ROS are thought to contribute to aging. Thus, the antioxidants in vegetables inhibit the action of undesirable ROS. This is also true for most types of fruits.

American farmers are important producers of soybeans, but in the past, most of the soy products were exported to the Orient.[33] In Japan and in China, many dishes use soy foods that are also rich in antioxidants. Soy milk, rich in essential micronutrients, and marketed with additional vitamins B,. D, E and calcium is a healthy substitute for milk. In part, the Japanese and Chinese have fewer of the chronic diseases besetting the Western world. There, the exception is a former high incidence of hypertension and stomach cancer because of their old tradition of excessive salt use.[15,20] There is now a national plan in Japan to teach people to reduce salt intake.[16]

Another excellent source of antioxidants is the beverage tea, derived from the plant *Camellia sinensis*.[32,37] Again, in China, Japan, or Korea, there is a custom of drinking green tea frequently during the day, inhibiting the effect of ROS. For example, there are more men in Japan smoking, but the mortality from lung cancer is lower than in the Western world.[38] One hypothesis is that they eat less fatty foods and include fish containing beneficial ω-3 oils. Moreover, the extensive tea use probably accounts for the lower cancer risk. Experiments in laboratory animals have demonstrated that green tea decreases the incidence of lung cancer in rats given a tobacco carcinogen. The same protection has been observed with black tea. Green and black teas are both derived from the leaves of the same plant.[37] They differ by the manufacturing process after collecting the leaves. Upon harvest, steaming or otherwise heating inactivates an enzyme, polyphenol oxidase, present in the leaf, which thus, leads to green tea. Harvesting of the newly formed buds and top leaves of the plants can produce white tea, upon steaming. On the other hand, if the leaves are ground, the polyphenol oxidae in the leaf oxidizes the original polyphenols present, to other types of polyphenols typical of black teas. Many studies have shown that green and black tea have basically similar health promoting attributes, because the associated polyphenols are rich in antioxidants, even though they have a different chemical structure.[37,38] In addition, the tea polyphenols when consumed by animals or humans increase the titer of defensive detoxifying enzymes, which play a role in protecting against the action of carcinogens.[35] Furthermore, the tea polyphenols decrease the growth rate of cancer cells, without affecting the regular growth of normal cells.

In the United States, only about 18% of people drink tea regularly and this excellent habit is even lower among ethnic minorities. Because Canada is part of the former British Empire, there are more tea drinkers in Canada, particularly the English-speaking Canadians, but less so in Quebec, demonstrating once more that local habits have long traditions. Recent data show that Americans consume about 144 servings of tea per year per person, in Japan, 500, in the United Kingdom, 1 000, and in Ireland, 1 180. Note that in the latter two countries, it is also customary to add substantial amounts of milk, that is, depending on the ratio tea:milk, this custom may block the antioxidant activity and associated beneficial effects of tea. In our research, we found that addition of the International Organization of Standards recommended amounts, 1.85% milk in black tea, inhibition of mammary gland and colon cancer in rats by tea was not affected.[4,32] We recommend a daily intake of 5 to 10 cups of tea, as a realistic means of disease prevention. Tea is inexpensive and a pleasant beverage, without calories. Other studies suggest that tea increases the body's metabolic rate, furthering weight control.[54-56] This might be due to the underlying mechanisms involved in control of the genes affecting formation of leptin, protein hormone with important effects in regulating body weight, metabolism, and reproductive function.[57]

HEALTHY AGING

Another important source of ROS is exercise. There are sound, important public health recommendations that people should exercise regularly, with

TABLE 8. Highest and Lowest Death Rates, Per Country[60]

	Colon and rectum		Lung		Stomach		Breast	Prostate
	Male	Female	Male	Female	Male	Female	Female	Male
Highest	Czech Republic	New Zealand	Hungary	Denmark	Russia	Russia	Denmark	Trinidad & Tobago
Lowest	Mexico	Mexico	Trinidad & Tobago	Azerbaijan	USA	USA	China	Turkmenistan

Note that "Colon and rectum" includes values for ascending, transverse, and descending colon. The highest levels are the sum of the three colon cancers with distinct etiologies, but most likely the colon cancers in the descending colon may be the prevalent type. Breast cancer includes deaths from premenopausal plus postmenopausal diseases, also with distinct risk factors. Nonetheless, the occurrence and clinical management probably reflect deaths in each geographic area.

emphasis on the intensity of the activities to foster an appreciable increase of air intake and thus, of oxygen uptake which leads to an increased formation of ROS in cells. It is also known that smokers have increased levels of ROS in lung, and that reactive oxygen radicals appear to be produced with the consumption of the food carcinogens, heterocyclic amines, in fried or broiled meats. For these reasons, it is important for all people to consume foods and beverages that are good sources of antioxidants such as vegetables, fruits, soy products, and tea.[4,35] ROS also leads to premature aging, which can be avoided by frequent intake of antioxidant-rich foods and beverages. This could possibly account for the fact that in Asia, there are many older people in good health, and Alzheimer's disease is also less frequent.[35]

CONCLUSION

Biomedical research in the last 40 years has been an excellent investment. Regrettably, the knowledge achieved regarding the relevance of nutrition, as the definitive means of cancer prevention has not been effectively transmitted to the public.[19] Thus, the important task remains to communicate to the public at large that their own lifestyle choices could be associated with important disease risk, or on the contrary, with good health to an old age. We need to convey to people that they are in danger of being affected by major chronic diseases and premature aging unless they alter their lifestyle, including nutritional and exercise habits[35,58]. The methods of geographic pathology have revealed areas in the world with high or low mortalities due to specific cancers, providing the background to investigate the relevant underlying mechanisms through marker studies in humans, or through laboratory investigations[59] (Table 8). Research on the rationale for areas with low mortality can also provide additional information on locally prevailing lifestyles and nutritional habits that are protective.[58,61] For example, a most recent study of the World Health Organization has explored many of the environmental factors associated with disease risk, rather than lifestyle and nutrition related factors, as we emphasize in this discussion.[62]

ACKNOWLEDGEMENTS

I am indebted to Dr. Rhonda Moore for her helpful, constructive suggestions in developing this chapter, and to Ms. Nancy Rivera for her continuing, able, technical, and administrative support.

REFERENCES

1. Jemal A, Murray T, Samuels A, et al. Cancer statistics, 2003. *CA Cancer J Clin*. 2003;53:5-26.
2. Parkin DM, Pisani P, Ferlay J. Global cancer statistics. *CA Cancer J Clin*. 1999;49:33-64.
3. Pisani P, Bray F, Parkin DM. Estimates of the world-wide prevalence of cancer for 25 sites in the adult population. *Int J Cancer*. 2002;97:72-81.
4. Weisburger JH. Lifestyle, health and disease prevention: the underlying mechanisms. *Eur J Cancer Prev*. 2002;11(suppl 2):S1-S7.
5. Blot WJ. Alcohol and cancer. *Cancer Res*. 1992;52(suppl):2119-2123.
6. Seitz HK, Simanowski UA, Garzon FT, et al. Possible role of acetaldehyde in ethanol-related cocarcinogenesis in the rat. *Gastroenterology*. 1990;98:406-413.
7. Loeb KR, Loeb LA. Significance of multiple mutation in cancer. 2000;21:379-385.
8. Hirohashi S, Loeb LA, Sugimura T, Terada M, Tlsty TD, eds. Genomic instability and carcinogenesis. *Proceedings Princess Takamatsu Cancer Research Fund*, 1998.
9. Hainaut P, Hollstein M. P53 and human cancer: the first ten thousand mutation. *Adv Cancer Res*. 2000;77:81-137.
10. Shibata D, Aaltonen LA. Genetic predisposition and somatic diversification in tumor development and progression. *Adv Cancer Res*. 2001;80:83-114.
11. King MC, Motulsky AG. Human genetics. Mapping human history. *Science*. 2002;298:2342-2343.
12. Robbins DH, Itzkowitz SH. The molecular and genetic basis of colon cancer. *Med Clin North Am*. 2002;86:1467-1495.
13. Lipkin M, Higgins P. Biological markers of cell proliferation and differentiation in human gastrointestinal diseases. *Adv Cancer Res*. 1988;50:1-24.
14. Cleaver JE. Ultraviolet photobiology: its early roots and insights into DNA repair. *DNA Repair*. 2002;1:977-979.
15. Howson CP, Hiyama T, Wynder EL. Decline of gastric cancer: epidemiology of an unplanned triumph. *Epidemiol Rev*. 1986;8:1-27.
16. Sugimura T. An overview of cancer prevention. *Eur J Cancer Prev*. 1996;5:1-8.
17. La Vecchia C, Negri E, Franceschi S, Decarli A. Case-control study on influence of methionine, nitrite and salt on gastric carcinogenesis in northern Italy. *Nutr Cancer*. 1997;27:65-68.
18. Chen W, Weisburger JH, Fiala ES, et al. Gastric carcinogenesis: 2-chloro-4-methylthiobutanoic acid, a novel mutagen in salted, pickled Sanma Hiraki fish or similarly treated methionine. *Chem Res Toxicol*. 1996;9:58-66.
19. Baquet CR, Horm JW, Gibbs T, Greenwald P. Socioeconomic factors and cancer incidence among blacks and whites. *J Natl Cancer Inst*. 1991;83:551-557.
20. International Agency for Research on Cancer. *IARC Monographs on the Evaluation of Carcinogenic Risks to Humans: Some Naturally Occurring Substances: Food Items and Constituents, Heterocyclic Aromatic Amines and Mycotoxins*. Vol. 56. Lyon, France: IARC; 1993:41-113.
21. International Agency for Research on Cancer. *IARC Monographs on the Evaluation of Carcinogenic Risks to Humans: Some Naturally Occurring Substances: Food Items and Constituents, Heterocyclic Aromatic Amines and Mycotoxins*. Vol. 56. Lyon, France: IARC; 1993:245-395.
22. Weisburger JH. Comments on the history and importance of aromatic and heterocyclic amines in public health. *Mutation Res*. 2002;506-507:9-20.
23. International Agency for Research on Cancer. *IARC Monographs on the Evaluation of Carcinogenic Risks to Humans: Tobacco Smoking*. Vol. 38. Lyon, France: IARC; 1986.

24. Suzuki Y, Yuen SR. Asbestos fibers contributing to the induction of human malignant mesothelioma. *Ann NY Acad Sci.* 2002;982:160-176.

25. Chiueh CC, ed. Reactive oxygen. *Ann NY Acad Sci.* 2000;89:1-426.

26. Weisburger JH, Williams GM. The distinction between genotoxic and epigenetic carcinogens and implication for cancer risk. *Toxicol Sci.* 2000;57:4-5.

27. McCann J, Ames BN. Detection of carcinogens as mutagens in the Salmonella/microsome test: assay of 300 chemicals: discussion. *Proc Natl Acad Sci USA.* 1976;73:950-954.

28. Williams GM. Methods for evaluating chemical genotoxicity. *Annu Rev Pharmacol Toxicol.* 1989;29:189-211.

29. Weisburger JH, Williams GM. Critical effective methods to detect genotoxic carcinogens and neoplasm-promoting agents. *Environ Health Perspec.* 1991;90:121-126.

30. Williams GM, Iatropoulos MJ, Wang CX, et al. Nonlinearities in 2-acetylaminofluorene exposure responses for genotoxic and epigenetic effects leading to initiation of carcinogenesis in rat liver. *Toxicol Sci.* 1998;45:152-161.

31. Ito N, Tamano S, Shirai T. A medium-term rat liver bioassay for rapid *in vivo* detection of carcinogenic potential of chemicals. *Cancer Sci.* 2003;94:3-8.

32. Weisburger JH. Prevention of cancer and other chronic diseases worldwide based on sound mechanisms. *BioFactors* 2000;12:73-81.

33. Messina M. Modern applications for an ancient bean: soy-beans and the prevention and treatment of chronic disease. *J Nutr.* 1995;125:567-569.

34. Weisburger JH. Dietary fat and risk of chronic disease: mechanistic insights from experimental studies. *J Am Dietetic Assoc.* 1997;97(suppl):S16-S23.

35. Weisburger JH. Eat to live, not live to eat. *Nutrition.* 2000;16:767-773.

36. Twombly R. Global Cigarette Consumption, 1880–2000. *J Natl Cancer Inst.* 2003;95:12.

37. Hara Y. *Green Tea: Health Benefits and Applications.* New York, NY:Marcel Dekker, Inc.; 2001:240-251.

38. Weisburger JH, Chung F-L. Mechanisms of chronic disease causation by nutritional factors and tobacco products and their prevention by tea polyphenols. *Food Chem Toxicol.* 2002;40:1145-1154.

39. Peto R, Chen ZM, Boreham J. Tobacco—the growing epidemic. *Nature Med.* 1999;5:15-17.

40. Brawley OW. Some perspective on Black-White cancer statistics. *CA A Cancer J Clin.* 2002;52:322-342.

41. Ghafoor A, Jemal A, Cokkinides V, et al. Cancer statistics for African Americans. *CA A Cancer J Clin.* 2002;52:326-341.

42. Ruiz B, Correa P, Fontham ETH, et al. Ascorbic acid, *Helicobacter pylori* and Lewis phenotype among blacks and whites in New Orleans. *Cancer Lett.* 1994;83:323-329.

43. Tuyns A, Pequignot G, Abbatucci JS. Esophageal cancer and alcohol consumption. Impotance of type of beverage. *Int J Cancer.* 1979;23:443-447.

44. Silverman DT, Hoover RN, Brown LM, et al. Why do Black Americans have a higher risk of pancreatic cancer than White Americans? *Epidemiology.* 2003;14:45-54.

45. International Agency for Research on Cancer. *IARC Monographs on the Evaluation of Carcinogenic Risks to Humans: Some Naturally Occurring Substances: Food Items and Constituents, Heterocyclic Aromatic Amines and Mycotoxins.* Vol. 56. Lyon, France: IARC; 1993:165-242.

46. Nagao M, Sugimura T, eds. *Food Borne Carcinogens: Heterocyclic Amines.* New York, NY: Wiley, 2000:1-373.

47. Snyderwine EG, Sinha R, Ferguson LR, eds. Proceedings, 8th International Conference on Carcinogenic/mutagenic N-substituted Aryl Compounds. *Mutation Res.* 2002;506-507:1-249.

48. Butler LM, Sinha R, Milikan RC, et al. Heterocyclic amines, meat intake, and association with colon cancer in a population-based study. *Am J Epidemiol.* 2003;157:434-445.

49. Felton JS, Fultz E, Dolbeare FA, Knize MG. Reduction of heterocyclic amine mutagens/ carcinogens in fried beef patties by microwave pretreatment. *Food Chem Toxicol.* 1994;32:897-903.

50. Slattery ML, Potter JD, Mak N, Caan BJ, Leppert M, Samowitz W. Western diet, family history of colorectal cancer, NAT2, GSTM-1 and risk of colon cancer. *Cancer Causes Control.* 2000;11:1-8.

51. Reddy BS. Novel approaches to the prevention of colon cancer by nutritional manipulation and chemoprevention. *Cancer Epidemiol Biomarkers Prev.* 2000;9:239-247.

52. Lipkin M, Reddy BS, Newmark H, Lamprecht SA. Dietary factors in human colorectal cancer. *Ann Rev Nutr.* 1999;19:545-586.

53. Stark AH, Madar Z. Olive oil as a functional food: epidemiology and nutritional approaches. *Nutr Rev.* 2002;60:170-176.

54. Conney AH, Lu Y-P, Lou YR, Huang MT. Inhibitory effects of tea and caffeine on UV-induced carcinogenesis relationship to enhanced apoptosis and decreased tissue fat. *Eur J Cancer Prev.* 2002;11(suppl 2):S28-S36.

55. Bell SJ, Goodrick GK. A functional food product for the management of weight. *Crit Rev Food Sci Nutr.* 2002;42:163-178.

56. Anderson RA, Polansky MM. Tea enhances insulin activity. *J Agric Food Chem.* 2002;50:7182-7186.

57. Friedman JM. The function of leptin in nutrition, weight, and physiology. *Nutr Rev.* 2002;60:S1-S14.

58. International Agency for Research on Cancer. *IARC Handbooks of Cancer Prevention: Weight Control and Physical Activity.* Vol. 6. Lyon, France: IARC; 2002:1-315.

59. Williams GM. Mechanisms of chemical carcinogenesis and application to human cancer risk assessment. *Toxicology.* 2001;166:3-10.

60. Greenlee RT, Murray T, Bolden S, Wingo P. Cancer Statistics, 2000. *CA Cancer J Clin.* 2000;50:7-33.

61. Greenwald P. From carcinogenesis to clinical interventions for cancer prevention. *Toxicology.* 2001;166:37-45.

62. World Health Organization. *The World Health Report 2002: Reducing Risks, Promoting Healthy Life.* Geneva, Switzerland: World Health Organization; 2002.

CHAPTER 8

Cross-Cultural Aspects of Cancer Care

Samuel Mun Yin Ho, Pierre Saltel, Jean-Luc Machavoine,
Nathalie Rapoport-Hubschman, and David Spiegel

Life and death, emotion and social support, stress and disease are universal human concerns. The diagnosis of cancer induces a human dread that is grounded in our biological being. Nonetheless, the experience of cancer and its treatment is inevitably influenced by cultural, ethnic, economic, and religious differences. In some cultures, the diagnosis of cancer conveys a greater sense of shame than others. Only recently have Japanese cancer patients been willing to make public declarations of their disease status, forming heretofore unheard of support groups such as "Akai Bono Kai." Cultural concerns about modesty and sexuality, or cultural acceptance of a fatalistic approach to life may inhibit screening activities in certain cultures, such as among Chinese and Latina women.[1-3] Direct talk about the future that might make an American cancer patient feel respected and involved in treatment could seem to a Chinese cancer patient a self-fulfilling prophesy of doom. De Toqueville described Americans as a "nation of joiners." We tend to be relatively direct and open, inclined to discuss problems and try to solve them. At the same time, we do not like to admit to having problems, and often lose ourselves in work and other activities when confronted with threats to health. Our desire for openness and shared decision-making in medical care is not entirely consistent with our belief in success, in transcending any obstacle and our reluctance to "give in" to illness or failure. Thus, while the problems associated with cancer are universal: fear of death, loss of social roles and physical abilities, and treatments that can cause mutilation, fatigue, cognitive impairment, nausea, menopause, and weight changes, the ramifications of these problems are magnified or mitigated by cultural and social context. The treatments that have been developed to provide social and emotional support in one cultural context cannot automatically be assumed to work in a different cultural context. In some cases, the differences are primarily in the process of engaging the patient in treatment. For example, Latina women with cancer are reluctant to enter a program of treatment without initial review and approval of their husbands, while European and American women would resent such a process of initiation. In other cultural situations, elements of intervention must be added or deleted to respect feelings or redress specific cultural problems.

Our approach in this chapter is to examine one intensive and well-studied program of psychosocial support for cancer patients, Supportive/Expressive group therapy,[4] and contrast and compare its utilization in two rather different cultures: China and France. The supportive/expressive approach to helping cancer patients has been tested in a number of different cultures: France, Canada, Australia, and Hong Kong, China among others.[4-7] While there are important differences in these cultures in the propensity to openly discuss problems, or even admit to having cancer, this approach has been found to work in reducing distress and pain. The fundamental human need to surround oneself with support, express the strong emotions associated with illness, confront existential concerns, reorder priorities in life, improve family support, clarify communication with physicians, and control symptoms such as pain and anxiety transcends cultural differences. Nonetheless, important cultural differences in how to introduce, conduct, and evaluate the effects of supportive/expressive group therapy require further research. We first present the model as developed in the United States over the past 25 years,[8-10] and then place it in cultural context by exploring differences in the model in contrasting cultures. This approach is designed to construct a dialectic between the synchronic, or relatively invariant components of intervention, and the diachronic, or relatively culturally specific elements, analogous to the approach of Levi-Strauss.[11]

ESSENTIALS OF SUPPORTIVE-EXPRESSIVE PSYCHOTHERAPEUTIC INTERVENTION DEVELOPED IN THE UNITED STATES

Our supportive/expressive intervention model has been extensively tested among women with breast cancer and women and men with HIV infection, and has been utilized by families of cancer patients as well.[4] The intervention is a semistructured group therapy program that involves meetings for 90 minutes once a week, led by two co-therapists. Interventions for early stage cancer patients have been structured to last for 12 weeks, while those for people with more advanced disease have run for years as open groups, with new members being added as others leave or die. The therapists are trained to encourage discussion of the major themes listed below, but to avoid didactic presentations. There is no order or plan to discuss certain themes on certain days. There are initial introductions and explanations early in the group history, and termination when it concludes. Otherwise, the focus is on conducting a here-and-now interpersonal group directed at social, emotional, existential, interpersonal, and symptom management issues. The power of such group support derives from its immediacy: issues of emotion, relationship, and meaning are explored in the present as they currently affect the women in the room, in accord with classical principles of group psychotherapy.[12] Supportive/expressive group therapy consists of seven basic components:

1. Social Support

Psychotherapy, especially in groups, can provide a new social network with the common bond of facing similar problems.[13] Just at a time when cancer removes one from the flow of life, when many others withdraw out of awkwardness or fear, psychotherapeutic support provides a new and important social connection. Indeed, having cancer, the very thing that damages other social relationships is the ticket of admission to such groups, providing a surprising intensity of caring among members from the very beginning. Thus, constructing new social networks for cancer patients and their families via support groups and other means is doubly important: it comes at a time in life when natural social support may erode, and when more is needed.[14]

2. Emotional Expression

The expression of emotion is important in reducing social isolation and improving coping.[15-18, 74] Yet it is often an aspect of cancer patient adjustment that is overlooked or suppressed. Emotional suppression and avoidance are associated with poorer coping.[19-22] At the same time, there is much that can be done in both group and individual psychotherapies to facilitate the expression of emotion appropriate to the disease. Doing so seems to reduce the repressive coping strategy that reduces expression of positive as well as negative emotion. Emotional suppression also reduces intimacy in families, limiting opportunities for direct expression of affection and concern. Indeed, there is evidence that those who are able to ventilate strong feelings directly cope better with cancer.[19-24]

The use of the psychotherapeutic setting to deal with painful affect also provides an organizing context for handling its intrusion. When unbidden thoughts involving fears of dying and death intrude, they can be better managed by patients and families who know that there is a time and a place during which such feelings will be expressed and addressed. Furthermore, disease-related dysphoria is more intense when amplified by isolation, leaving the patient to feel that she is deservedly alone with the sense of anxiety, loss, and fear that she experiences. Being in a group where many others express similar distress normalizes their reactions, making them less alien and overwhelming. There is recent evidence that participation in supportive/expressive group therapy results in significant alterations in emotional control, with reduced suppression of emotion at the same time that patients experience a greater sense of self-efficacy in managing their emotions.[15]

Death anxiety in particular is intensified by isolation, in part because we often conceptualize death in terms of separation from loved ones. Feeling alone, especially at a time of strong emotion, makes one feel already a little bit dead, setting off a cycle of further anxiety. This can be powerfully addressed by psychotherapeutic techniques that directly address such concerns.

3. Detoxifying Dying

This component of the therapy involves looking the threat of death right in the eye rather than avoiding it. The goal is to help those facing the threat of death see it from a new point of view. When worked through, life-threatening problems can come to seem real but not overwhelming.[4,25] Following a diagnosis of cancer, a variety of coping strategies come into play, including positive reappraisal and cognitive avoidance.[73] However, denial and avoidance have their costs, including an increase in anxiety and isolation. Facing even life-threatening issues directly can help patients shift from emotion-focused to problem-focused coping,[4,26,27] moving from accepting the emotional reality to finding active means of coping with various aspects of the process of dying. Indeed, the process of dying is often more threatening than death itself. Direct discussion of death anxiety can help to divide the fear of death into a series of problems: loss of control over treatment decisions, fear of separation from loved ones, anxiety about pain. Discussion of these concerns can lead to means of addressing if not completely resolving each of these issues. Thus, even facing death can result in positive life changes.

Even the process of grieving can be reassuring at the same time that it is threatening. The experience of grieving others who have died of the same condition constitutes a deeply personal experience of the depth of loss that will be experienced by others after one's own death. Similarly, spouses come to face their potential losses by watching others grieve, and at the same time they learn that such losses can be borne and worked through.[25,26,28]

4. Reordering Life Priorities

The acceptance of the possibility of illness shortening life carries with it an opportunity for re-evaluating life priorities. When cure is not possible, a realistic evaluation of the future can help those with life-threatening illness make the best use of the remaining time. One of the costs of unrealistic optimism is the loss of time for accomplishing life projects, communicating openly with family and friends, and setting affairs in order. Facing the threat of death can aid in making the most of life.[4,9,24] This can help patients take control of those aspects of their lives they can influence, while grieving and relinquishing those they cannot. Having such a domain of control can be quite reassuring, redefining the meaning of the illness and one's life in the context of a "life project."

5. Family Support

Psychotherapeutic interventions can also be quite helpful in improving communication, identifying needs, increasing role flexibility, and adjusting to new medical social, vocational, and financial realities. There is evidence that an atmosphere of open and shared problem solving in families results in reduced anxiety and depression among cancer patients.[29,30] Thus, facilitating the development of such open addressing of common problems is a useful therapeutic goal. The group format is especially helpful for such a task, in that problems expressing needs and wishes can be examined among group members as a model for clarifying communication in the family.

In addition to enhancing communication, group participants are encouraged to develop role flexibility, a capacity to exchange roles or develop new ones as the pressures of the illness demand. One woman, for example, who became unable to carry out her usual household chores, wrote an "owner's manual" to the care of the house so that her husband could better help her and carry on after her death. Others wrote letters to friends asking them to cook an extra bit of dinner on one evening a month to share with them, thereby relieving them of the pressure of cooking.

6. Communication with Physicians

Support groups can be quite useful in facilitating better communication with physicians and other health care providers. Groups provide mutual encouragement to get questions answered, to participate actively in treatment decisions, and to consider alternatives carefully. Such groups must be careful not to interfere with medical treatment and decisions, but rather to encourage clarification and the development of a cooperative relationship between doctor and patient.

7. Symptom Control

Cognitive techniques such as self-hypnosis are taught to manage symptoms such as pain and anxiety. These include learning to identify emotions as they develop, analyze sources of emotional response, and move from emotion-focused to problem-focused coping. These approaches help the patient take a more active stance toward the illness. Rather than feeling overwhelmed by an insoluble problem, they learn to divide problems into smaller and more manageable ones.

Specific coping skills can be demonstrated and taught which are designed to help patients reduce cancer-related symptoms such as anxiety and pain. Techniques used include specific self-regulation skills such as self-hypnosis.[31]

OUTCOME

Supportive/expressive group psychotherapy for cancer patients has been shown to reduce psychological distress,[9,32-34] improve coping responses,[9] and reduce pain.[31] This approach has also been shown to result in longer survival time among women with metastatic breast cancer.[35] The effect of psychosocial treatment on survival time has been demonstrated in half of the published randomized trials.[36-40] In comparing supportive expressive group therapy with cognitive-behavioral group treatment of HIV-infected individuals, Kelly and colleagues[41] found the supportive expressive intervention more effective. While no formal randomized trials have been conducted of the application of this model to couples, we have conducted both spouse and couples' groups over the past two decades, and found them to be well-accepted and helpful to them in addressing existential concerns, managing overwhelming affect, and improving family relationships.

In order to examine the cross-cultural salience of this approach, colleagues in Hong Kong and France have contributed their experience applying the same model to their rather different cultural settings.

PSYCHOSOCIAL SUPPORT IN HONG KONG

There are reasons why the supportive expressive mode of psychotherapy is a challenge in Hong Kong. Many Chinese cancer patients think that psychotherapy is irrelevant to their illness, and that only the mentally unsound need psychotherapy.[42] The suggestion of entering into a psychotherapeutic group may offend them (as a sign of weakness, inferiority compared to other patients, and the like). Besides, many cancer therapeutic and support groups in China (including Hong Kong) use bodily activities and creative art forms, from either Western models or traditional Chinese wellness exercises (eg, Tai Chi and Qi Gong), to promote expression and social support and as a form of distraction (pleasurable activities in contrast to the torturous cancer experience).[43,44] A therapeutic group that focuses almost exclusively on verbal sharing and face-to-face interaction may pose a threat to the patients—and perhaps the therapists as well (control difficulties, worries about participation, or lack of structure and therapeutic efficacy). To complicate the situation further, Chinese cancer patients are not used to expressing their emotions in direct ways. They tend to use passive-aggressive coping that is characterized by a "short-circuit open-conflict" approach—the use of indirect language, intermediaries, and face-saving ploys to handle their anxiety and emotions.[45] The mere anticipation of talking about one's feelings among a group of strangers may be a highly uncommon and threatening experience.

On the other hand, there are indications of the enormous needs of the Chinese patients in having access to therapeutic group interventions. Chinese cancer patients may have little social support outside the therapeutic context. Within the family, members may hesitate to start conversations to comfort patients. They believe that consolation possibly brings up themes of suffering or dying with tremendously painful and unbearable treatment processes, and thus brings additional worries and burdens to the patient. Moreover, the patients may not be willing to share their emotional turmoil with other family members, not because they think that the other family members are unsupportive, but because they do not want to impose burdens and suffering on their loved ones. The opportunity to "pour out" of one's emotional angst without having to worry about bothering and burdening others, especially family members, can be highly valuable once the group format is accepted. This interpersonal focus among Chinese people has been well discussed in the literature[46,47] and has a profound effect on patients' adjustments to suffering and illness.[48,49] Chinese cancer patients often prefer distraction coping (eg, sweet memories and telling jokes) to avoid addressing the overwhelming stress that is related to pain and death. The ability to tolerate momentary upsets, unhappiness, and emotional disturbances is even considered a virtue.[42] Seeking help from outside the family, especially from mental health professionals, may be regarded with shame. In addition, many Chinese still believe that current sufferings are the consequences (the *karma*) of past actions.[50] It has been shown that the attribution of illness to an external and stable causal factor (*karma*) can make the misery more bearable[51] and may have a positive effect on the adjustment to cancer.[52] However, this unscientific conclusion devalues the patient's personal self-evaluation and self-appreciation, and as a result, Chinese feel shame at sharing feelings with others. This *stigmatization* effect may lead to dehumanization, threat aversion, low self-esteem, and social isolation.[53] Worse still, cancer is thought to be an infectious disease by some people in China. The true story below from a Chinese cancer patient illustrates this point.

> One time when I was out having dinner with my friend, I recognized my friend was not willing to eat the food my chopsticks touched. She even requested using another pair of chopsticks for us. I just find myself very offended. What does she mean requesting another chopsticks separate from mine? Is she thinking that I will spread cancer to her? That's totally ridiculous. I can clearly identify she will not be my friend anymore.

This story can be explained by inadequate medical knowledge and misconceptions about cancer. This stigmatization is a barrier to developing a supportive atmosphere in which patients can express their feelings, and therefore inhibits their emotional expression. Evidence suggests that emotional control is associated with higher perceived stress as well as anxiety and depressive symptoms among Chinese women cancer survivors.[54] Potential stigmatization and efforts toward avoidance may often deprive a patient of corrections to their distorted beliefs.

Many Chinese cancer patients thus cope with the disease in isolation. We have reason to believe that a supportive expressive mode of psychotherapy may be potentially beneficial to them. In Hong Kong, the first therapeutic group for breast cancer women that followed the supportive expressive model[4,55] was conducted between February 7 and March 28, 2003, after David Spiegel's training workshop in Hong Kong in November 2002. This first group aimed to examine the feasibility of conducting the supportive/expressive group therapy among Chinese and to explore what adaptations were needed for Chinese cancer patients. We adopted a closed group format for this brief support group. This format facilitated the equal exposure of every member in the group as well as enabling the therapist to have a sharper focus on the themes to be covered within the allotted time. The group was conducted by one of us (S.H.)—a male clinical psychologist with more than 10 years of experience in cancer psychotherapy and research—without a co-facilitator. A co-therapist was not included because of the pioneering nature of this project. Moreover, a conscious effort was made to follow the guidelines described in the manual for supportive/expressive group therapy[56] as closely as possible. There were seven women in the group, which is approximately equal to the optimal size for a psychotherapy group.[12] The following paragraphs describe our experience in conducting the group and highlight some of the characteristics of conducting the supportive expressive mode of psychotherapy among Hong Kong Chinese. Here we focus on the adaptations made that allowed the group to function well in the cultural setting of Hong Kong.

The Supportive Expressive Group

Lee et al.[42] described their experience in providing psychological care to a Chinese woman with breast cancer in Hong Kong, and suggested that therapists should focus on dealing with the patients' concrete daily life and role function difficulties in the initial sessions of intervention before focusing overtly on emotional difficulties. They further suggested that many Chinese cancer patients may not be motivated to participate in psychotherapy because they do not understand the rationale behind the treatment. Participants assume that the therapist will give them direct and concrete advice during therapy; it will be frustrating to Chinese participants if these expectations are unmet in the initial stage of therapy. Appropriate psychoeducational information was given as a means of reducing the stigma associated with participation and meeting expectations, especially at the initial stage of the group therapy. Our experience indicated that, more often than not, Chinese cancer patients used these educational materials to generate a more fruitful discussion in the group therapy, as illustrated below.

Based on this rationale, a conscious effort was made to address the concrete daily life problems of the patients and to facilitate instrumental support among members instead of moving to emotional sharing too soon in the initial sessions. In Chinese culture, instrumental support implies constructive contributions to caring and brings comfort to each person, which may pave the way for emotional sharing in future sessions. At the beginning of the first psychotherapy session, it was emphasized to members that the group could serve as a pool of collective wisdom and resource sharing. All participants were encouraged to describe their experience and coping skills, so that others could use them for reference if they encountered similar problems or challenges in the future. It turned out that all participants could gain mutual support in the initial stage of therapy and began to develop a supportive atmosphere for emotional sharing toward the end of the third session. A woman in the group finally resolved her interpersonal conflicts. It was the open and fruitful discussion among group members that made this successful outcome possible.

Rosary was diagnosed with breast cancer as her father underwent dialysis for kidney problems. Because of her own disease, she could not take her father for medical check-ups and kidney dialysis. She did not reveal her disease to her father for fear of giving him an additional emotional burden. She felt extremely guilty as a result, and always had the feeling that she should take responsibility for her father's death. Her guilt was also taken as a reason for her present suffering and the behavioral problems of her child (refer to the concept of *karma* mentioned above).

> *Rosary:* Even now that my father is dead, I tell myself I did something wrong. One day, my son kept blaming his father when I was riding on a bus with him. It reminded me of my wrongdoings to my own father. How could I blame my son for not being nice to me and my husband when I myself didn't take care of my own father?

Rosary had somehow mixed up her feelings toward her father, her son, and her present illness. In a discussion about active coping strategies in the third session, I was asked to talk about the stress and coping from a psychological point of view. The group was briefed on basic stress and coping principles in psychology and it was emphasized that one should try to separate the effects of different stressful events in order to cope better. Before the close of this session, group members used the materials to talk about Rosary's situation.

> *Mary:* You always link your emotions together—your grief towards your father and your feelings towards your son. You thought that you did something wrong to your father, that's why your son treated you badly. That doesn't make sense at all. Sometimes you are talking about your mother-in-law; it's not good to mix up your emotions. Everyone experiences unhappiness, if you mix up your emotions, then you further burden yourself. The fact that your father is dead, you shouldn't think too much about that. If you find your son is naughty, why don't you think about his lovely face when he was small? A kid always takes adults as models, if you always say he is naughty, then his behavior is turning even worse.

This timely feedback from other participants turned out to be very powerful, and Rosary became much better after this session. In fact, because of the relational orientation of Chinese,[46,57,58] participants may rely on group norms (the validation and approval of their feelings by the others) to evaluate their feelings and thinking. It is not uncommon for an individual to suppress emotions in order to achieve validation from others. Some patients may not want to impose unhappiness on their doctors and choose not to talk about their emotional problems in front of physicians. This is in fact the case of Jenny.

> *Jenny:* Sometimes it depends on whom you talk to, some physicians do feel the same way you are. I feel sorry to make the physician unhappy, it seems like they look even unhappier than me.

The above example, on the other hand, reflects the fact that doctor-patient communication is essential. Sometimes the lack of communication may be due to poor communication skills on the part of the doctor, yet at other times, it may simply be due to the lack of time available during a typical consultation or follow-up session. Chinese patients have a lot of respect (and fear) toward medical doctors but are seldom willing to initiate a contact themselves:

Mary described her anxiety about not receiving a call from her doctor. In the third session, she indirectly revealed that she recognized changes to her body. She assumed that it was due to the poor prognosis or a possible relapse.*

> *Mary:* I feel very tired. I don't feel rested even if I sleep a lot. I started feeling this way almost a week ago. I didn't even have such a feeling after the surgery. Personally, I think I am a very tough and routine person. If I feel I am very tired, there must be something wrong. This feeling is even worse than what I felt before the surgery. You know, I couldn't even walk one time when I was in the street.

Mary felt very physically uncomfortable and emotionally unstable. She also indicated that she planned to reveal her health condition to her family as she thought she possibly had a relapse. In the fifth session, Mary continuously revealed that she worried about her doctor not calling her, and strongly suspected that it was due to her relapse. These were just her thoughts, she admitted, without any confirmation from her physicians.

> *Mary:* As I told you before, it was only my thoughts. The physicians didn't tell me that I had a relapse.

---

* The linkage of "not calling" from her physician and a relapse could be another example of interpersonal orientation among the Chinese—Mary assumes (automatically) that her physician didn't want to hurt her (by not calling) because of her poor medical examination results!

At this junction, two group members, Maria and Susan, shared their experience of calling their doctors for information. They even gave Mary necessary numbers to call and encouraged her to take the initiative to call the physician right after the session.

> *Maria*: Why don't you call your doctor?
> *Mary*: I don't know which doctor or hospital I should call.
> *Susan*: You may call the hospital. According to what I know, if the doctor didn't call you up, that means you have no problem. If you have a relapse, the doctor must call you up for a medical check.
> *Maria*: You should take the initiative. You can actually call the doctor. You must take the action.

Mary did call her doctor directly. In the seventh session, she was very happy to describe her conversation with her doctor. Her doctor did try several times to reach her about the result in the past weeks but could not find her. The medical result turned out to be uneventful and the woman felt great relief.

> *Mary*: I finally called the doctor. The doctor said he did call me several times, but he couldn't reach me as I seldom stayed in Hong Kong during the daytime.

The theme of doctor-patient communication in supportive expressive psychotherapy is particularly relevant to Chinese patients. As the psychotherapist is also considered a medical health professional and often attracts the same respect (and fear) from the patients, it is not uncommon for participants to seek validation of their worries and fears from the group therapist. As the therapist and only male in the group, I was asked to tell them about how a husband would feel toward a wife with a mastectomy. While encouraging the women to ask their husbands directly, I gave the following response.

> *Therapist*: If your husband marries you because of your appearance or outlook, even if you don't have cancer, he won't stay with you long. There may be extra-marital relationship problems. You should have something else other than your appearance that is attractive to your husband.

My rationale was that, because of the taboo against talking about sex and body image in the social context, these women might not have another chance to seek acceptance and validation from another male outside the therapeutic context. My response could allay their worries and enable them to seek further clarification from their husbands.

Not only is sex and body image in the social context a taboo subject; whether one should reveal her illness to families also poses threat to an individual in a Chinese community. I purposefully chose to adopt metaphorical expression to review this point during the therapy. In addition, Chinese people tend to use metaphorical expressions and rhetorical figures to communicate ideas. The Chinese language is rich in metaphor, and many Chinese characters (word symbols) originated from collective mental representations of phenomena. It has been suggested that the use of metaphor may help Chinese people to express difficult emotions related to suffering and death.[59] The participants also had the tendency to use other experiences and metaphors to talk about their cancer experience. In one session, the women were very interested in talking about whether their husbands had extramarital relationships. Almost everyone was involved in the conversation, except for one woman who was not married. I allowed them to discuss this "noncancer" subject freely, as if they were gossiping. The group finally came to a conclusion that even if a woman knew about the extramarital relationship of her husband, it was still better to keep it a secret in the family.

> *Susan*: Even if you know that your husband is going out with a mistress outside the family, sometimes it's better not to talk. You don't want to fight all the time at home.
> *Therapist*: Aren't you feeling very uncomfortable?
> *Susan*: Yeah, very uncomfortable in fact, but there's nothing I can do. I know that he has a mistress outside the family, but still it's better not to talk.

When such "noncancer" subjects arise in the group, the therapist should not discourage the participants from talking about it first, but should bear in mind that they should somehow relate it to cancer.[4] The therapist should then make every effort to try to relate the subjects to the themes of the group later in the therapeutic session. The therapist made the following comment in response to the above sharing.

> *Therapist*: The topic we just discussed—whether you should openly talk to your husband if you suspect that he has an extra-marital relationship. Put it into other words, it just like catching cancer in the sense of whether you will reveal your illness to your families, isn't it?

Since I noticed that Marleen, the only single woman in the group, who kept silent during the whole sharing, I asked how she felt about the discussion. After this comment, Marleen expressed her decision to get married and described her anxiety about her future life. Even though she had a close relationship with her boyfriend, she struggled to tell her potential mother-in-law (who didn't know that the woman had cancer!) about her disease. The group members helped her to resolve her worries related to the marriage and her future relationship with her boyfriend's mother.

> *Marleen*: I worry the most that I probably won't have a baby due to my disease. I also worry about not telling his mum about my disease.

The group then encouraged Marleen to share her worries with the fiancé. Marleen reported the following experience in the next session.

> *Marleen*: I had a long, deep, and heart-touching conversation with my boyfriend after the last session. I even asked him if he did mind about my disease. I felt extreme relief because we have such a long conversation, for we now know each other more and reassure our confidence to get marry.

She felt extreme relief even though they both decided to keep the secret. Most importantly, she felt reassured about their decision to get married.

OUTCOME

The verbal feedback from the participants was generally very positive. The following quotations from Mary, the woman who thought that she had a relapse because her physician did not call, summarize the experience of most participants:

> *Mary*: It's good to express emotions to others, I feel happier than before. Now, I can sleep easily without many dreams almost every night. I am very happy that I finally sense family warmth, which I have never experienced before. Last time, I treated my family to dinner in a restaurant. We ate too much and we all felt love towards each other.
> Since the 3rd session, I can sense that this group is basically for sharing. The therapist doesn't seem to comment on our thoughts. We share how we cope with problems, so that we can learn from each other and we can report the progress in the next session.

I find this group very helpful. Sometimes you think that you are right, but if you hear the opinions of others, you may discover a new way of thinking. That's the reason I find this group very exciting.

Rosary, the woman with unresolved grief (see above), compared her experience in the supportive expressive group with her previous experience in joining groups that focused on activities, and mentioned that the present therapeutic group could enhance her understanding of her problems.

> *Rosary:* In the previous group, they used a rope to tie the participants together before they asked us to cut the rope with scissors. I knew that I had messed up something and should disconnect them—but what had I messed up? This group teaches me that I always connect all sorts of emotions together—about my grief towards my dad and my current feelings towards my son. I didn't even notice that. In fact, I didn't even think that I link up all things together. Now, I know what my problem was.

SUMMARY

Conducting the supportive expressive mode of psychotherapy is a challenge to both the participants and the therapist, mainly because Chinese people are not used to talking about their emotions and participating in a "doing-nothing-but-talking" group. Several adaptations were made for this first group of supportive expressive psychotherapy in Hong Kong, although not always consciously. The main adaptations included the focus on concrete daily problems and instrumental support in the initial sessions of the therapy, the awareness of the interpersonal orientation of the participants, and the metaphorical use of "noncancer" subjects. Supportive expressive psychotherapy will provide another model of psychological care for cancer patients in Hong Kong and China, and will enhance our existing model of care. The feasibility of long-term open groups should be explored further in Hong Kong.

Thus, key similarities and differences between American and Chinese cultures were highlighted by this experience. In both cultures, the social context is highly valued, more so in China where the role of the individual is defined more in terms of his or her place in the social environment. This makes gathering together in groups redefined by a common problem natural. However, at the same time, the high valence placed upon social structure makes Chinese cancer patients very sensitive to any expression of feelings that might threaten their position in the group, offend others, or cause them to lose face. Thus, the initial work of the group involves greater effort to make frank discussion of problems and open expression of emotion less threatening. This can be accomplished by initially emphasizing information transfer more and emotional expression less, by fostering discussion of common problems that are real but less threatening than cancer, and by using indirect and metaphorical issues as a means of allowing patients to "test the waters."

Teaching patients common means of assertiveness is even more important in Hong Kong than in the United States, where a certain amount of self-assertion is considered a normal part of the patient "role" and a valued attribute. This applies both to communication with physicians, and to means of handling cancer-related problems with family and friends.

In Hong Kong, there are often concerns that frank discussion of cancer-related problems, including fears regarding dying and death, amount to "bad luck," or creating rather than discussing problems. In the United States, irrational fears regarding "causing cancer" emotionally or "making it spread" more often involve inner misattribution of some emotional "need" for cancer in the individual's psyche, rather than communication about it. In other words, it is the individual rather than communication in a social group that has irrational power. In both cases, the group can serve a healing function in desensitizing such fears, as concerns about making matters worse are ventilated and dispelled, with the group observing that such fears are not realized, and that the increased closeness and greater range of affect experienced, positive as well as negative, is therapeutic.[15,16] Thus, the major synchronic themes observed involve the importance of social relationships, the value of assertiveness, the use of metaphorical speech, and the meaning of emotional expression. Attention to these differences in valence across cultures seems to facilitate the achievement of more universal goals of shared experience, giving as well as receiving help, and feeling included in a close social world despite the effects of cancer and its progression.

PSYCHOSOCIAL SUPPORT IN FRANCE

Cultural Differences between France and the United States

While French and American cancer patients share many similar experiences, the cultural context in which they live modifies their way of coping with the illness. Similarly, when cancer patients participate in supportive expressive group therapy, their personal experience reflects both who they are as persons and as members of a cultural group. Several studies have compared Americans to Japanese on dimensions relevant to group psychotherapy for cancer patients such as self-disclosure, emotional expression, and the like.[60,61] To the best of our knowledge, no studies comparing French to Americans exist with respect to health and psychology characteristics salient to receiving emotional support during treatment for cancer.

At a general level, psychological aspects of health care have a more central position in the public imagination in American society than in France. The pragmatism of Americans and their enthusiasm for problem-solving, apparent in the large American self-help and do-it-yourself literature, is reflected in the general American interest in management of their response to illness, and gives a specific coloration to the way people live and cope with cancer, and hence to the manner in which psychological interventions are received. These influence the cognitions and behaviors of cancer patients. Indeed, the traditional Cartesian dualism of mind and body is still prominent in the French culture, and mind-body theories have not had in France the large influence they have known in the United States; consequently such approaches have not influenced patients' conceptions of illness, and personal control over the disease is not an important dimension of the French conception of health. Thus, the general level of involvement in developing coping strategies is therefore higher among the American than the French public.

Psychosocial Intervention in France

In France, psychiatrists and psychologists who came to the field of psychosocial cancer care in the 1970s focused their attention on the specific characteristics of doctor-patient relationships. They tried to help nurses and physicians fully take into account the specific needs of patients, drawing from theoretical frameworks emerging from the psychoanalytic model. The work of the Hungarian psychoanalyst Balint,[62] who emigrated to England, made available through his method of casework a description of the psychological determinants at work in the medical encounter. His famous book, *The Doctor, His Patient and the Illness*,[62] had a major impact on French health care professionals interested in problems related to medical illness, familiarizing them with concepts such as defense mechanisms. A few years later, psychologists influenced by Winnicott emphasized the essential function of the holding process, and the importance of health professionals' warmth and availability in their contact with cancer patients. Psychologists and psychiatrists contributed to a positive evolution of the quality of care, especially nursing care, by emphasizing the importance of the relationship between doctors and other health care professionals and patients. The effort was to use the caregiving relationship to limit the negative psychological consequences of the evolution of modern oncology, which included painful and mutilating treatments, and complex decision-making processes that had the potential to result in a dehumanization of care because of extremely technical methods, and highly standardized procedures and protocols. At the beginning of the 1990s, the involvement of mental health professionals made possible the adoption in French society of new conceptions of palliative care, in particular those of Cicely Saunders from the London St Christopher Hospice. This led to a variety of psychological interventions in the framework of palliative care mobile teams. These teams meet with hospitalized patients and offer their help which consists of listening, being present, being attentive to emotional, social, relational, or medical patients needs, helping in the process of decision making, and educating about the illness. Such interventions have been increasingly directed at patients who are not in a terminal phase of care.

However, planning for how to provide psychological help to cancer patients and their families outside of the hospital setting has not been a top priority in France. Interventions have been limited to the period of emotional crisis, or alternatively to classical psychopathological evaluation in the context of consultation/liaison hospital psychiatry.

The advent of studies indicating the possibility that psychosocial support might lead to improved survival time[35] prompted French health professionals to propose psychological interventions for cancer outpatients. The characteristics of the French health care system, which offers to almost everyone free medical and psychological services in hospitals, is clearly an obstacle to psychological interventions provided outside the hospitals, which must be paid for by patients themselves. Therefore, in France, psychological interventions are most often linked to hospital care and referrals are most often made by a physician or a nurse.

The French medical model is still based on paternalism, with patients expecting their doctors to give them advice and necessary support for them. Patients rarely initiate first steps for supplemental care by themselves. Thus, a good deal of control of the development of psychosocial services is, in France, in the hands and built on the cultural orientations of health care professionals rather than members of the public.

However, the last few years have seen an important change and many patients insist now on receiving psychological help. This trend has been promoted by powerful patients and volunteers associations such as "La Ligue Nationale Contre Le Cancer" that have advocated in the media in favor of psychological help for cancer patients. Recently, the President made the fight against cancer a priority in his political program, and a national budget has been allocated to the field of psycho-oncology.

Psychological support is more often provided in an individual format, by psychologists or volunteers, but the number of patients and the efficacy of group approaches tend to make them more frequently implemented. For example, in Marseilles, an educational program focused on nutrition for cancer patients has been built along the supportive expressive model by Mouysset.[63] Chabert from Chambery, implemented a weekly group lead by a psychologist and a radiotherapy technician[64] for radiotherapy patients, very close in its approach to the supportive expressive model, even though the duration of the group is much shorter—two months.

The French tradition in psychiatry and psychology is not to conduct quantitative research, but rather to clinically evaluate interventions' efficacy and patients' satisfaction. Therefore, this type of practice rarely results in published studies, but nonetheless, the clinicians who work mostly exclusively in the field of psycho-oncology are without any doubt able to attest to the efficacy of supportive/expressive groups. Nowadays in France, a majority of oncologists are in favor of the participation of their patients to such groups, they do not feel that their position is threatened anymore by the groups. By contrast, the initial reluctance of cancer patients to be confronted by other patients' painful experiences represents an obstacle of importance.

Experience with Supportive Expressive Group Therapy in France

Two psychologists, Schwab (Paris) and Machavoine (Caen) were, starting in 1995, the first to implement supportive expressive group therapy for women with metastatic breast cancer in comprehensive cancer care centers. Machavoine's study focuses on this first experience with chemotherapy metastatic breast cancer patients.[65,66] Recruitment difficulties impeded the realization of a randomized comparative study, therefore a single semi-open group (involving 5 to 6 members) was held weekly. After 2 1/2 years and 87 sessions, the study reports an important emotional investment and satisfaction from the patients. A psychological evaluation conducted every 6 months by a psychiatrist, shows intense but brief (less than 2 weeks) depressive episodes, no augmentation of anxiety, and emotional reactions appropriate to anxiety-provoking situations, such as medical tests and treatments.

Building Bonds

To a foreign observer of supportive expressive group therapy, the bonding process seems to occur very rapidly in American groups. In a French group setting, the early process of bonding and sharing of emotional experiences may be delayed. Interestingly, French breast cancer patients seem to discuss shared and rather personal problems, but at the same time to maintain a certain polite formality, referring to one another by surnames rather than first names, as would be common in the United States. American culture puts more emphasis than the French culture on the importance of being part of a group in general. As compared to French, Americans socialize easily in various types of groups (professional, sports, schools, churches, and the like). They also seem to have less difficulty in mixing the professional sphere and the familial one, something that happens very rarely in France where the two worlds almost never meet. The individual nature of the French culture may make it more difficult for French patients to first adjust to the group process and later, as encouraged in the supportive-expressive model, to build outside support composed of group members.

Other features of the supportive expressive model will also be received differently in France. Instrumental support is more frequent in the American society than it is in the French society. For example, cooking for a friend or running errands for her can seem natural in an American context and will be part of the instrumental support that members of the group will receive from their social network. Such behaviors are unknown to the French who tend to rely during times of illness on well-developed governmental institutions.

Emotional Expression

Comparing supportive expressive group therapy in different cultural contexts may highlight some characteristics in American culture that appear salient to French clinicians. The rationale for supportive expressive therapy is based on strategies that tend to build group support and encourage patients to explore their experiences and express their emotions.[4] These two fundamental components of supportive expressive group therapy may be more difficult to initiate in a French context. For example, the types of emotion one is willing and able to express are clearly related to culture. Studies comparing Americans to Japanese found that Americans elaborate, highlight, or emphasize more positive feelings than negative feelings more than do Japanese.[61] The French may be at the other end of the spectrum. French culture does not emphasize emotional expression, in general, or expression of positive emotions, in particular. Therefore, in a group setting, the harder task of a French group leader might be at first to promote emotional expression at all. In addition, while supportive expressive therapy has sometimes helped patients move out of the "prison of positive thinking,"[4] French patients have not been immersed in the widely disseminated popular idea that "positive thinking" will help them fight cancer.

In addition, some studies suggest that cultures influence disclosure to others. Americans, when compared to Japanese, reported significantly higher levels of self-disclosure.[60] As for the French, self-disclosure, in general, and self-disclosure of a diagnosis of illness, in particular, are less common for French patients than for American patients. While it seems that self-disclosure of the diagnosis enables patients to take an active stance and to cope better with the illness, it is still unusual in France, and patients tend to hide cancer diagnosis from their social environment, thereby preventing the provision of emotional and instrumental support by relatives and friends.

Detoxifying Dying

Six members of the group have died during the 2 1/2 years of the group. One year after the end of the group, three patients were still alive. Patients who died during the group benefited at the end of their lives from the sincere expression of support and solidarity from the other group members. They in turn, continuing their participation in the group, had the opportunity to become more familiar with illness progression and the end of life through watching others, to cope with death anxiety, and to anticipate their own future. Nurses attested of more peaceful deaths among the members of the group and physicians reported that members of the group communicate better with them, had a better understanding of the information provided to them and of the process they were going through. For the group, going through such a difficult time together enhanced the bonding process. A phase of intense emotional reaction was followed by a strong desire to live beyond the threat of death, by investing anew in their social and affective lives. Similar to experience in the United States and Hong Kong, anticipating death did not have a traumatic effect. On the contrary, it was an opportunity for living in a more authentic manner. One patient said: "I understood that it was a disease that could finally kill, I knew it, but only intellectually, in an abstract way." Detoxifying dying was a shared experience for these patients and their group leaders, a psychologist and a trained oncology nurse.

The group has been understood to work as a "skills and resources reservoir".[65,66] Through imitation and identification, every member can try new and useful behaviors, and experience psychological changes that will foster autonomy, even in the face of death. Similar to observations in the United States and Hong Kong, processes such as exchanges of information, of experiences, shared expression of feelings, meaning making, fighting loneliness, and finding a new feeling of dignity that happened in this group. To be able to fight together against the illness seems to represent a universal component of the human capacity to cope.

SUMMARY

The supportive expressive model originated in the United States and some of its features are clearly adapted to the American culture. Some specific cultural characteristics, salient in the context of health/illness may appear when confronting the practice of supportive expressive therapy in the two countries. In a French cultural setting, some of the processes that typically unfold during supportive expressive group therapy may be delayed or altered. The notable differences between American and French cancer patients during supportive expressive group therapy have to do with issues such as perceived control, emotional expression, bonding process, self-disclosure, and social support.

Some variations or alterations in conducting supportive expressive group therapy may be required in France. However, despite some modifications that may appear in the evolution of group processes, the core features of the model will without any doubt, and as attested by the French studies mentioned above, apply to the universality of the cancer experience. The French people remember what Jean Paul Sartre, the famous philosopher, said in "Critique de la Raison Dialectique" about being a member of a group: "I am for you what you are for me, a reciprocity that goes beyond the imaginary."

CONCLUSIONS

Clearly cultural, economic, and political differences mark the application of supportive care principles in widely differing cultures. Yet universal human dimensions of emotion, social support, existential threat, and a desire for meaning infuse the process of providing psychosocial support in the three different cultures examined here. Yalom[73] notes four "ultimate concerns" of human existence: death, freedom, meaning, and isolation. We will summarize the synchronic and diachronic aspects of this cross-cultural supportive care journey according to these themes.

Death is a universal and ultimate concern. The dread of nonbeing is experienced everywhere, but differently. In China, talking about death is sometimes seen as inviting it or condemning oneself to it. The approach taken to discussing it involves indirection, addressing less-threatening problems first, testing the waters. Death threatens Americans in a different way—it is seen as a failure—of optimism or ambition or will—a human failing rather than a human necessity. The approach to discussing it that seems to work best involves defining an area related to death that invites active participation—the process of dying. Thus, one can succeed in dying with dignity even if one cannot will away the inevitable. In France, death creates inconvenient public intimacy, calling for stronger reactions than people are comfortable with. It is seen as an uncomfortable fact to be avoided, yet can be approached for discussion because the private anxiety about it is even more isolating and threatening. That people can benefit from confronting the threat of death together is seen in all three cultures—the paths to doing this vary.

Freedom is a powerful aspect of human existence, emphasizing choice. This is a particular virtue in America, where these are highly valued, nurturing the reliance on individualism. Yet freedom can be a burden as well, leading to expectations that any path could be taken at any time, and making people feel irrationally responsible for a disease they did not cause. Group support usefully emphasizes limitations on freedom—facing the inevitable free of unnecessary guilt. In China, freedom is less highly prized, while one's role in the social environment is more valued. Being free is less important than being a responsible part of the social order, so hesitation to discuss cancer and its implications has more to do with effects on the network of family and friends. In France also, medical care is more authoritarian, making choices about care and support more of a departure from the norm.

Meaning is intensified in the context of threatened death. In a socio-centric culture such as China, the idea that one can be a more effective family member by coping better is an important tool to elicit emotional involvement by cancer patients. In the United States, the idea that one has responsibilities to others even in the process of dying is less natural but even more helpful. It makes dying patients feel less irrelevant, more a part of some meaning structure that goes beyond themselves. This is not dissimilar from the experience of French cancer patients.

Isolation is a concern in all cultures, but much less so in Eastern ones. However, the price of feeling embedded in a social context is often constraint on expression of emotion or thought so as to avoid disrupting social ties. Getting cancer can create shame and stigma. Discussing common fears and concerns in a group can powerfully reduce the stigma, but doing so has risks. This is more the case when social norms militate against expression of strong emotion, which is naturally associated with serious illness and the threat of death. Finding culturally appropriate means of inviting and managing emotional expression despite cultural restrictions such as saving face in China, losing the appearance of strength in America, or appearing inappropriately informal in France, can be a challenge. Nonetheless, the threat of death intensifies isolation, which is a powerful symbol for death itself—being removed from loved ones. Shared emotional expression and bonding in groups can help cancer patients mange their illness in a way that allows them to reapproach their social connections taking their altered social status into account.

Each culture has its strengths and weaknesses, sets of beliefs, and natural supportive mechanisms. Psychosocial support for cancer patients can work best by utilizing cultural idiosyncrasies to address fundamental human needs.

ACKNOWLEDGMENT

Dr. Ho would like to express his sincere thanks to Professor Peter W.H. Lee, Department of Psychiatry, University of Hong Kong, for giving valuable comments on the first draft of this chapter.

REFERENCES

1. Mo B. Modesty, sexuality, and breast health in Chinese-American women. *West J Med.* 1992;157:260-264.
2. Perez-Stable EJ, Sabogal F, Otero-Sabogal R, Hiatt RA, McPhee SJ. Misconceptions about cancer among Latinos and Anglos [see comments]. *JAMA.* 1992;268:3219-3223.
3. Saint-Germain MA, Longman AJ. Breast cancer screening among older Hispanic women: knowledge, attitudes, and practices. *Health Educ Q.* 1993;20:539-553.
4. Spiegel D, Classen C. *Group Therapy for Cancer Patients: a Research-Based Handbook of Psychosocial Care.* New York: Basic Books; 2000.
5. Goodwin PJ, Leszcz M, Ennis M, et al. The Effect of Group Psychosocial Support on Survival in Metastatic Breast Cancer. *N Eng J Med.* 2001;345:1719-1726.
6. Goodwin PJ, Leszcz M, Koopmans J, et al. Randomized trial of group psychosocial support in metastatic breast cancer: the BEST study. Breast-Expressive Supportive Therapy study. *Cancer Treat Rev.* 1996;22(Suppl A):91-96.
7. Bloch S, Kissane D. Psychotherapies in psycho-oncology. An exciting new challenge *British J Psychiatry.* 2000 August; 177:112–116.
8. Classen C, Butler LD, Koopman C, et al. Supportive-expressive group therapy and distress in patients with metastatic breast cancer: a randomized clinical intervention trial. *Arch Gen Psychiatr.* 2001;58:494-501.
9. Spiegel D, Bloom JR, Yalom I. Group support for patients with metastatic cancer. A randomized outcome study. *Arch Gen Psychiatr.* 1981;38(5):527-533.
10. Spiegel D, Yalom I. A support group for dying patients. *Int J Group Psychotherapy.* 1978;28:233-245.
11. Levi-Strauss C. *Structural Anthropology.* New York: Basic Books; 1963.
12. Yalom ID. *The Theory and Practice of Group Psychotherapy.* New York: Basic Books; 1995.
13. Spiegel D. Psychosocial intervention in cancer. *J Nat Cancer Inst.* 1993;85(5):1198-1205.
14. Mulder C, van der Pompe G, Spiegel D, Antoni M. Do psychosocial factors influence the course of breast cancer? A review of recent literature methodological problems and future directions. *Psychooncology.* 1992;1:155-167.

15. Giese-Davis J, Koopman C, Butler L, et al. Change in emotion-regulation strategy for women with metastatic breast cancer following supportive-expressive group therapy. *Journal of Consulting and Clinical Psychology* 2002;70:916-925.
16. Giese-Davis J, Spiegel D. Emotional expression and cancer progression. In: Davidson RJ, Scherer K, Hill Goldsmith H, eds. *Handbook of Affective Sciences.* Oxford: Oxford University Press; 2003.
17. Gross J. Emotional expression in cancer onset and progression. *Soc Sci Med.* 1989;28:1239-1248.
18. Mouysset JL, Baciuchka-Palmaro M, Ichou M, et al. Les ateliers de nutrition en oncologie medicale: une experience pilote. *Bulletin DU Cancer.* 2001;88:959-94.
19. Greer S. Psychological response to cancer and survival. *Psychol Med.* 1991;21(1):43-49.
20. Greer S, Morris T, Pettingale KW. Psychological response to breast cancer: effect on outcome. *Lancet.* 1979;2(8146):785-787.
21. Giese-Davis J, Sephton SE, Spiegel D. Repression associated with a physiological risk factor for shorter survival in women with metastatic breast cancer. Paper submitted for presentation at: Annual Meeting for the Society of Behavioral Medicine Research; 2000b; Nashville, TN.
22. Giese-Davis J, Spiegel D. Emotional expression and cancer progression. In: Davidson RJ, Scherer, K, Hill Goldsmith H, eds. *Handbook of affective sciences.* Oxford: Oxford University Press, 2003.
23. Greer S, Moorey S, Baruch J, et al. Adjuvant psychological therapy for patients with cancer. *Br Med J.* 1992;304:675-680.
24. Spiegel D. Essentials of psychotherapeutic intervention for cancer patients. *Support Care Cancer.* 1995;3:252-256.
25. Spiegel, D. *Living Beyond Limits.* New York: Ballantine/Fawcett; 1994.
26. Spiegel D. Facilitating emotional coping during treatment. *Cancer.* 1990;66(Suppl 6):1422-1426.
27. Moos RH, Schaefer, JA. The crisis of physical illness: an overview and conceptual approach. In: Moos RH ed. *Coping with Physical Illness 2: New Perspectives.* New York: Plenum; 1987:3-25.
28. Spiegel D, Bloom J, Gottheil E. Family environment of patients with metastatic carcinoma. *J Psychosoc Oncol.* 1983a;1:33-44.
29. Spiegel D, Bloom JR, Gottheil E. Family environment as a predictor of adjustment to metastatic breast carcinoma. *J Psychosoc Oncol.* 1983b;1(1):33-44.
30. Giese-Davis J, Hermanson K, Koopman C, Weibel D, Spiegel D. Quality of couples' relationship and adjustment to metastatic breast cancer. *J Fam Psychol.* 2000a;14(2):251-266.
31. Spiegel D, Bloom JR. Group therapy and hypnosis reduce metastatic breast carcinoma pain. *Psychosom Med.* 1983;45(4):333-339.
32. Classen C, Butler LD, Koopman C, et al. Supportive-expressive group therapy reduces distress in metastatic breast cancer patients: A randomized clinical intervention trial. *under review.* 2000.
33. Spiegel D, Morrow GR, Classen C, et al. Group psychotherapy for recently diagnosed breast cancer patients: a multicenter feasibility study. *Psycho-Oncology.* 1999;8:482-493.
34. Spiegel D, Morrow GC, Riggs C, et al. Effect of group therapy on women with primary breast cancer. *Breast J.* 1996;2(1):104-116.
35. Spiegel D, Bloom JR, Kraemer HC, Gottheil E. Effect of psychosocial treatment on survival of patients with metastatic breast cancer. *Lancet.* 1989;2(8668):888-891.
36. Blake-Mortimer J, Gore-Felton C, Kimerling R, Turner-Cobb JM, Spiegel, D. Improving the quality and quantity of life among patients with cancer: a review of the effectiveness of group psychotherapy. *Eur J Cancer.* 1999;35(11):1581-1586.

37. Compas BE, Haaga DA, Keefe FJ, Leitenberg H, Williams, DA. Sampling of empirically supported psychological treatments from health psychology: smoking, chronic pain, cancer, and bulimia nervosa. *J Consult Clin Psychol.* 1998;66(1):89-112.

38. Edelman S, Lemon J, Bell DR, Kidman AD. Effects of group CBT on the survival time of patients with metastatic breast cancer. *Psychooncology.* 1999;8(6):474-481.

39. Fox BH. Some problems and some solutions in research on psychotherapeutic intervention in cancer. *Support Care Cancer.* 1995;3(4):257-263.

40. van der Pompe G, Antoni M, Visser A, Garssen, B. Adjustment to breast cancer: the psychobiological effects of psychosocial interventions. *Patient Educ Couns.* 1996;28(2):209-219.

41. Kelly JA, Murphy DA, Bahr GR, et al. Outcome of cognitive-behavioral and support group brief therapies for depressed, HIV-infected persons. *Am J Psychiatry.* 1993;150(11): 1679-1686.

42. Lee PW-h, Wu LY-f, Fung AS-m. Psychological care in oncology. In: Fielding R, Chan CL-w, eds. *Psychosocial Oncology & Palliative Care in Hong Kong. The first decade.* Hong Kong: Hong Kong University Press; 2000:29-54.

43. Chan CL-w, Law MY-y, Leung PP-y. An empowerment group for Chinese cancer patients in Hong Kong. In: Fielding R, Chan CL-w, eds. *Psychosocial Oncology and Palliative Care in Hong Kong. The first decade.* Hong Kong: Hong Kong University Press; 2000:167-187.

44. Chang FM-y, Tsang SK-m. From expression to empowerment: using creative arts as self-healing media for cancer patients. In: Fielding R, Chan CL-w. eds. *Psychosocial Oncology and Palliative Care in Hong Kong. The First Decade.* Hong Kong: Hong Kong University Press; 2000:189-211

45. Ho SMY, Shiu WCT. Death anxiety and coping mechanism of Chinese cancer patients. *Omega J Death Dying.* 1995;31(1):59-65.

46. Ho DYF. Relational counseling: an Asian perspective on therapeutic intervention. Paper presented at: The 55th Annual Convention International Council of Psychologists; 1995; Graz, Austria.

47. Markus HR, Kitayama S. Culture and the self: implications for cognition, emotion, and motivation. *Psychol Rev.* 1991;98:224-253.

48. Ho SMY, Chow AYM, Chan CL-w, Tsui YKY. The assessment of grief among Hong Kong Chinese: a preliminary report. *Death Stud.* 2002;26:91-98.

49. Ho SMY, Ho JWC, Chan CLW, Kwan K, Tsui YKY. Decisional consideration of hereditary colon cancer genetic test results among Hong Kong Chinese adults. *Cancer Epidem Biomar.* 2003;12(5):426-432.

50. Leslie J. The implications of the physcial body: health, suffering and *Karma* in Hindu thought. In: Hinnells J R, Porter R eds. *Religion, Health and Suffering.* New York: Columbia University Press; 1999:23-45.

51. Yang, K-s Theories and research in Chinese personality: An indigenous approach. In: Kao H S R, Sinha D eds. *Asian Perspectives on Psychology* Vol 19. New Delhi: Sage Publications; 1996:237-262.

52. Ho SMY, Wong KF, Chan, CL-w, Watson M, Tsui YKY. Psychometric properties of the Chinese version of the Mini Mental Adjustment to Cancer (Mini-MAC) Scale. *Psycho-Oncology.* 2003;12(6):547-556.

53. Dovidio JF, Major B, Crocker J. Stigma: introduction and overview. In: Heartherton T f ed. *The Social Psychology of Stigma* New York: Guildford Press; 2000:1-28

54. Ho RTH, Chan CLW, Ho SMY. Emotional control in chinese female cancer survivors; in submission.

55. Classen C, Butler LD, Koopman C, et al. Supportive expressive group therapy and distress in patients with metastatic breast cancer: a randomized clinical intervention trial. *Arch of Gene Psychiatr.* 2001;58:494-501.

56. Classen C, Diamond S, Soleman A, Fobair P, Spira J, Spiegel D. *Brief Supportive-Expressive Group Therapy for Women with Primary Breast Cancer: a Treatment Manual.* Stanford, CA: Stanford University School of Medicine; 1993.

57. Ho DYF. Selfhood and identity in Confucianism, Taosim, Buddhism, and Hinduism: contrasts with the West. *J Theory Social Behav.* 1995;25(2):115-139.

58. Ho DYF. Indigenous psychologies. Asian perspectives. *J Cross Cult Psychol.* 1998;29(1):88-103.

59. Ho SMY, Cheung WS. Death metaphors - another dimension of death. Paper presented at: the Death and the Life-World, The Chinese University of Hong Kong; March 27, 2002; Hong Kong.

60. Asai A, Barnlund D. Boundaries of the unconscious, private, and public self in Japanese and Americans: a cross-cultural comparison. *Int J Intercultural Relations.* 1998;22(4):431-452.

61. Kitayama S, Markus HR, Kurokawa M. Culture, emotion, and well-being: good feelings in Japan and the United States. *Cognition Emotion.* 2000;14(1):93-124.

62. Balint M. The medecin, his patient and the illness. *Int.* University press; 1957.

63. Mouysset JL, Backiuchka-Palmorro M, Dudoit E. Les ateliers de nutrition, une expérience de 4 années *Communication Congrès national de la Société Française de Psycho-Oncologie* CAEN; 2001.

64. Chabert A, Ganot J, Intrup J. Un groupe de parole à l'hôpital pour des femmes en cours de *traitement* radiothérapique du cancer du sein. *Rev Francoph Psycho-onco.* 2002;3-4:61-64.

65. Machavoine JL, Labarre N, Simonet M, et al. Besoins partagés, demandes exprimées: expérience d'un groupe de soutien psychothérapique dans un centre de lutte contre le cancer *Actes du Congrès National de la Société Française de Psycho-oncologie-* PARIS; 1999.

66. Machavoine JL, Labarre N, Simonet M, et al. (2001) Expérience d'un Groupe de Soutien Psychothérapique dans un Centre de Lutte Contre le Cancer Communication *XVIII ème Congrès de la Société Française de Psycho-oncologie, Caen, 4–6, octobre 2001.*

67. Saltel P, De Raucourt D, Derzelle M, et al. Standards, options et recommandations pour une bonne pratique en psycho-oncologie. *Bull Cancer.* 1995;82(10):847-864

68. Diamond S, Gore-Felton C, Gale DA, Classen, C, & Spiegel, D. *Supportive-expressive group therapy for persons with HIV infection: A treatment manual.* Psychosocial Treatment Laboratory, Department of Psychiatry and Behavioral Sciences, Stanford University School of Medicine, Stanford, CA, 1995.

69. Temoshok L. Biopsychosocial studies on cutaneous malignant melanoma: psychosocial factors associated with prognostic indicators, progression, psychophysiology, and tumor-host response. *Soc Sci Med.* 1985;20(8):833-840.

70. Spiegel D. *Living Beyond Limits: New Help and Hope for Facing Life-Threatening Illness.* New York: Times Books/Random House; 1993.

71. Jarrett SR, Ramirez AJ et al. Measuring coping in breast cancer. *J Psychosom Res* 1992; 36(6):593–602.

72. Spiegel D, Kimberling R. Group psychotherapy for women with breast cancer: Relationships among social support, emotional expression and survival. *Emotion, Social Relationships, and Health.* B. Singer, ed., Oxford University Press, 2001:97–123.

73. Yalom, ID *Existential Psychotherapy.* 1980. New York: Basic Books.

Part III

Symptoms and Their Management across Cultures

CHAPTER 9

The Cultural Experience
of Cancer Pain

Judith A. Paice and Joseph F. O'Donnell

> *Every system is perfectly designed to get the results*
> *it gets.*
>
> DONALD BERWICK[1]

INTRODUCTION

Kleinman has described health care systems as forms of social reality where everyday life is enacted, where social roles are defined and performed, in which people through discourse and actions negotiate with each other in established relationships under a system of cultural rules.[2] For these reasons, health care systems greatly affect the way cancer pain is addressed. As a symptom that requires interdisciplinary care and is "owned" by no one discipline, organizations must support the structure and communication necessary to provide cancer pain relief. Because systems are made up of the individuals who are members of the organization, each health care professional must understand the cultural impact of systems, barriers to adequate pain control, pain syndromes common in cancer, the components of a thorough assessment, as well as an ability to communicate available treatment options. Furthermore, because cancer pain often occurs within a cluster of associated symptoms, knowledge regarding the care of these phenomena is necessary.

ORGANIZATION OF HEALTH CARE SYSTEMS IN THE UNITED STATES AND UNITED KINGDOM

Health care systems are complex, complicated, and constantly in flux. There is no "perfect" health care system and each seems to evolve to fit the "culture" and reflect the "values" of the society it serves. The US and UK healthcare systems represent different approaches to the delivery of health care in these highly developed and affluent western societies. Each has its own strengths and weaknesses. These two nations that some say are made up of "two peoples divided by a common language" (an extremely superficial comparison) have evolved health systems that are quite different from each other (Table 1).[3]

TABLE 1. Comparison of Population Demographics of the US and UK

	US	UK
Population	272 639 608	59 113 439
Age structure (yrs)		
0–14	22%	19%
15–64	66%	65%
65+	12%	16%
Life expectancy	76.23 yrs	77.37 yrs
Males	72.95 yrs	74.73 yrs
Females	79.67 yrs	80.15 yrs
Race/ethnic groups		
Caucasian	83.5%	93.8%
African American	12.4%	
Asian	3.3%	0.6%
Native American	0.8%	
Indian		1.6%
Pakistani		1.0%
Black Caribbean		0.9%
Black African		0.6%
Black Other		0.5%
Bangladeshi		0.4%
Literacy[a]	97%	99%
Population below poverty	12.7%[b]	17%
Cancer incidence	189.2/100 000	247.8/100 000

[a] 1978 estimate.
[b] 1998 estimate.

The "modern" UK system has been in place since the founding of the National Health Service (NHS) in 1948. Healthcare in the United Kingdom is thought of as a public service or a social good. Though patients with resources may purchase extra care, governmental funding through taxes finances health care. This percentage of public funding is approximately 90%. Coverage is universal with no one uninsured and the cost is free at the point of service, at a cost of 7% of the gross national product (GNP).[4]

The UK system is based on an emphasis on primary care providers (GPs) as the access point. GPs usually see patients in ambulatory settings. Specialists or consultants provide in-hospital care. The recruitment of clinicians into generalist careers is an increasingly difficult problem.[5] There is a limited role for the "for profit" sector of healthcare in the United Kingdom. During Prime Minister Thatcher's administration, the government tried to impose what they termed as "quasi market" strategies to help control costs. It seems that in the United Kingdom there is more of a fear of real markets, a resistance to competition and a tolerance for bureaucratic central control. For instance, the Blair government in 1997 toned down the market strategies of the Thatcher regime.[6] Overall, the NHS strategy is to maximize the "collective good," and this may sometimes conflict with the care of an individual patient. Nonetheless, there is general satisfaction with this strategy, but often there may be periods of unrest in the public when "lines get too long" or hospital beds are felt to be "not available." Care in the United Kingdom is sometimes delayed, generally restrained and characterized by more "wait and see" with patients encouraged to have a "stiff upper lip."[4]

In the United States, coverage is employer based, though 40% to 50% of the funding comes through governmental programs (ie, Medicare, Medicaid, Veterans Administration). This market-based system creates the unfortunate and unwanted problem that up to 44 million citizens are uninsured, many more are underinsured, and these numbers are rising each year. In addition, 30 million citizens live in designated medically underserved areas.[7] Some would categorize the health care industry in the United States as more of a "business opportunity," rather than a social good.5 The United States uses 14% of the GNP for health care (and this is rising faster than inflation). Coverage is very complicated with many variations of health insurance policies, each with their own deductibles or co-payment requirements. The Medicare regulations have more than 137 000 pages of complicated rules. (Contrast this with the tax code, which has about 10 000 pages). Despite efforts to increase the role of primary care, specialty and tertiary care dominate the US system. Clinicians spend time both in and move between the hospital and ambulatory setting. There seem to be more incentives for doing more rather than less (or even what is known to work). Deeply ingrained beliefs in market principles, entrepreneurship, and the competitive value of innovation drive US medicine. The US system seeks to provide "patient centered" individualistic health care with a premium on intervention and innovation. There is a general dissatisfaction among the public with the system as it now exists, although most patients are more satisfied with their individual clinician.[8] There is also a great deal of "resistance to change" inbred in this complicated system with many interested parties wanting to preserve the status quo. There are periodic attempts to switch to a "single payer" system, the most recent being the ill-fated Clinton Health Plan that failed due to political pressure. Also, at the state level, there are additional innovative attempts to control costs, increase coverage (especially to vulnerable populations), and ensure quality (eg, Oregon and Vermont).

Most people, both from inside and outside the United States believe that the country provides the most advanced health care in the world. It is a system that values discovery, application, and innovation. Yet within this US "system" are in fact many subsystems of care and many of these have results comparable to those in countries that are far less technologically advanced than the United States. There is considerable evidence that the "U.S. Healthcare system does not provide consistent high quality medical care to all people."[9] For instance, despite the high level of spending, the US ranks far below the top nations on such indicators as infant mortality, life expectancy, and many other indicators. The health statistics for African Americans actually worsened in the decade of the 1980s and in 1993, the gap in health status was reported to have widened between the affluent and poor.[10] As a consequence, there has been a recent call for a redesign of the system, one with the following characteristics: safety, effectiveness, patient centeredness, timeliness, efficiency, and equity.

Both systems in the United States and the United Kingdom face considerable challenges. Several are listed in Table 2. All of these issues are placed in a system that is growing increasingly complex, with more and more stakeholders creating more and more demands. These are only a few of the challenges that each system is trying to meet.

PREVALENCE OF CANCER PAIN

Cancer is a common disease; about one in three people living in the United Kingdom or the United States will eventually have cancer and it is the second leading cause of death. In the global context, pain remains a common symptom for patients with cancer and pain control remains a significant problem despite widespread and aggressive educational campaigns. By applying already known principles of pain management, more than 90% of

TABLE 2. Challenges Facing Health Care Systems within the US and UK

- *Control of costs:* Costs continue to rise and cost control measures, which have most recently taken the form of "managed care," have failed to bring control. Leaders in each system spend an increasing proportion of their energy and time on this problem with no easy solutions in sight.
- *The explosion of scientific discovery:* The recent scientific revolution is the most impressive in human history, The understanding of the root causes and development of targeted treatments and prevention strategies for diseases have never been more hopeful. Yet, the path from bench to bedside is still difficult and systems to incorporate and utilize discovery are needed. It is almost impossible for the individual clinician to keep up to date with this knowledge explosion.
- *The role of the informatics revolution:* We have powerful new ways of storing, analyzing, and communicating data that we have never had before. This power needs to be harnessed and utilized to improve outcomes. We are only at the beginning of realizing this potential.
- *The quest for quality:* We need to know what works, what works best and at the same time is most cost effective. It is a tragedy that so much of what is done in medicine lacks the "evidence base" to support it. The application of outcome measures will help this situation.
- *The loss of stature of the professional:* There is no question that some of the prestige has been lost for clinicians in medicine. Ethical scandals, business motives, mistakes (which are far too common), and the erosion of compassion have tarnished the practice of medicine. There is a great deal of attention being paid to the restoration of professional values by medical organizations. Much needs to be done to restore trust in the system
- *The challenges of globalization:* We live in a global village. Infectious agents can travel at the speed of aeroplanes. No longer is the practice of medicine just a local phenomenon. In addition, a healthy workforce is an important element to be able to compete in the global market.
- *The changing disease burden:* At the turn of the 20th century, most illness was acute and death occurred at a much younger age. As infections came under better control, the lifespan increased and the illness burden shifted to more chronic diseases like cancer, heart disease, and diabetes, and these required prolonged intervention and continuity of care over the long term.
- *The challenges of diversity:* The United States is a nation of immigrants. The percentage of people from different parts of the world continues to change the ethnic composition of the United States. These different ethnic groups bring with them their cultural traditions, their worldviews, their values, and their language. This adds tremendous complication to the medical encounter as we struggle to try to understand each other.

---

pain can be controlled and through referral to specialized pain centers with specialized knowledge and techniques, most of the remaining may be controllable also.[11] It is estimated that 30% to 45% of patients with cancer will have moderate to severe pain at diagnosis or in the intermediate stages of their illness. On average, 75% of patients with advanced cancer have pain. Of those patients with cancer and related pain, 25% to 30% describe it as moderate to severe and 25% to 35% describe it as severe.[12]

Cancer Pain in Minorities

Patients from minority groups have higher incidence and death rates at younger ages for certain cancers, more exposure to risk factors predisposing to cancer, they tend to be diagnosed later with more advanced stage tumors, and may experience less aggressive care.[13] The tragedy is that the gap seems to be widening rather than closing in the United States. As an example, African Americans are less likely offered curative surgery for breast, colon, and lung cancer.[14] As an important symptom in cancer, pain is much more likely to be inadequately assessed, treated, and controlled in minority patients.[15]

Multiple studies have shown inadequate treatment of cancer-related pain in minority populations. Cleeland and colleagues[16] found that outpatients with cancer pain who were treated in clinics that served ethnic and racial minority patients were three times more likely to be undermedicated with analgesics when compared to patients in other settings. In a later study, this group[17] reported that 65% of minority patients left an office visit with an inadequate medication prescription for control of their pain versus 50% of nonminority patients (the latter statistic a large enough problem in its own right). The dose of narcotics prescribed in patient-controlled anesthesia varied in different ethnic groups.[18] Minority patients with bone fractures were twice as likely to receive inadequate doses of analgesics in the emergency room compared to nonminority patients.[19] These inequities also have been documented in nursing homes and cancer centers.[20] Numerous studies document inadequate end-of-life care in minority populations.[21]

There have been numerous reports and calls to action because of the great disparities in health care outcomes that occur throughout the United States.[22] The Clinton Administration in their Initiative on Race in America (http://www.wsws.org/public_html/iwb6-30/edit.htm) instituted a number of ongoing initiatives including the upgrading of the office of Minority Health to a Center for Minority Health and Health Disparities at the National Institutes of Health (NIH). This signaled an important message: a center is more influential in setting policy, in influencing budgetary expenditures, and can award grants. For example, the National Cancer Institute's Office of Education is updating its materials on pain and symptom management to make them more accessible, culturally and educationally appropriate and useful to underserved groups.[23] The American Cancer Society has as one of its primary goals to eliminate disparities in cancer outcomes. The Intercultural Cancer Council is bringing together organizations and individuals to collaborate around issues of minority health and disparities in outcomes (http://icc.bcm.tmc.edu/), and the Institute of Medicine (IOM) recently issued a landmark report on eliminating disparities, which has documented inequities and sought solutions.[24] The IOM also has a task force reviewing the structure of the NIH. The NIH has less than 1% of its grants going to investigators from underserved minority groups and only 23 million of a 3 billion NCI budget goes to issues of resolving disparities.[25]

Equity of care is a foundational principle in the NHS. In 1999, the UK Department of Health (DOH) commissioned Ziggi Alexander to study ethnic minority issues in health care. Significant disparities were found in the care of Black, Asian, and other minority groups including differences in disease prevalence and mortality rates, access to care, quality of services, and delivery of services. There was a lack of research on minority groups and in fact, there were NHS policies excluding minority participants from trials. There was an under representation of minority leaders in the NHS and DOH. Yet, one DOH and NHS priority is to reduce these disparities. In response to Alexander's report, the DOH acknowledged that it is "working to mainstream these issues in everything we do as part of our program of modernisation and specific priorities for action."[26]

In addition, there are compelling data on the role of socioeconomic status that transcend the effects of race.[27] Poorer people are sicker and tend to present to the health care system at more advanced stages of disease. They have been shown to have inadequate access and inadequate resources for self-care. Even when controlled for risk factors and access, poorer people have been shown to have increased mortality for similar diseases.[28] Higher levels of education, especially for women, are also associated with better health outcomes.[29]

Barriers to Cancer Pain Management

Many of the reasons for inadequate pain control and the barriers to adequate pain relief have been identified and reviewed in the pain literature.[11] Barriers include those attributed to the health care professional, to the patient, and to the system. These same barriers are present in minority populations to an even greater degree.

Although it is inappropriate to promote stereotypes for a group, there are certain characteristics that do seem to be more common in individuals from minority groups. These individuals tend to come from poorer socioeconomic groups, to be more often un-or underinsured, to have less formal educational achievement, and to come from poorer neighborhoods. However, numerous studies have shown that minority patients may not be offered the same level of intervention no matter what their health or economic status, so these issues go beyond those associated with just poverty.[28]

Patient and family barriers include a reluctance to report pain in the fear of jeopardizing aggressive disease-oriented treatment, fear that pain means the disease is progressing, concern about not being perceived as a "good" patient, reluctance to take medications for fear of addiction or stigmatization, worries about side effects and tolerance. Minority patients tend to experience even greater barrier to adequate pain control. Language, underlying cultural belief systems and the ability to understand "the other" remain challenging. Patients from some minority populations may show less outward behavior related to pain causing observers to underestimate the pain.[29]

African Americans and Mexican Americans tend to believe in the "dignity" that is associated with suffering and may report later in the course of their illnesses to clinicians or tend to minimize discomfort.[30] Minority patients tend to lack trust in a system that has not treated them fairly.[31] This is felt to be due to a historical accumulation of social injustices making the system and its motives seem suspect. Patients know the statistics of morbidity and mortality in minorities and may fear being "undertreated" rather than receiving aggressive disease specific care. For many, "quantity of life equals quality of life." Minority patients are more likely to live in poverty and to have poorer health in general. They are more likely to have to attend to the stresses and survival needs of daily existence than to have time and energy for self-care. Their insurance coverage is likely to be less. Maslow found that 31% of minority patients had no health insurance vs 14% of Caucasians.[24] Even when employed, minority workers were less likely to be covered (56% vs 66%).[24] Fifteen percent of minority patients openly said that they would get better care if they were members of a different race.[24]

Another set of barriers are those of clinicians and they include a lack of up-to-date knowledge, inadequate assessments in time limited encounters, fear of prescribing powerful drugs with regulatory concerns about their licenses, fear of promoting addiction in patients, or producing difficult to manage side effects.[32] Minorities again face more significant barriers. The maldistribution of services makes areas populated by large numbers of minority patients have fewer clinicians and fewer choices. Overall access to care is harder and even when in the "system," minority patients make fewer visits. Minority patients have fewer available clinicians and fewer choices. Clinics in these areas are more likely to be understaffed and busier. Minority patients have less access to specialists (8% of minorities vs 18% of nonminorities get referrals).[33] Minority patients have less participatory visits with clinicians.[34]

Most importantly, racial stereotypes still exist. The IOM report described these in great detail. Nonminorities are more likely to believe that minorities "live off welfare, are more prone to violence, are less intelligent and lazy."[35] This may cause projection of a stereotype that undervalues a patient's participation in medical decision-making. Often this is thought to be unintentional and unconscious but it is readily perceived by the patients. Studies have shown that clinicians make different and less aggressive recommendations to minority standardized patients who are playing roles with the same levels of illness as nonminorities.[36] There are also not enough minority clinicians in the workforce despite valiant efforts to raise the numbers.[37] Presently, there are ongoing efforts in medical schools and residencies to address issues of cultural competency training, but there is still a long way to go in this area.[38]

System issues that have been identified include a low priority given to pain management, inadequate reimbursement, restrictive regulation policies and problems with availability of the medications, and limited access to pain specialists. Despite large gains in equity, institutional racism still exists. Racial stereotypes are listed above and views like these may pervade institutions. Experts now say that the old version of "Jim Crow" overt racism has turned to a subtle "laissez faire" version and that people are not even conscious of it.[39] It can be identified in hiring policies, leadership policies (who are the advocates for these patients?), the fact that managed care shies away from minority patients with greater risk, and is less likely to employ and more likely to terminate minority clinicians.[40] Our system tolerates poorer health outcomes in the poor, and we see hospitals and clinics either not locating in or moving from minority neighborhoods. Even with cost and lack of access as huge barriers and even if a minority patient gets "in" the system and gets a prescription for pain medicines, the pharmacies in the neighborhoods are less likely to stock the drugs because of fear of robbery and violence.[41] In addition, we do not have enough data now, nor do we collect it, to know the extent of problem. Experts suggest that regulatory organizations require reporting of such health care disparities as a first step in beginning to correct them.[42]

All is not bleak though. There exist jewels of programs that may serve as models to better address these issues. The Harlem Palliative Care Network, a collaborative project between Memorial Sloan-Kettering Cancer Center, North General Hospital, and the Visiting Nurse Service of New York is such a jewel worth emulating.[43]

CANCER PAIN SYNDROMES

To provide relief from cancer pain, clinicians must be aware of the multidimensional nature of pain, particularly the concept of suffering. Furthermore, an awareness of the common pain syndromes, their etiology and presentation is necessary when conducting a thorough pain assessment and developing a treatment plan.

Suffering

Dame Cicely Saunders, founder of the hospice movement, coined the term "total pain" to define the pain experience.[44] Pain is more than a simple biological construct since it is more than the biological damage that may occur in a nerve or a tissue or an organ. Pain is both the stimulus and the person's response to it since it includes psychological, social, emotional, financial, spiritual, and existential dimensions. It varies from person to person from the stoic, "keep it all inside" person to the emotional and expressive person.[12]

Suffering is a broader term. It is probably one of the most common symptoms that accompany illness. It refers to loss of the personhood, a threat to the identity and future of the person, and it constitutes a threat to the self-image, a perceived lack of options for coping, a sense of personal loss, and a lack of a basis for hope.[45] Suffering is most eloquently discussed in the work of Eric Cassell. Cassell states that: "the test of medicine should be its adequacy in the face of suffering...modern medicine fails that test. In fact, the central assumptions in which twentieth century medicine is founded provide no basis for an understanding of suffering. For pain, difficulty in breathing, or other difficulties of the body, superbly yes: for suffering, no."[45]

Michael Kearney, an Irish palliative care physician, has written extensively about this topic.[46,47] He states that the "medical model" is excellent in attending to the physical aspects of the pain experience. Physical pain, which is damage or perceived damage to a cell or a tissue or an organ, can often be "controlled" through attention to careful assessment, to treating the underlying process, and by careful applications of interventions from "without," such as medications or procedures with careful assessment and adjustments to make sure they work. The other physical symptoms like anxiety, depression, social concerns, and other co-existent symptoms may also be approached by interventions from without.[46,47]

Kearney further proposes that the medical model remains unable to deal with the nature of suffering including the threatened loss of integrity of the person. As a remedy, he suggests that we invoke a different model, given that most of our ideas in Western, "evidence based" medicine are inherited from the school of Hippocrates. Kearney informs us that at the time of Hippocrates, there were actually many schools of medicine. One was called the Aescalapian school or "temple medicine."[47] Aescalapius is the Greek God of healing and the staff of Aescalapius is the symbol of medicine. The Aescalapian School attended to people with illnesses that often could not be dealt with by other schools, including incurable diseases. Patients in this tradition would go to the temples, located in beautiful places and be attended by people called Therapeutes (from which the term therapeutic is derived). They would bathe, rest, meditate, eat well, and at some point in their "stay," go to sleep in the temple. At this time, there they would have some type of personal experience, for example, a dream, and perhaps, they would leave the temple on the next day "healed." The Aescalapian tradition believed that healing was not ours to give, it came from within, or from the earth (like the snake crawling up the staff).[47]

Kearney suggests we take a similar approach to suffering, since "our job is to create a safe space where healing can happen." We do this best by listening, "witnessing," and validating our patient's plight. He uses terms from psychotherapy. We must "contain and hold" the space, "stay with and support" the patient so their own healing powers from within can have a chance to work.[47] There is a tremendous benefit to patients to feel "listened to." Moreover, the patients may be able to teach the clinicians how to approach the care of suffering. For example, the African American spiritual tradition of "witnessing" should be very helpful to the relief of suffering. Kearney also uses tools from psychotherapy like dream analysis to draw deep into the psyche to deal with suffering which he also calls "soul pain."[47] Much of what is seen in the Aescalapian tradition is also reflected in some aspects of alternative or complementary medicine, which seems to focus more on the "care of the self" with things like nutrition, meditation, aromatherapy, massage, and laying down of the hands.[47]

It has been said that the most powerful tool in the clinician's armamentarium is the physician him/her self. Kearney teaches the therapeutic use of self and his writings are important tools in the approach to and relief of suffering.[47] And perhaps it was Dame Cicely Saunders who said it best when she stated that: "The way we care can reach the most hidden places" and "the real presence of another person is a sense of security."[44]

Common Syndromes in Cancer Pain

Cancer pain can result from three primary etiologies. The majority of pain experienced by individuals with cancer originates directly from the tumor.[48] Pain can also occur as a result of therapy aimed at reducing the tumor, including surgery, chemotherapy, radiation therapy, and other treatments. For example, surgery produces incisional pain, some chemotherapeutics can produce painful neuropathies, and hormonal therapy often leads to an acute onset of generalized bone pain in those being treated for prostate cancer. Finally, people with cancer can experience pain totally unrelated to

TABLE 3. Pain Syndromes Common in Cancer

Pain associated with the tumor
Bone metastases
Invasion of sacral, brachial, or other nerve

Pain associated with the treatment
Surgery related
    Procedural pain after surgery, diagnostic procedures, invasive techniques
    Post-surgical syndromes
        Post-mastectomy syndrome
        Post-thoracotomy syndrome
        Phantom limb pain
Chemotherapy related
    Mucositis
    Painful flare
    Peripheral neuropathy secondary to chemotherapy
        Vinca alkaloids, cisplatin, oxaliplatin, thalidomide, taxol
Radiation related
    Skin reaction

Pain unrelated to cancer or its treatment
Arthritis
Diabetic neuropathy

the cancer or its treatment, such as arthritis, diabetic neuropathy, or ischemic vascular disease (see Table 3).

The prevalence of these syndromes and the extent of pain intensity in different cultural groups have not been extensively explored. Laboratory studies using experimental pain models (including heat, cold, and pressure) suggest that African Americans report greater sensitivity to these stimuli when compared with Caucasians and that women report greater responses than men.[49,50] Clinical studies of acute and chronic pain states are inconsistent in their findings when examining racial or cultural disparities.[51–54] These differences have not been explored in a cancer population, although a study of patients with HIV demonstrated higher levels of pain reported by African Americans.[55] Racial and ethnic differences may be due to biological, social, psychological mechanisms, and the cultural context of care.[49]

MEASUREMENT, ASSESSMENT, AND COMMUNICATION REGARDING CANCER PAIN

Understanding the nature of the patient's pain is critical. This information is obtained through the pain history, supplemented with information obtained through the physical examination and additional diagnostic workup, when indicated.[56] The pain history includes the location (or as often occurs in cancer, multiple locations are involved), the pain intensity, the terms used to describe the quality of the pain, as well as factors that aggravate or alleviate the pain. Past experiences with pain and pain treatment provides clues regarding the meaning of pain and responses (favorable and unfavorable) to pharmacologic and nonpharmacologic therapies.

Unidimensional Tools

Instruments used to quantify aspects of the pain assessment range from unidimensional measures, such as tools that determine pain intensity, to multidimensional scales that attempt to capture physical, affective and other domains.[57,58] Pain intensity scales include the numerical rating scale (NRS), where 0 indicates "no pain" and 10 denotes the "worst pain imaginable." The NRS can be used as a paper and pencil scale or can be administered verbally without visual cues, and they have been translated into numerous languages. Histogram representation of the 0 to 10, with the smallest bar indicating 1 and increasing incrementally to the tallest bar denoting 10, is under study in non-English speaking and low literacy populations who might have difficulty with the verbal 0 to 10 scale.[59] Visual analog scales (VAS) illustrate pain as a 10 cm (or 100 mm) linear continuum, anchored with the same descriptors used in the NRS. The patient is asked to make a mark on a point on the line that best represents their pain intensity. This requires visual and motor acuity, and some studies suggest that elders or cognitively impaired persons have difficulty completing the VAS.[60] Hybrid forms of the NRS and VAS have been used, where a vertical or horizontal line is anchored with descriptor and numbers. Other tools include verbal descriptor scales (VDS), where patients are asked to rate their pain intensity using such terms as "no pain, mild, moderate, severe, excruciating."[61] Although these pain intensity scales have demonstrated validity and reliability, care must be taken when selecting descriptors that are clearly understood by the patient. And those descriptors must be used consistently, otherwise, change in pain or response to treatment will be difficult to ascertain.

Despite the seeming simplicity of these unidimensional pain intensity tools, at least one study has demonstrated that when nurses have a different "mother tongue" than the patient, they are more likely to report disparities in pain intensity when compared to the patient's rating.[61] Thus, culture and ethnicity can affect simple pain intensity ratings.

Pediatric tools include a faces scale, illustrating a range of emotions from happy to very distressed, the Oucher scales, which include pictures of children in various states of discomfort (employing children of different gender and ethnic backgrounds), and the Eland color scale, which uses four colors on a gender-neutral figure drawing to indicate the intensity and location of pain. A comprehensive review of pediatric pain measures can be found in several texts.[62,63]

Multidimensional Instruments

Comprehensive, multidimensional tools include the McGill Pain Questionnaire (MPQ) and the Brief Pain Inventory (BPI). In a study using the MPQ for cancer pain, investigators found no differences in the sensory component of pain amongst various ethnic groups. However, patients who identified their ethnic origin as England, Germany, Scandinavia, or Italy scored lower on the affective subscale of the MPQ, although the reasons for these differences are unclear.[64] The BPI includes pain intensity measures and a functional impairment subscale, where patients are asked to indicate the degree (0 to 10) to which pain has interfered with their activity, mood, ability to walk, work, relations with others, sleep, and enjoyment with life.[65] The BPI has been translated into a large number of languages, including French, Mandarin, Spanish, Vietnamese, and many others. In a study of Taiwanese patients, the BPI was valid only in those with higher educational level, suggesting that terminology may need to be modified for those with fewer years of formal education.[66]

Physical Assessment

While conducting a comprehensive assessment, it is critical to consider that behavioral responses are unreliable indicators of pain. "He does not look as if he is in pain" is a common response heard by clinicians. Cultural issues account for much of the disparity seen in these behavioral expressions. Some cultures believe that pain is a necessary part of life and that denying expression of pain is a sign of dignity and strength. These beliefs have been attributed to Mexican Americans, Hispanics, and Latin Americans, as well as the Japanese and Chinese,[67,68] although more research must be completed to verify these findings. Many stoic patients, including the elderly, are even reluctant to use the term "pain," in part because the meaning of the pain or the reluctance to be a "bad patient." Some worry that admitting to pain must imply the cancer has returned. Skilled clinicians will continue questioning when these patients deny pain, using alternate terms such as discomfort or hurt.[32]

   The comprehensive physical examination indicated in identifying the etiology of cancer-related pain is described in detail in several textbooks.[48,69] Little research has been conducted in relationship to cultural influences and pain-related physical assessment. Clearly, sensitivity to modesty concerns within various ethnic and religious groups is warranted while conducting this examination.[70] For example, many Islamic women and women of Chinese descent prefer to be examined by a female health care professional. Religious beliefs may also require that clothing remain in place during the evaluation or that family members be present. Optimally, if the clinician does not speak the same language as the patient, a professional translator will be present, although separated to provide privacy.

After conducting a thorough pain history and physical examination, a plan of care is developed, optimally with the patient and their family. This requires effective communication on the part of all involved.

Communication

The expression of pain is a form of communication, and cultural differences in emotional expression and stereotypes about pain also influence the clinician's interpretation and expectations regarding pain severity. This is possibly due to the conscious and unconscious bias on the part of the clinician and patient, or the subtle differences in cultural expressive cues (ie, body language) that the individual can more readily recognize emotion expressed in the style in which they are accustomed.[71,72] Given the problems with communication and treating cancer-related pain, guidelines for effective pain communication are receiving more attention than ever in medical education. It has been designated one of the core competencies that the Accreditation Council for Graduate Medical Education (ACGME) has said that all residency graduates must possess (www.acgme.org/outcome/comp/compFull.asp).

Communication may be verbal, in writing, or even by "sign" and it may utilize techniques from simple words or gestures to sophisticated media. Body language (or para communication) can portray even more information than is carried in words. No matter what the medium, each message involves a sender, a receiver, and a code, and is done in a particular context. The message of the sender and what is heard by the receiver can be affected by such things as age, sex, culture, language, education, physical impairments, and emotional states.

Communication about pain involves words, expectations and behaviors. Words may have different meanings (eg, words like "pain, hurt, or ache" may be used and interpreted differently by both the sender and the receiver). Body language and behaviors indicating pain may be much less pronounced in certain minority groups causing clinicians to underestimate their pain.[29]

A typical history of pain should include the quality, quantity, duration or frequency, onset, location, radiation to other sites, precipitating factors, aggravating and alleviating factors, and associated symptoms. It is important to ascertain the time line of the pain and when the patient last was pain free, how it interferes with daily life, how it has been treated (including any over the counter or "folk" remedies) and what are the complications of the pain itself and what it is being treated with. It is also important to ascertain information about co-morbid conditions and any social, emotional, or other things contributing.[70,73]

Useful questions might include: What keeps you from doing what you want to do? Where is the pain? Does it interrupt your sleep? Is it predictable? How long does it last? If it goes away after you take medicines, how long does it take? (This helps determine if short-acting analgesic doses are adequate.) How long does the relief last? (This helps determine if the dosing interval of the short-acting drug is appropriate or if the dose of long-acting drugs is appropriate.)

One useful model of the interview is the Cohen-Cole three-component model.[74] According to this model, the purpose of the interview is to develop rapport, to gather information and to negotiate a plan of further steps to achieve realizable therapeutic goals. Developing rapport happens best when there is mutual respect. A model for building this respect comes from the work of Dr. Ned Cassem.[75]

Cassem suggests that all illness (pain included) is a threat to the personhood. He tells his residents who are seeing patients with heart attacks that: "On the same day your patient suffers a myocardial infarction, he or she also suffers an ego infarction and it takes the ego much longer to recover." As a remedy, Cassem suggests that we need to try to "rescue our patients from the anonymity that accompanies illness." We need to find out: "Who is this person? Who were they at the top of their game?" What defines him/her?" Thus, rather than subordinating the patient's narrative of illness to the dominant biomedical narrative, we need to connect our stories with theirs.

Suffering in the context of cancer and pain can serve to create a disparity between whom the person was, who they are, and if they have a future.[76] According to Cassem's model, care and repair of the self can begin by asking three categories of questions: (a) What are their accomplishments? (eg, prowess in acting, music, awards won, sports, rank in military, status in the neighborhood, etc.) He also suggests we ask about things that they are ambivalent about or even "naughty" stories. (b) Who is really important to them? (eg, who loves them? whom do they love? who are they closest to? what are their big stories? even who are their enemies?) (c) What are their favorite things? (Cassem's favorite topic, eg, music, books or poems, newspapers, movies, stars, hobbies, sports teams, restaurants, food, and cars) Also, do they have any aversions? Any addictions? Somewhere in these questions may come a closeness, a respect, a "connection" and once the patient knows that we care, he or she is more likely to let us into "hidden" places and may indeed even let us know what might help them.

Stewart[77] has argued: "Without some agreement about the nature of what is wrong, it is difficult for a doctor and a patient to agree on a plan of management that is acceptable to both of them. It is not essential for the physician actually to believe that the nature of the problem is as the patient sees it, but the doctor's explanation and recommended treatment must at least be consistent with the patient's point of view." These points of view differ not only across ethnic differences but also across socioeconomic, gender, sex, age, religious, and occupational differences. Perhaps the greatest challenge is to understand patients across cultural barriers. To do so, one must acquire a set of skills, knowledge, and attitudes that enhance the understanding of and respect for a patient's values, beliefs and expectations, awareness of one's own assumptions and values (as well as those of the medical system), and the ability to adapt care to be congruent with the patient's expectations.[70,73,78] Some dimensions of culture include; health and illness beliefs (what paradigm is used to explain illness/healing?); decision-making style (does decision-making rest with the individual patient, the group/family, or community peers?): healing traditions (what are the alternative/complementary approaches used?); locus of control (do the individuals believe that they are responsible for their own destiny or is it predetermined [fate]?); status/hierarchy (is the status of head of household conferred by age, gender, or kinship?); privacy (is privacy at the level of the individual or family?): communication (is there a preferred mode of communication, eg, written, verbal, sign? Is there a preferred language? Is an interpreter needed?: Socioeconomic status (is social status in the community conferred based on family, vocation, wealth, or education?); and immigrant status (are there acculturation and generational issues at play?).

Kleinman[2] suggests asking the following questions to ascertain the patient's explanatory model for their illness: (a) What do you call the problem?; (b) What do you think caused the problem?; (c) Why do you think it started when it did?; (d) What do you think the sickness does? How does it work?; (e) How severe is the sickness? Will it have a long or a short course?; (f) What kind of treatment do you think you should receive?; (g) What are the most important results you hope to receive from this treatment?; (h) What are the chief problems the sickness has caused?; (i) What do you fear most about the sickness? The approach to a patient presenting with pain may be summarized by the RESPECT model (Table 4).[77]

It has been shown that more accurate information is obtained when there is not a language barrier. On occasion, a translator may be necessary

TABLE 4. Respect Model

R = Rapport
Connect on a social level
See the patient's point of view
Consciously attempt to suspend judgment
Recognize and avoid making assumptions

E = Empathy
Remember that the patient has come to you for help
Seek out and understand the patient's rationale for his/her
 behavior or illness.
Verbally acknowledge and legitimize the patient's feelings.

S = Support
Ask about and try to understand barriers to care and compliance
Help the patient overcome barriers
Involve family members if appropriate
Reassure the patient you are and will be available to help

P = Partnership
Be flexible with regard to issues of control
Negotiate roles when necessary
Stress that you are working together to address medical
 problems

E = Explanations
Check often for understanding
Ask for clarification

C = Cultural competence
Respect the patient and his/her culture and beliefs
Understand that the patient's view of you may be defined
 by ethnic or cultural stereotypes
Be aware of your own biases and preconceptions
Know your limitations in addressing medical issues across cultures
Understand your personal style and recognize when it
 may not be working with a given patient

T = Trust
Self-disclosure may be an issue for some patients who are
not accustomed to Western medical approaches
Take the necessary time and consistently work to establish trust.

---

and this may make communication even more difficult. Some suggestions
when using an interpreter include: encourage the interpreter to meet the
patient before the interview if possible and try to meet with the interpreter
yourself, ask the interpreter to provide feedback, tell the interpreter your
goals, ask the interpreter if they have any concerns, introduce the interpreter
to the patient, look at the patient, watch for nonverbal communication,

avoid jargon, encourage the interpreter to repeat verbatim what the patient said, ask the patient to repeat your instructions at the end of the visit to check for understanding, and be patient.[15] It is advisable not to use family members if at all possible.

TREATMENT OF CANCER PAIN

Drug therapy is the primary treatment for the management of cancer pain. Nonpharmacologic techniques are often useful, particularly as a complement to pharmacologic interventions. Three general categories of drugs are used in the management of cancer pain, including nonopioids, opioids, and adjuvant analgesics. Furthermore, in certain circumstances, cancer therapies can be useful in reducing tumor burden, thereby reducing pain.[11]

Nonopioids

Nonopioids include nonsteroidal anti-inflammatory drugs (NSAIDs) and acetaminophen. NSAIDs interfere with the enzyme cyclooxygenase (prostaglandin synthetase), which blocks the conversion of arachidonic acid to prostaglandins (PGE_1), prostacyclins (PGI_2), and thromboxane (TXA_2). Inhibition of prostaglandin synthesis leads to relief of inflammation and pain.[78] The toxicities associated with NSAIDs include gastrointestinal effects ranging from dyspepsia to hemorrhage, prolonged bleeding time, renal dysfunction, and hypertension.[79–81] Risk factors include age, history of ulcer, concomitant use of corticosteroids or anticoagulants, higher NSAID doses, and may include cigarette and alcohol use.[82,83] Prevention of gastrointestinal toxicity includes the administration of prostaglandin analogs, such as misoprostol, or proton pump blockers. The prolonged bleeding times are reversible once the drug is cleared from the plasma, except for aspirin, which has an irreversible effect on platelet aggregation. Thus, aspirin may be discontinued approximately 1 week before planned invasive procedures. In most cases, renal dysfunction resolves once the NSAID is cleared from the plasma.[80]

The new generation of NSAIDS, called cyclooxygenase-2 or COX-2 inhibitors or selective NSAIDs, have efficacy approximately equal to traditional NSAIDs. Once considered safer than nonselective NSAIDs, controversy exists regarding their safety and whether gastrointestinal toxicities are truly decreased.[84,85] Cost-benefit ratios must be considered when choosing between these agents.

Acetaminophen has both analgesic and antipyretic properties, with little anti-inflammatory activity. Maximum daily doses should not exceed 4 g or 4000 mg,[86] a concern when administering admixtures of opioids and acetaminophen, particularly if patients are taking additional over-the-counter preparations containing acetaminophen.

Opioids

Opioids are the mainstay of treatment for the majority of cancer pain syndromes. They are safe and effective when used appropriately. Unfortunately, their use carries significant stigma, largely due to misunderstandings regarding the terms tolerance, physical dependence, and addiction. Tolerance is "a state of adaptation in which exposure to a drug induces changes that result in a diminution of one or more of the drug's effects over time.[87] Because there is no maximum dose or ceiling effect of agonist opioids, tolerance can be overcome, if it occurs at all, through careful titration. The dose necessary to relieve pain is highly variable and should be based on the patient's self-report of pain severity. Physiologic dependence is "a state of adaptation that is manifested by a drug class specific withdrawal syndrome that can be produced by abrupt cessation, rapid dose reduction, decreasing blood level of the drug, and/or administration of an antagonist."[87] Opioid withdrawal signs include agitation, abdominal cramping and diarrhea, rhinorrhea, piloerection, and pain.[87] Physiologic dependence is not addiction, and should not be a clinical problem. If opioids are no longer necessary, gradual reduction in the dose (by approximately 25% to 50% daily) is sufficient to prevent the abstinence syndrome.[87]

Psychological dependence, or addiction, has been defined as "a primary, chronic, neurobiological disease with genetic, psychological, and environmental factors influencing its development and manifestations ... characterised by behaviours that include one or more of the following: impaired control over drug use, compulsive use, continued use despite harm and craving."[87] Fear of addiction is unjustified and should not serve as a barrier to adequate cancer pain relief. Unfortunately, due in part to excessive media attention to drug diversion, patients and family members fear the development of addiction due to the use of opioids.[88,89] Women, and those from lower socioeconomic groups are more likely to suffer from the stigma associated with opioids and the misperceptions surrounding these terms.[17] Studies repeatedly demonstrate that these patients are provided lower doses of opioids while hospitalized, and have greater difficulty obtaining opioids from pharmacies that serve their neighborhoods.[41] For example, one study documents that women with cancer were prescribed less than half the amount of opioid analgesics when compared with men. Controlling for weight failed to eliminate this disparity.[90]

Opioid Selection

The choice of opioid is based upon the patient's previous response to a particular agent, including both analgesia and adverse effects, as well their need for alternate routes of delivery. Opioids work to relieve a wide variety of pain syndromes, including both nociceptive and neuropathic pain. Erroneously referred to as "opioid-nonresponsive pain," analysis of existing studies suggests that opioids are effective in relieving neuropathic pain.[91,92] However, higher doses of opioids may be needed. Scheduled dosing is preferred over as-needed administration, beginning with a low dose and gradually titrating upward.[93,94] Failure to respond to one opioid should result in rotation to another, due to the wide variability in response to individual opioid agonists.[95] A wide variety of opioids are available for clinical use in various formulations, including immediate-release tablets, long-acting pills and capsules, liquids, suppositories, and parenteral solutions.

Meperidine, propoxyphene, and mixed agonist-antagonists are not recommended in cancer pain. Meperidine is metabolized in the liver to normeperidine, which is then excreted renally. Renal dysfunction leads to accumulation of normeperidine, resulting in central nervous system (CNS) toxicity such as seizures.[96,97] Furthermore, meperidine has poor oral bioavailability; 50 mg of oral meperidine is approximately equianalgesic to two aspirin tablets (650 mg). Propoxyphene, which is metabolized to norpropoxyphene, also demonstrates the potential for CNS toxicity and overall has poor analgesic effects.[88] Mixed agonist-antagonists, such as butorphanol, produce psychotomimetic effects, have a ceiling dose, and can produce abstinence symptoms if given to patients currently receiving pure agonist opioids.

Opioid-Related Adverse Effects

Adverse effects to opioids often can be prevented, and in most cases, easily managed. Clear communication and education is needed to offset patient- and clinician-related barriers effecting the management and treatment of cancer pain.

Constipation Constipation is an almost universal complication of narcotic analgesics. Tolerance to this side effect does not usually occur and it may get worse as therapy continues. It should be managed aggressively beginning with the initiation of opioids.[98] There are also many other conditions that may interfere with bowel function (eg, obstruction, hypercalcemia, neuropathy, and decreased food and water intake) and these should be assessed and addressed.

Ducosate (Colace) and a senna compound should be started with the initiation of opioids. Senna compounds are preferred since they are stimulating and cathartic. Stool softeners or emollient laxatives (Colace) may work less well when used alone. If constipation persists, bisacodyl (Ducolax) tablets (2 to 3) at night or metoclopramide 10 to 20 mg four times a day may be indicated. If constipation persists, and no impaction is found to be present, magnesium citrate (8 oz) may be added. Other options are Fleet Phospho-soda oral solution, mineral oil enemas, Ducolax suppositories, or Fleet Phospho-soda enemas. Lactulose solution can be used orally, but it may cause cramps and flatulence.[98]

If impacted, carefully disimpact, following with enemas until clear. Enemas may include Fleet (containing 150 ml sodium phosphate), which stimulates peristalsis and a rectal colic reflex, or saline enemas that use high volumes of salt water (these are felt to be safe but often uncomfortable). Tap water or soapsuds enemas may cause electrolyte disturbances and should be avoided. For resistant constipation, metoclopramide infusions have been used.

Sedation   Lethargy often accompanies the onset of opioid usage. However, lethargy or sedation may be diminished after the first few days of opioid therapy. If persistent, management may include changing the opioid dose intervals so that lower doses are given more frequently or changing the medication to another equianalgesic preparation. Sleep hygiene needs to be assessed including latency, awakening during sleep, total hours, snoring, partner reports of sleep apnoea and whether the patient feels refreshed.

Caffeinated beverages or caffeine tablets may be helpful. Some patients may benefit from the addition of methylphenidate (Ritalin). It is suggested to begin with 5 mg in the AM, and adjust as tolerated. Some patients may require up to 1.5 mg/kg/d in divided doses. Modafinil (Provigil) 200 to 400 mg/day and pemoline (Cylert) 18.75 mg (1 to 5 tablets in the AM) have also been used but beware of hepatic toxicity with the latter. These agents may also improve the cognitive function of patients on opioids.[99,100]

Nausea and Vomiting   Nausea and vomiting are frequent complications of opioids, particularly in opioid naïve patients. Constipation may exacerbate this and should be treated aggressively. The clinician must assess the other potential causes (eg, obstruction, hypercalcemia, and CNS metastases). Changing opioids may provide relief. If there is a vestibular component (vertigo or positional symptoms), meclizine (12.5 to 25 mg up to qid) may be useful as well as promethazine (25 mg po/pr/iv) up to qid or scopolamine patches. Other agents used are metoclopramide, prochlorperazine (Compazine), perphenazine (Trilafon), or haloperidol. Ondansetron (4 to 8 mg po) is a powerful antiemetic, but is also very expensive. Patients on phenothiazines should be monitored for extrapyramidal side effects. The addition of diphenhydramine (Benadryl) may help if these occur. If nausea begins when the opioid is first started, it may be helpful to give concomitant antiemetics on a fixed schedule.[94,101]

Myoclonus Myoclonus (muscle jerks) may be seen, especially with higher doses of opioids and at end of life. It can be managed by decreasing the dose, changing the preparation or adding a benzodiazepine. The longer acting agents, such are clonazepam, are preferred.[102]

Delirium Anxiety, delirium, and hallucinations are potential adverse effects associated with opioids. Other co-morbid conditions may contribute, especially infection, alcohol withdrawal, CNS disease, or when another CNS active drug is added. Metabolic causes like hypercalcemia, hyponatremia, uremia, hypoxemia, or hepatic dysfunction should be excluded. Delirium sometimes can be managed by changing to an alternate opioid. Haloperidol may also be useful.[103]

Diaphoresis Sweating is commonly seen in chronic opioid use. It can be managed by adding glycopyrrolate (Robinol) 1 to 3 mg at bedtime or hyoscymine (Levsin) 125 to 250 mg up to qid.

Pruritus Itching may be dose dependent. It can be managed by moistening the skin or by adding an antihistamine like diphenhydramine (Benadryl) or an H2 blocker like cimetidine or ranitidine.[94]

Edema Edema/myositis may occur especially in the lower extremities. It has been seen with oxycodone, morphine, fentanyl, hydromorphone, and hydrocodone. It may develop when doxepin, citalopram, fluozitine, and possibly trazadone have been added to stable doses of opioids. To check for myositis, CPK levels need to be done. If present, switch opioids or discontinue any new medicine added.

Urinary Retention Urinary hesitancy or urinary retention may occur with opioids, particularly with spinal administration, but other mechanisms such as an enlarged prostate must be considered. Tricyclic antidepressants often exacerbate this, as may constipation. Bladder catheterization might be temporarily indicated. Terazocin (Hytrin) 1 to 3 mg at night or tamsulosin (Flomax) 0.4 mg 1/2 hr after meals may be helpful.

Sexual Dysfunction Sexual dysfunction and altered libido are common in chronic opioid use. Low testosterone levels may be contributory in both men and women and replacement may be effective. For men, the replacement dose is 200 mg testosterone cypionate intramuscularly every 2 weeks. For women, the dose is 15 mg intramuscularly every 2 weeks. There are topical gels also. After attaining normal levels, erectile problems may persist in men and may be treated with bupropion (Wellbutrin) 75 to 100 mg 1 hr pre-erections or sildenafil (Viagra) 50 to 100 mg 1/2 hr pre-relations. Bupropion (Wellbutrin) may be effective for ejaculatory dysfunction.[104,105]

Respiratory Depression Respiratory depression is a feared complication but it is rarely seen. Patients on long-term dosages usually develop tolerance to this symptom. Physical stimulation is the first maneuver to try if this occurs. Opioid antagonists like naloxone should be given cautiously, as this will lead to rapid onset of the abstinence syndrome and complete return of pain. If antagonists are indicated for severe respiratory depression, low dose of naloxone should be tried first (eg, 0.4 mg in 10 ml of saline, pushing 0.5 to 1 ml of this solution every few minutes).[94]

Adjuvants

Adjuvant analgesics include a variety of agents approved for other purposes, but have been found to provide pain relief. These are of particular benefit in neuropathic pain syndromes, which can be particularly complex and difficult to relieve pain syndromes.

Corticosteroids

Corticosteroids have long been used to treat a variety of neuropathic pain states, particularly those related to cancer.[106] Dexamethasone has the least mineralocorticoid effect and due to the long duration of effect, dosing can be scheduled once per day. Unfortunately, immunosuppressant and endocrine effects limit long-term use.

Tricyclic Antidepressants

Tricyclic antidepressants block the reuptake of biogenic amines including serotonin and norepinephrine.[106,107] Amitriptyline may not be well tolerated, particularly in the elderly, due to its significant anticholinergic effects. Alternative agents include nortriptyline or desipramine.[108] A low dose should be started, usually at bedtime, and titrated every 3 to 7 days based upon the patient's response. Newer serotonin selective reuptake inhibitors, such as fluoxetine, appear to have little efficacy in relieving neuropathic pain.

Anticonvulsants

Anticonvulsants, particularly carbamazepine, phenytoin, or valproate, were used extensively to treat neuropathic pain. Potential toxicities required regular screening, particularly for neutropenia, megaloblastic anemia, and others. Gabapentin, approved for treatment of complex partial seizures, has been shown to demonstrate analgesic properties in both animal and human models of neuropathic pain.[109,110] Using doses of up to 3600 mg/day in randomized controlled multicenter studies of patients with postherpetic neuropathy and diabetic neuropathy, mean daily pain intensity scores decreased significantly and other secondary outcome measures, such as sleep and mood, improved when compared to the placebo groups. The most common side effects, dizziness and sedation, appear to be reduced with slower dose titration. As a result of gabapentin's efficacy and limited adverse effects, it has become the first line therapy in most neuropathic pain states.

Local Anesthetics

Lidocaine (5%) patches effectively reduce pain related to postherpetic neuropathy without any significant plasma levels of drug found with application of up to three patches.[111] Oral lidocaine analogs, such as mexiletine, have been shown to be effective in some patients. Intravenous lidocaine infusions are gaining acceptance in a variety of pain management settings, from pain clinics to hospices. A bolus intravenous dose lidocaine of 1 to 2 mg/kg is given over 15 to 30 mins. If this is effective, it may be followed by a continuous infusion of 1 to 2 mg/kg/hr.[112] An early warning sign of potential toxicity is perioral numbness. Hepatic dysfunction and significant cardiac conduction abnormalities are contraindications to the treatment. Epidural or intrathecal administration of a local anesthetic, alone or in conjunction with an opioid, may allow relief in patients who are not candidates for systemic delivery.[113]

Others

Ketamine and dextromethorphan are N-methyl-D-aspartate (NMDA) receptor antagonists that are being explored for their use in neuropathic pain. To date, adverse effects (including hallucinations) have limited ketamine's use.[114] Although one study of post-surgical neuropathic pain supports the use of topical capsaicin, other studies suggest the pain associated with application of this drug precludes its use.[115,116] Ablative procedures and nerve blocks may be of benefit in some patients with localized pain syndromes.[117]

Pharmacogenetics

Variances in the amount of opioids administered to patients of various ethnic backgrounds were often attributed to perceived physiologic differences. In fact, the amount of opioid administered to a patient may be related to cultural influences such as the patient's pain expression (stoic patients may not report pain) or clinicians' biases about drug use (eg, Blacks and Hispanics received lower doses of opioids than Whites in one study of postoperative pain).[16–20,118] Additionally, gender differences in opioid prescription and administration persist, despite the lack of sufficient evidence that females need lower doses.[91] Elder patients are often given lower doses of opioids, although the prevalence of chronic pain states is significantly elevated in this population.[119]

Thus, beliefs regarding ethnicity, gender, age, and other cultural variables likely influence the majority of the variance seen in opioid and analgesic administration.[36,49] However, a newer field of study, pharmacogenetics, scientifically explores the influence of genetics on drug metabolism.[120] Genetics shape protein expression, particularly influencing enzyme expression. Enzymes are critical to the absorption, metabolism, and excretion of drugs. The cytochrome P450 (CYP) system is a major factor in drug metabolism, consisting of more than 20 families of enzymes. Enzymes critical to drug metabolism include CYP 1A2, CYP 2D6, CYP 2C9, and others. Several of these enzymes demonstrate genetic polymorphism. Approximately 5% to 10% of White patients, and 1% to 2% of African Americans and Asians, lack the CYP 2D6 enzyme.[120] Patients lacking this enzyme are unable to metabolize certain drugs. For example, codeine requires metabolism to morphine and other products to produce analgesia. Patients lacking CYP 2D6 may be unable to obtain relief when given codeine.[121,122] Their claims of poor pain relief when given codeine often resulted in labels of drug seeker by health care professional, when in fact, the lack of analgesia was due to this missing enzyme. Other analgesics metabolized by this enzyme include dextromethorphan (an NMDA antagonist), mexiletine (an analogue of lidocaine), and secondary tricyclic antidepressants.[123]

Gender does not seem to affect CYP 2D6 expression, although the activity of other enzymes in the CYP system is affected by sex. Because women were excluded from phase I and II clinical trials until 1993, limited pharmacokinetic information exists. Beierle and colleagues provide a comprehensive review of current knowledge.[124] Increasing age is associated with decreases in CYP enzymes. However, the clinical implications in relationship to drug dosing are not well known. Enzyme deficiencies also explain many drug-drug interactions that can be seen in the management of cancer pain and other symptoms.[123]

Cancer Therapies and Other Treatment Options

Therapies directed against the tumor, including surgery, chemotherapy, hormonal therapy, radiation therapy, may provide relief through reducing tumor burden.[125] Unfortunately, little research has evaluated the analgesic effect of various chemotherapeutic regimens, instead focusing primarily on tumor regression.[126,127] Radiation therapy is extremely effective in the management of several pain states, particularly pain associated with bone metastases.[128] Approximately 75% of all patients treated for pain due to bone metastases obtain some level of relief, and almost half become pain free.

Bisphosphonates (pamidronate, zoledronate) can be useful in relieving bone pain.[129,130] Intrathecal or epidural opioids in combination with local anesthetics produce effective analgesia with minimal side effects.[108] Neuroablative techniques such as chemical or surgical rhizotomy likewise can be effective in resistant cancer pain.[131,132]

Nonpharmacologic Therapies

Cognitive behavioral techniques such as guided imagery, relaxation, and distraction provide temporary relief of cancer-related pain.[133] These therapies have not been expansively studied in the cancer population, and no studies exist regarding cultural differences in their application, nor in their acceptability by different cultural groups. One study of patients with rheumatoid arthritis revealed that African American women were more likely to use pain coping behaviors such as distraction and praying, while Caucasians reported higher use of ignoring the pain.[134]

CONCLUSION

Cancer pain is a complex phenomenon, influenced greatly by the underlying biology, cultural factors (including those of the patient/family and the clinician), as well as the health care system. To be effective in relieving pain, each health care professional must understand the causes of cancer pain, appropriate assessment techniques, and therapeutic options. Furthermore, the professional must practice culturally competent health care as it relates to cancer pain. Additional research is needed to understand the way cultural differences affect the pain experience for individuals with cancer.

REFERENCES

1. Massoud RK, Reinke AJ, Franco LM, et al. *A Modern Paradigm for Improving Healthcare Quality.* Bethesda, MD: The Quality Assurance Project, U.S. Agency for International Development; 2001.
2. Kleinman A. *Patients and Healers in the Context of Culture.* Berkeley, CA: University of California Press; 1980.
3. Ajdari Z, Fein O. Primary care in the United Kingdom and United States: are there lessons to learn from each other? *Arch Fam Med.* 1998;7:311-314.
4. Onion DK, Berrington RM. Comparisons of UK general practice and US family practice. *J Am Board Fam Pract.* 1999;12:162-172.
5. Davies HT, Marshall MN. UK and US health systems: divided by more than a common language. *Lancet.* 2000;355:336.
6. Thai KV, Wimberly ET, McManus SM, eds. *Handbook of International Health Systems.* New York, NY: Marcel Dekker, Inc.; 2002.
7. Schifrin E. An overview of women's health issues in the United States and United Kingdom. *Womens Health Issues.* 2001;11:261-281.
8. Reinhardt U, Hussey P, Anderson G. Cross national comparisons of health systems using OCED data, 1999. *Health Aff.* 2002;21:169-181.
9. Institute of Medicine. *Crossing the Quality Chasm: A New Health System for the 21st Century.* Washington, DC: National Academy Press; 2001.
10. Pappas G, Queen S, Hadden W, Fisher G. The increasing disparity between socioeconomic groups in the US 1960 and 1986. *N Engl J Med.* 1993;329:103-109.
11. *Clinical Practice Guideline Number 9: Management of Cancer Pain.* Rockville, MD: Agency for Health Care Policy and Research, US Dept of Health and Human Services; 1994. AHCPR Publication 94-0592.
12. Fitzgibbon DR. Cancer pain: management. In: Loeser JD, Butler SH, Chapman CR, Turk DC, eds. *Bonica's Management of Pain.* 3rd ed. Philadelphia, PA: Lippincott Williams & Wilkins; 2001:659-703.
13. Blendon RJ, Aiken LH, Freeman HE, Corey CR. Access to medical care for black and white Americans: a matter of continuing concern. *JAMA.* 1989;261:278-281.
14. Bach PB, Crenner C, Warren JL, Begg CB. Racial differences in the treatment of early stage lung cancer. *N Engl J Med.* 1999;341:1198-1205.
15. Krakauer EL, Crener C, Fox K. Barriers to optimal end-of-life care in minority patients. *J Am Geriat Soc.* 2002;50:182-190.
16. Cleeland CS, Gonin R, Hatfield AK, et al. Pain and its treatment in outpatients with metastatic cancer. *N Engl J Med.* 1994;330:592-596.
17. Cleeland CS, Gonin R, Baez L, Loehrer P, Pandya KJ. Pain and treatment of pain in minority patients with cancer: the Eastern Cooperative Oncology Group minority outpatient pain study. *Ann Intern Med.* 1997;127:813-816.
18. McDonald DD. Gender and ethnic stereotyping and narcotic analgesic administration. *Res Nurs Health.* 1994;17:95-99.
19. Todd KH, Lee T, Hoffman JR. The effect of ethnicity on physician estimates of pain severity in patients with isolated extremity trauma. *JAMA.* 1994;271:925-928.
20. Benabei R, Gambosi G, Lapane K. Management of pain in elderly patients with cancer. *JAMA.* 1998;279:1877-1882.

21. Crawley L. Palliative care in African American communities. *J Palliat Med.* 2002;5:775-779.
22. Hogue CJR, Hargraves MA, Collins KS. *Minority Health in America: Findings and Policy Implications from the Commonwealth Fund Minority Health Survey.* Baltimore, MD:Johns Hopkins University Press; 2000.
23. Foley K, Gelband H, eds. *Improving Palliative Care for Cancer, Institute of Medicine and National Research Council,* Washington, DC: National Academy Press; 2001.
24. Institute of Medicine. *Unequal Treatment: Confronting Racial and Ethnic Disparities in Health Care.* Washington, DC:National Academy Press; March 2002.
25. Institute of Medicine. *The Unequal Burden of Cancer: An Assessment of NIH Research and Programs for Ethnic Minorities.* Washington, DC: National Academy Press; 1998.
26. Alexander Z. *The Department of Health: Study of Black, Asian and Other Minority Issues.* Available at: www.doh.gov.uk/race_equality. Accessed 2000.
27. Love RR. Determinants of health and global cancer strategies. *Cancer Strategy.* 1999;1:8-10.
28. Williams D, Rucker T. Understanding and addressing racial disparities in health care. *Health Care Financ Rev.* 2000;21:75-90.
29. Todd KH. Pain assessment and ethnicity. *Ann Emerg Med.* 1996;27:421-423.
30. Bolling J. Guinea across the water: the African American approach to death and dying. In: Perry JK, Ryan AJ, ed. *A Cross-Cultural Look at Death, Dying and Religion.* Chicago, IL: Nelson-Hall Publishers; 1995:145-149.
31. DeSpelder L, Strickland A. *The Last Dance: Encountering Death and Dying.* 6th ed. Boston, MA: McGraw Hill Higher Education; 2002.
32. Anderson KO, Ruhman SP, Hurley J, et al. Cancer pain management among underserved minority outpatients: perceived needs and barriers to optimal control. *Cancer.* 2001;94:2295-2304.
33. Reed WL, Darity W, Roberson NL, eds. *Health and Medical Care of African Americans.* Westport, CT, and London: Auburn House; 1993.
34. Cooper-Patrick L, Gallo J, Gonzales J, et al. Race, gender and partnerships in the patient-physician relationship. *JAMA.* 1999;282:583-589.
35. Davis JA, Smith TW. *General Social Survey 1972-1990, Chicago.* National Opinion Research Center; 1990.
36. Bonhom V. Race, ethnicity and pain treatment: striving to understand the causes and solutions to the disparities in pain treatment. *J Law Med Ethics.* 2001;29:52-68.
37. Minorities continue to be underrepresented in medicine. *Am Med News.* 1998;11.
38. Like RC, Steine RP, Rubel AJ. Recommended core curriculum in culturally sensitive and competent health care. *Fam Med.* 1996;27:291-297.
39. Bobo L, Kluegel JR, Smith RA. Laissez-faire racism: the crystallization of a "kinder, gentler" anti-black ideology. In: Tuck SA, Martin JK, eds. *Racial Attitudes in the 1990s—Continuity and Change.* Westport, CT: Praeger; 1997.
40. Lavizzo-Mourey R, Clayton LA, Byrd M, Johnson G III, Richardson D. The perceptions of African American physicians concerning their treatment by managed care organizations. *J Natl Med Assoc.* 1996;88:210-214.
41. Morrison RS, Wallenstein S, Natale DK, Senzel RS, Huang LL. We don't carry that failure of pharmacies in predominantly non white neighborhoods to stock opioid analgesics. *N Engl J Med.* 2000;342:1023-1026.
42. Bierman A, Lurie N, Collins KS, Eisenberg J. Addressing racial and ethnic barriers to effective health care: the need for better data. *Health Aff.* 2002;21:91-102.
43. Payne R, Payne TR. The Harlem Palliative Care Network. *J Palliat Med.* 2002;5:781-792.
44. Saunders C. *The Management of Terminal Disease.* London, England: Edward Arnold; 1978.
45. Cassel E. The nature of suffering and the goals of medicine. *N Engl J Med.* 1982;306:639-645.
46. Kearney M. *Mortally Wounded, Stories of Soul Pain, Death and Healing.* Dublin, Ireland: Marino Books; 1996.

47. Kearney M. *A Place of Healing.* New York, NY: Oxford Press; 2000.

48. Cherny NI, Portenoy RK. Cancer pain: principles of assessment and syndromes. In: Wall PD, Melzack R, eds. *Textbook of Pain.* 4th ed. Edinburgh, NY: Churchill Livingstone; 1999:1017-1064.

49. Edwards CL, Fillingim RB, Keefe F. Race, ethnicity and pain. *Pain.* 2001;94:133-137.

50. Mogil JS, Yu L, Basbaum AI. Pain genes?: natural variation and transgenic mutants. *Ann Rev Neurosci.* 2000;23:777-811.

51. White SF, Asher MA, Lai SM, et al. Patients' perceptions of overall function, pain, and appearance after primary posterior instrumentation and fusion for idiopathic scoliosis. *Spine* 1999;24:1693-1699.

52. Sheffield D, Biles PL, Orom H, et al. Race and sex differences in cutaneous pain perception. *Psychosom Med.* 2000;62:517-523.

53. McCracken LM, Matthews AK, Tang TS, et al. A comparison of blacks and whites seeking treatment for chronic pain. *Clin J Pain.* 2001;17:249-255.

54. Todd KH, Deaton C, D'Amato, et al. Ethnicity and analgesic practice. *Ann Emerg Med.* 2000;35:11-16.

55. Breitbart W, McDonald MV, Rosenfeld B, et al. Pain in ambulatory AIDS patients. I: pain characteristics and medical correlates. *Pain.* 1996;68:315-321.

56. Abrams BM. History taking in the patient in pain. In: Raj PP, ed. *Practical Management of Pain.* 3rd ed. St. Louis, MA: Mosby; 2000:333-338.

57. McCaffery M, Pasero C. *Pain: Clinical Manual.* 2nd ed. St. Louis, MA: Mosby; 1999.

58. Chapman CR, Syrjala KL. Measurement of pain. In: Loeser JD, Butler SH, Chapman CR, Turk DC, eds. *Bonica's Management of Pain.* 3rd ed. Philadelphia, PA: Lea & Febiger; 2001:310-328.

59. Melzack R, Katz J. Pain measurement in persons with pain. In: Wall PD, Melzack R, eds. *Textbook of Pain.* 4th ed. Edinburgh, NY: Churchill Livingstone; 1999:409-426.

60. Herr KA, Garand L. Assessment and measurement of pain in older adults. *Clin Geriatric Med.* 2001;17:457-478.

61. Harrison A, Busabir AA, al-Kaabi AO, et al. Does sharing a mother-tongue affect how closely patients and nurses agree when rating the patient's pain, worry and knowledge? *J Adv Nurs.* 1996;24:229-235.

62. McGrath PJ, Unruh AM. Pain in children. In: Wall PD, Melzack R, eds. *Textbook of Pain.* 4th ed. Edinburgh, NY:Churchill Livingstone; 1999:1463-1477.

63. Goldschneider KR, Mancuso TJ, Berde CB. Pain and its management in children. In: Loeser JD, Butler SH, Chapman CR, Turk DC, eds. *Bonica's Management of Pain.* Philadelphia, PA: Lippincott Williams & Wilkins; 2001:797-812.

64. Greenwald HP. Interethnic differences in pain perception. *Pain.* 1991;44:157-163.

65. Daut RL, Cleeland CS, Flanery RC. Development of the Wisconsin brief pain questionnaire to assess pain in cancer and other diseases. *Pain.* 1983;17:197-210.

66. Ger LP, Ho ST, Sun WZ, et al. Validation of the Brief Pain Inventory in a Taiwanese population. *J Pain Symptom Manage.* 1999;18:316-322.

67. Gordon C. The effect of cancer pain on quality of life in different ethnic groups: a literature review. *Nurse Pract Forum.* 1997;8:5-13.

68. Lipson JG, Dibble SL, Minarik PA. *Culture and Nursing Care: A Pocket Guide.* San Francisco, CA: UCSF Nursing Press; 1996.

69. Loeser J. Medical evaluation of the patient with pain. In Loeser JD, Butler SH, Chapman CR, Turk DC, eds. *Bonica's Management of Pain.* Philadelphia, PA: Lippincott Williams & Wilkins; 2001:267-278.

70. Galanti G-A. *Caring for Patients from Different Cultures: Case Studies from American Hospitals.* 2nd ed. Philadelphia, PA: University of Philadelphia Press; 1997.

71. Dedier J, Penson R, Williams W, Lynch T. Race, ethnicity, and the patient-caregiver relationship. *Oncologist.* 2002;7(90002):43-49.

72. Selby M. Ethical dilemma: dealing with racist patients. *BMJ.* 1999;318:1129.

73. Luckmann J. *Transcultural Communication in Health Care.* Albany, NY: Delmar Thomson Learning; 2000.

74. Cohen-Cole, Stephen A. *The Medical Interview: The Three Function Approach.* St. Louis, MA: Mosby Year Book; 1991.

75. Holland JC (Chair), Cassem EH (Speaker), Mount B (Speaker), Simmons P. Dealing with loss, death, and grief in clinical practice: spiritual meaning in oncology. *American Society of Clinical Oncology Education Book.* Alexandria, VA: American Society of Clinical Oncology; 2002:198-205.

76. Chapman CR, Gavrin J. Suffering: the contributions of persistent pain. *Lancet.* 1999;353:2233-2237.

77. Stewart M, Brown JB, Weston WW, McWilliam CL, Freeman TR. *Patient Centered Medicine: Transforming the Clinical Method.* Thousand Oaks, CA: Sage Publications; 1995.

78. Mutha S, Allen C, Welch M. *Toward Culturally Competent Care: A Toolbox for Teaching Communication Strategies.* San Francisco, CA: Centre for Health Professions, University of California, San Francisco; 2002.

79. Miyoshi HR. Systemic nonopioid analgesics. In: Loeser JD, Butler SH, Chapman CR, Turk DC, eds. *Bonica's Management of Pain.* 3rd ed. Philadelphia, PA: Lea & Febiger; 2001:1667-1681.

80. Mercadante S. The use of anti-inflammatory drugs in cancer pain. *Cancer Treat Rev.* 2001;27:51-61.

81. Garcia RLA. Nonsteroidal antiinflammatory drugs, ulcers and risk: a collaborative meta-analysis. *Semin Arthritis Rheum.* 1997;26(Suppl):16-20.

82. Wolfe MM, Lichtenstein DR, Singh G. Gastrointestinal toxicity of nonsteroidal anti-inflammatory drugs. *New Engl J Med.* 1999;340:1888-1899.

83. Perez Gutthann S, Garcia Rodriguez LA, Raiford DS, Duque Oliart A, Ris Romeu J. Nonsteroidal anti-inflammatory drugs and the risk of hospitalization for acute renal failure. *Arch Intern Med.* 1996;156:2433-2439.

84. Mukherjee D, Nissen SE, Topol EJ. Risk of cardiovascular events associated with selective COX-2 inhibitors. *JAMA.* 2001;286:954-959.

85. Juni P, Rutjes AWS, Dieppe PA. Are selective COX 2 inhibitors superior to traditional nonsteroidal anti-inflammatory drugs? *BMJ.* 2002;324:1287-1288.

86. Schiodt FV, Rochling FA, Casey DL, et al. Acetaminophen toxicity in an urban county hospital. *N Engl J Med.* 1997;337:1112-1117.

87. *Definitions Related to the Use of Opioids for the Treatment of Pain: A Consensus Document from the American Academy of Pain Medicine, the American Pain Society, and the American Society of Addiction Medicine.* Skokie, IL: American Pain Society; 2001.

88. Pargeon KL, Hailey BJ. Barriers to effective cancer pain management: a review of the literature. *J Pain Symptom Manage.* 1999;18:358-368.

89. Paice JA, Toy C, Shott S. Barriers to cancer pain relief: fear of tolerance and addiction. *J Pain Symptom Manage.* 1998;16:1-9.

90. Schumacher KL, Koresawa S, West C, et al. The usefulness of a daily pain management diary for outpatients with cancer-related pain. *Oncol Nurs Forum.* 2002;29:1304-1313.

91. Cherny NI, Thaler HT, Friedlander-Klar H, et al. Opioid responsiveness of cancer pain syndromes caused by neuropathic or nociceptive mechanisms. *Neurology.* 1994;44:857-861.

92. Rowbotham MC, Twilling L, Davies PS, et al. Oral opioid therapy for chronic peripheral and central neuropathic pain. *N Engl J Med* 2003;348:1223-1232.

93. Max MP, Payre R, Edwards WT, Subshire A, Inturrisi CE. *Principles of Analgesic Use in the Treatment of Acute Pain and Cancer Pain.* 4th ed. Skokie, IL: American Pain Society; 1999.

94. Cherny NI. The management of cancer pain. *CA Cancer J Clin.* 2000;50:70-116.

95. Indelicato RA, Portenoy RK. Opioid rotation in the management of refractory cancer pain. *J Clin Oncol.* 2002;20:348-352.

96. Szeta HH, Inturrisi CE, Houde R, et al. Accumulation of normeperidine, an active metabolite of meperidine, in patients with renal failure or cancer. *Ann Intern Med.* 1977;86: 738-741.

97. Kaiko RF, Foley KM, Grabinski PY, et al. Central nervous system excitatory effects of meperidine in cancer patients. *Ann Neurol.* 1983;13:180-185.

98. Mercadante S. Diarrhea, malabsorption, and constipation. In: Berger A, Portenoy RK, Weissman D, eds. *Principles and Practice of Supportive Oncology.* Philadelphia, PA: Lippincott-Raven Publishers, 1998:191-205.

99. Rozans M, Dreisbach A, Lertora JJL, et al. Palliative uses of methylphenidate in patients with cancer: a review. *J Clin Oncol.* 2001;20:335-339.

100. Teitelman E. Modafinil for narcolepsy. *Am J Psych.* 2001;158:970-971.

101. O'Mahony S, Coyle N, Payne R. Current management of opioid-related side effects. *Oncology.* 2001;15:61-77.

102. Ferris DJ. Controlling myoclonus after high-dosage morphine infusions. *Am J Health Syst Pharm.* 1999;56:1009-1010.

103. Breitbart W, Cohen K. Delirium in the terminally ill. In: Chochinov HM, Breitbart W, eds. *Handbook of Psychiatry in Palliative Medicine.* New York, NY: Oxford University Press; 2000: 75-90.

104. Abel EL. Opiates and sex. *J Psychoactive Drugs.* 1984;16:205-216.

105. Paice JA, Penn RD, Ryan WG. Altered sexual function and decreased testosterone in patients receiving intraspinal opioids. *J Pain Symptom Manage.* 1994;9:126-131.

106. Portenoy RK. Adjuvant analgesics in pain management. In: Doyle D, Hanks GWC, MacDonald N, eds. *Oxford Textbook of Palliative Care.* Vol 2. New York, NY: Oxford University Press; 1998:361-390.

107. Sindrup SH, Jensen TS. Efficacy of pharmacological treatments of neuropathic pain: an update and effect related to mechanism of drug action. *Pain.* 1999;83:389-400.

108. Max MB, Lynch SA, Buir J, et al. Effects of desipramine, amitriptyline, and fluoxetine on pain in diabetic neuropathy. *N Engl J Med.* 1992;42:131-133.

109. Backonja M, Beydoun A, Edwards KR, et al. Gabapentin for the symptomatic treatment of painful neuropathy in patients with diabetes mellitus: a randomized controlled trial. *JAMA.* 1998;280:1831-1836.

110. Rowbotham M, Harden N, Stacey B, et al. Gabapentin for the treatment of postherpetic neuralgia: a randomized controlled trial. *JAMA.* 1998;280:1837-1842.

111. Galer BS, Rowbotham MC, Perander J, Friedman E. Topical lidocaine patch relieves postherpetic neuralgia more effectively than a vehicle topical patch: results of an enriched enrollment study. *Pain.* 1999;80:533-538.

112. Ferrini RL. Parenteral lidocaine for severe intractable pain in 6 hospice patients continued at home. *J Palliat Med.* 2000;3:193-201.

113. Staats PS, Dougherty PM. Spinal analgesics: present and future. In: Raj PP, ed. *Practical Management of Pain.* 3rd ed. St. Louis, MA: Mosby; 2000:513-522.

114. Mercadante S, Arcuri E, Tirelli W, et al. Analgesic effect of intravenous ketamine in cancer patients on morphine therapy: a randomized, controlled, double-blind, crossover, double-dose study. *J Pain Symptom Manage.* 2000;20:246-252.

115. Ellison N, Loprinzi CL, Kugler J, et al. Phase III placebo-controlled trial of capsaicin cream in the management of surgical neuropathic pain in cancer patients. *J Clin Oncol.* 1997;15:2974-2980.

116. Paice JA, Ferrans CE, Lashley F, et al. Topical capsaicin in the management of HIV-associated peripheral neuropathy. *J Pain Symptom Manage.* 2000;19:45-52.

117. Furlan AD, Lui P-W, Mailis A. Chemical sympathectomy for neuropathic pain: does it work? Case report and systematic literature review. *Clin J Pain.* 2001;17:327-336.

118. Ng B, Dimsdale JE, Shragg P, Deutsch R. Ethnic differences in analgesic consumption for postoperative pain. *Psychosom Med.* 1996;58:125-129.

119. Cleary JF, Carbone PP. Palliative medicine in the elderly. *Cancer.* 1997;80:1335-1347.

120. Steimer W, Potter JM. Pharmacogenetic screening and therapeutic drugs. *Clin Chim Acta.* 2002;315:137-155.

121. Fagerlund TH, Braaten O. No pain relief from codeine...? An introduction to pharmacogenetics. *Acta Anaesthesiol Scand.* 2001;45:140-149.

122. Sindrup SH, Brosen K. The pharmacogenetics of codeine hypoalgesia. *Pharmacogenetics.* 1995;5:335-346.

123. Bernard SA, Bruera E. Drug interactions in palliative care. *J Clin Oncol.* 2000;18:1780-1799.

124. Beierle I, Meibohm B, Derendorf H. Gender differences in pharmacokinetics and pharmacodynamics. *Int J Clin Pharmacol Ther.* 1999;37:529-547.

125. Janjan NA, Weissman DE. Primary cancer treatment: antineoplastic. In: Berger AM, Portenoy RK, Weissman DE, eds. *Principles and Practices of Supportive Oncology.* Philadelphia, PA: Lippincott, Williams & Wilkins; 1998:43-59.

126. Ellison NM. Palliative chemotherapy. *Am J Hosp Palliat Care.* 1998;15:93-103.

127. Doyle C, Crump M, Pintilie M, et al. Does palliative chemotherapy palliate? Evaluation of expectations, outcomes, and costs in women receiving chemotherapy for advanced ovarian cancer. *J Clin Oncol.* 2001;19:1266-1274.

128. Jeremic B. Single fraction external beam radiation therapy in the treatment of localized metastatic bone pain: a review. *J Pain Symptom Manage.* 2001;22:1048-1058.

129. Paterson AH. Bisphosphonates: biological response modifiers in breast cancer. *Clin Breast Cancer.* 2002;3:206-216.

130. Berenson JR, Rosen LS, Howell A, et al. Zoledronic acid reduces skeletal-related events in patients with osteolytic metastases. *Cancer.* 2001;91:1191-1200.

131. Furlan AD, Lui P-W, Mailis A. Chemical sympathectomy for neuropathic pain: does it work? Case report and systematic literature review. *Clin J Pain.* 2001;17:327-336.

132. Eisenberg E, Carr DB, Chalmers TC. Neurolytic celiac plexus block for treatment of cancer pain: a meta-analysis. *Anesth Analg.* 1995;80:290-295.

133. Syrjala KL, Donaldson GW, Davis MW, Kippes ME, Carr JE. Relaxation and imagery and cognitive-behavioral training reduce pain during cancer treatment: a controlled clinical trial. *Pain.* 1995;63:189-198.

134. Jordan MS, Lumley MA, Leisen JC. The relationships of cognitive coping and pain control beliefs to pain and adjustment among African-American and Caucasian women with rheumatoid arthritis. *Arthritis Care Res.* 1998;11:80-88.

CHAPTER 10

Complementary and Alternative Medicine in Patients with Cancer

Edzard Ernst and Clare Stevinson

DEFINITION

Complementary/alternative medicine (CAM) has been defined as "diagnosis, treatment, and/or prevention which complements mainstream medicine by contributing to a common whole, by satisfying a demand not met by orthodoxy or by diversifying the conceptual frameworks of medicine."[1] This definition tries to define CAM by what it is rather than using the approach of numerous other attempts to define CAM by what it is not, for example, CAM is not taught in medical schools, it is not backed up by science. This definition has partly been adopted by The Cochrane Collaboration.

THE PREVALENCE OF CAM IN CANCER PATIENTS

There are numerous surveys attempting to define the prevalence of CAM in cancer patients. A systematic review of all such investigations[2] published between 1977 and 1998 included 26 surveys conducted in 13 different countries. The average prevalence was 31% but variation was considerable. This is due to national differences but perhaps more importantly to the fact that different investigators include different therapies under the umbrella term CAM. Moreover, substantially different prevalence figures emerge depending whether one relies on standard history taking or specific questioning.[3]

Recent surveys have added to our knowledge. In Canada, CAM was used by 49% of patients with colorectal cancer,[4] and by 72% of patients with breast cancer.[5] The most commonly used therapies were psychological/spiritual interventions, vitamins, minerals, and herbal medicines. Sixty-eight percent of all CAM users informed their doctor about their CAM usage—a figure that was only 41% in New Zealand cancer patients.[6] Another survey yielded a lower prevalence figure (29%) and suggested that the most commonly used CAM therapies are vitamins, herbal medicines, and minerals.[7] American patients with breast cancer used CAM in 73% of cases[8] and for all gynecological cancers, the figure was 50%.[9] The most common sources of information on CAM were friends, family, and the media.[8]

A survey of all 1350 naturopaths practicing in the United States or Canada showed that 77% of them had provided naturopathic care for women with breast cancer.[10] Their therapies consisted most commonly of dietary counseling, herbal medicines, and other supplements. When we asked professional CAM organizations which therapy they thought was indicated for cancer, they listed aromatherapy, Bach Flower remedies, massage therapy, and reflexology.[11]

REASONS FOR POPULARITY

Given the growing popularity of CAM and the fact that the majority of this use is based on "out-of-pocket" expenditure,[12] the issue of why people use it is both relevant and intriguing. Although the question itself is a simple one, the answer is undoubtedly complex. One consistent finding is that the majority of CAM use does not occur instead of orthodox medical care, but in addition to it.[12-14] Patients report using orthodox medicine for some complaints and CAM for others, or they may choose to use CAM alongside conventional treatment.

Furnham[15] summarized the main hypotheses relating to why people use CAM. "Push" factors include dissatisfaction with orthodox medicine. Prior negative experiences or a general anti-establishment attitude may be the underlying cause. "Pull" factors include compatibility between the philosophy of certain therapies with patients' own beliefs and a greater sense of control over one's own treatment.

Astin[16] surveyed 1035 US residents about their use of CAM, health status, and attitudes to conventional medicine and showed that only philosophical congruence was predictive of CAM use. Rather than being "pushed," participants were "pulled" toward CAM because it was seen as more compatible with their values, worldview, spiritual/religious philosophy, or beliefs about health and illness. Those respondents who could be identified as "cultural creatives"[17] were more likely to be users of CAM. These individuals tended to be at the cutting edge of cultural change and innovation in society. They were characterized by their interests in environmentalism, feminism, globalism, esoteric forms of spirituality, self-actualization, altruism, self-expression, and their love of the exotic.

Kaptchuk and Eisenberg[18] have also suggested that certain fundamental premises of CAM contribute to its persuasive appeal: the perceived association of CAM with *nature, vitalism* ("life forces", "qi", or "psychic energy"), the *science, tradition, or philosophy* of CAM and *spirituality.* These factors often serve to bridge the gap between the domain of medical science with its search for truth and strict causality and the domain of religion with its moral freedom and self-chosen values.

Other possible explanations for the use of CAM refer to underlying reasons rather than specific patient motives. Patients using CAM may tend to experience greater levels of psychosocial stress, and may experience neurosis, and are thus drawn toward the touching/talking approach of CAM. Levels of neurosis have been shown to be high in patients visiting CAM therapists,[19] higher than those visiting a general practitioner (GP).[20] However, this may be little more than a reflection of the nature of the conditions being treated. CAM practitioners often see patients with chronic disorders in whom the incidence of neurosis is relatively high. An association has been demonstrated between poorer mental health and depression and use of CAM following surgery.[21] These findings suggest that those individuals with greater psychosocial stress may be more likely to turn to CAM.

A qualitative US study of 22 patients self-medicating with St. John's wort for depression addressed these questions directly.[22] The coherent motivations were: (a) desire to take control of own health; (b) perception that their condition was not serious enough to require medical treatment; (c) belief that St. John's wort was safer than prescribed antidepressants; (d) perception of St. John's wort as a relatively easily accessible therapeutic option.

A study from Honolulu shows that, in cancer patients, heavier CAM use is associated with lower doctor satisfaction and greater disease severity.[23] In prostate cancer patients, progressive disease is linked with more CAM use, and 90% of CAM users believe that CAM would help them to live longer and improve quality of life while 47% expected a cure.[24] Keenness to try all available options was also the most important reason for CAM use in a survey of 211 general practice patients from Austria, Germany, and England.[25] Using CAM as a "last hope" was another common answer in this study.

Patients who turned to CAM as a last resort could be clearly differentiated from those who embraced CAM for its compatibility with their own beliefs in a UK-based study.[26] Those patients who sought CAM as a last resort had similar scores to the general population on locus of control. Furthermore, they maintained faith in the principles of orthodox medicine and displayed little initial commitment to the values or philosophies of CAM. Other patients chose CAM because it matched their own beliefs about health and illness. These individuals showed a greater internal locus of control and skepticism for orthodox medicine.

This study also found that 68% of patients reported a better relationship with the CAM practitioner than with their own GP.[26] CAM practitioners were perceived as more friendly and personal, treated the relationship with their GP more like a partnership, and provided more time for the consultation. Satisfaction with the therapeutic encounter was also greater with CAM practitioners than GPs in a survey of UK arthritis sufferers using both CAM and conventional care in parallel.[27] Satisfaction with the time spent on the patient was higher with CAM practitioners, as it also was in a Spanish study of CAM use by patients with somatoform disorder.[28] Physicians using homeopathy spend more than twice as long on patient consultations than conventional physicians.[29] A clinical trial of homeopathy for premenstrual syndrome reported a response rate of 47% in a pretreatment placebo washout phase[30] which may have been due largely to the depth and intimacy of the homeopathic interview.

In general, CAM is rarely employed as a replacement of orthodox medical care but as an adjunct to it. CAM use has been described as "shopping for health."[15] Nonetheless, rather than being specifically "pushed" or "pulled" toward CAM, patients simply perceive it as one of a range of treatment options available to them and exercise their freedom of choice and discriminating power accordingly. The consistent finding that CAM use is associated with higher levels of income may support the concept of CAM as a commodity for individuals who can afford it. A strong positive correlation exists between sale data of BMW cars (a possible measure of affluence) and use of herbal remedies in the United States.[31]

Many CAM-users have an eclectic approach to health care, which could be described as "consumerist."[32] Perhaps it is more pertinent to ask why people do not use CAM. One UK study of 90 fibromyalgia patients showed that those patients who did not use CAM cited two reasons: lack of information and expense.[33] A Canadian study involving 36 breast cancer patients identified three main reasons for not using CAM: lack of information, skepticism about efficacy, and fear of harm of therapies.[34] Certain patients who wanted to use CAM did not actually do so because of the cost of therapies, lack of access, and lack of time to devote to the therapy.[35]

EFFECTIVENESS OF CAM THERAPIES AS CANCER CURES

Proponents of numerous CAM treatments claim to cure cancer, lower the tumor burden, or prolong the life of cancer patients. Many cancer patients also believe that this is true.[24] The evidence for or against such claims is, however, not so clearly in favor of this notion. Based on an 8-year follow up, Risberg et al. recently showed that CAM users had higher death rates than non-users (79% vs 65%).[36] While this finding was based on survey data, we clearly need clinical trials to determine the efficacy of so-called CAM "cancer cures."

Di Bella Therapy

The "Di Bella therapy" contains melatonin, bromocriptine, either somato-statin or octroctide, and retinoid solution (as well as cyclosphamide and hydroxyurea in some cases). Eleven independent, multicenter, uncontrolled phase II studies including 386 patients with advanced cancer were initiated in Italy.[37] None of the patients showed complete remission and only three patients had a partial remission. A retrospective comparison of 314 patients vs matched patients from Italian cancer registers showed a significantly shorter 5-year survival time for Di Bella's patients.[38]

Diet

Proponents of "alternative" diets sometimes claim that their approach can prolong the life of cancer patients. A review of the evidence found no con-vincing data in support of this hypothesis.[39] Unreplicated data apparently showing a six-fold increase in 5-year survival rates of melanoma patients treated with the Gerson diet[40] are unconvincing due to seriously flawed methodology. Similar claims for macrobiotic diets are also not supported by evidence from rigorous clinical trials. One third of cancer patients on a macrobiotic diet experience problems due to weight loss, the restrictive and unpalatable nature of the regimen, and the expense and inaccessibility of some ingredients.[41]

Herbal Medicine

Fifty patients with advanced solid malignant tumors for whom no effective standard anti-cancer therapy existed were treated in a controlled clinical trial (CCT), either with melatonin (20 mg/day) or with melatonin and aloe vera tincture (1 ml twice daily).[42] No response was seen in the former group while two partial responses were observed in the group treated with aloe vera. This result awaits confirmation from more rigorous trials.

"Destagnation" is a complex mixture of traditional Chinese herbs. An RCT with 188 patients suffering from nasopharyngeal carcinomas compared its efficacy with that of radiation therapy.[43] The 5-year success rate was 53% in the experimental and 37% in the control group. The difference was statistically significant.

Essiac is a herbal mixture which is popular in North America and consists of *Arctium lappa, Rheum palmatum, Rumex acetosella*, and *Ulmus fulva*. A systematic review did not find a single published clinical trial.[44] Several unpublished investigations were identified, and there was some indirect evidence for anti-cancer activity of several of the constituent herbs. Thus, there is insufficient evidence to recommend this herbal mixture.

Mistletoe *(Viscum album)* extracts are widely used by cancer patients.[45] They contain mistletoe lectins and viscotoxins. Both have been shown to modify intracellular protein synthesis, stimulate cytokine production, inhibit tumor colonization, and induce cell necrosis. Two independent systematic reviews on mistletoe,[46,47] found only a small number of clinical trials, none of which, due to significant methodological flaws, were conclusive. Kleijnen and colleagues therefore concluded: "we cannot recommend the use of mistletoe extracts in the treatment of cancer patients with an exception for patients involved in clinical trials."[47]

The herbal formula PC-SPES contains *Chrysanthemum morifolium, Gandoderma lucidium, Glycyrrhiza glabra, Isatis indigotica, Panax pseudoginseng, Robdosia rubesceus, Scutellaria baicalensis*, and *Serenoa repens*. No less than 116 clinical and other investigations have been published.[48] The mixture has potent estrogenic activity,[49] which could increase risk of breast cancer incidence or progression, and was shown to lower prostate specific antigen in patients with prostate cancer and to inhibit the growth of prostate cancer cells in vitro.[50] Recently it has been demonstrated that the preparation has been adulterated with prescription drugs and it was taken off the market.

Sho-saiko-to is a Chinese herbal mixture that contains extracts of seven medicinal herbs. Two hundred and sixty patients with hepatocellular carcinoma and cirrhosis were treated with 7.5 g of the mixture daily while the control group received conventional drugs only.[51] The 5-year survival rate showed a (nonsignificant) trend to be higher in the experimental group compared to the control group.

A hypericin extract from St John's wort *(Hypericum perforatum)* was administered intra-lesionally 3 to 5 times per week in patients with basal cell carcinoma or squamous cell carcinoma.[52] The lesions were subsequently irradiated with visible light. The authors claim that hypericin displayed selective tumor-targeting. Clinical remissions were observed after 6 to 8 weeks. These preliminary results require confirmation in a rigorous RCT.

Other Supplements

A systematic review[53] of all clinical trials of hydrazine sulfate included three RCTs from the US. Many studies were methodologically weak. None of the RCTs suggested positive effects. Therefore, it was concluded that "the value of hydrazine sulfate as an antitumor agent—specifically its capacity to stabilize tumor size, cause tumor regression and improve survival—remains uncertain."[53]

Laetrile, for example, has been tested in several rigorous clinical trials.[54] No clinically relevant benefit was found, either in terms of cure, survival, or stabilization of cancer growth, or improvement of symptoms.

Several studies have tested the efficacy of melatonin supplementation for slowing tumor progression.[55] One RCT, for instance, suggested that patients with brain metastases treated with melatonin experienced a longer survival time compared with patients who received supportive care only.[56]

The (partly) herbal mixture "714-X" containing camphor, ammonium chloride and nitrate, sodium chloride, ethyl alcohol, and water is being promoted for prostate cancers. A systematic review found several animal studies but no clinical trials that supported its benefit.[57] The author concluded that "side-effects appear to be minimal, but evidence of its effectiveness is limited." Shitake mushroom extract was tested in an uncontrolled study on 62 men with prostate cancer.[58] By 6 months, 23 patients had progression of the disease and none exhibited a positive clinical response. There was also no sign that this treatment lowered prostate-specific antigen in these patients.

Shark cartilage is claimed to have anti-angiogenesis effects that might inhibit malignant growth. Preclinical investigations supported this hypothesis to some extent[59] but the results of clinical trials were less encouraging. Sixty patients with advanced cancers of various types were treated with shark cartilage (1 g/kg/day) as the sole anti-cancer therapy in an uncontrolled pilot study.[60] No complete or partial responses were noted. The authors concluded that shark cartilage, as a single agent, did not prolong life and had no beneficial effect on quality of life. Thus, the claim that shark cartilage is beneficial for cancer patients is not supported by evidence.

Preclinical studies have demonstrated that bovine thymus extracts restore lymphocyte function, improve immunological variables, activating natural killer cells, and increase cytotoxic activity as well as mitogen-induced interferon levels in human lymphocytes. Animal experiments have suggested that thymus extracts inhibit tumor growth. A systematic review of all RCTs did not arrive at positive conclusions.[61] Injectable thymus preparations can cause severe allergic reactions and have the potential to transmit serious infections.

Support Group Therapy

The evidence to suggest that psychosocial support groups (usually including therapeutic elements like relaxation or self-hypnosis) prolong survival rates in cancer patients is far from uniform. One much quoted RCT showed that survival was 18 months longer in the experimental compared to the control group.[62] A recent review included 10 studies, of which 5 (total sample size = 580 patients) yielded a positive and 5 (total sample size = 672 patients) yielded a negative result.[63]

Complex Therapies

A hundred and two patients with lung cancer were randomized into one group treated conventionally and another receiving additional individualized treatments according to the principles of traditional Chinese medicine.[64] In the latter group, the 2-year survival rate was significantly greater than in the control group (56% vs 16%).

The Bristol Cancer Help Centre Study is an example of the confusion that may result from seriously flawed research.[65] This trial apparently demonstrated that the survival rate of those breast cancer patients who were treated by an adjunctive package of CAM modalities was significantly poorer than for controls. Yet the study was not randomized and thus baseline differences are a probable cause for the counter-intuitive result.

A matched-pair comparison was conducted of survival of cancer patients receiving standard care with those receiving a package of CAM (autogenous immune-enhancing vaccine, bacille Calmette-Guérin, vegetarian diets, and coffee enemas) as well as standard care.[66] There were no differences in survival times, but patients in the experimental group reported significantly poorer quality of life.

Eleven patients with inoperable pancreatic adenocarcinomas were treated with a package of CAM consisting of large oral doses of pancreatic enzymes, various nutritional supplements, "detoxification" procedures, and an organic diet.[67] The survival rates were 81% at 1 year, and 45% at 2 years. The authors point out that this is far better than expected according to the literature. Thus, this pilot study seems to warrant further, more rigorous study.

EFFECTIVENESS OF PALLIATIVE/SUPPORTIVE CAM THERAPIES

Many CAM modalities have the potential to not only increase but to also enhance the well-being of cancer patients. For these reasons, they are often used in palliative and supportive care for cancer patients. The following section summarizes the evidence regarding such approaches.

Acupuncture

A systematic review strongly suggests that acupuncture at the P6 point near the wrist has a useful role in reducing nausea induced by chemotherapy.[68]

Hypnotherapy

Several (mostly small) RCTs have demonstrated the usefulness of hypnotherapy in palliative cancer care. It has been shown to be effective in controlling pain and nausea/vomiting in various settings.[69,70] In children, hypnotherapy was more effective than attention controls in reducing nausea.[71,72]

Relaxation

The effectiveness of relaxation therapy has been repeatedly tested. In one RCT, for instance, the program consisted of breathing exercises, muscle relaxation, and imagery. This regimen was significantly superior in controlling pain of cancer patients than any such intervention.[73] In yet another RCT, 96 women with advanced breast cancer were randomized to receive either regular relaxation training and imagery or standard care only. The experimental group experienced better quality of life than the control group.[74]

Supplements

Alzoon is a herbal mixture of extracts of *petasites*, juniper, ferns, *brunellias*, and dandelions that has been treated with oxygen and UV-light. It is being promoted for the treatment of cancers. An uncontrolled study with 42 cancer patients suggested that 14% of the patients experienced a temporary improvement of quality of life and appetite.[75]

Oral mixtures of proteolytic enzymes (Wobe Mucos) are promoted for increasing the well-being of cancer patients. A systematic review included seven prospective clinical studies including 692 patients in total.[76] The authors concluded, "enzyme therapy has generally been found to be a well tolerated form of treatment for the relief of side-effects caused by other tumor therapies and for improving quality of life." Due to methodological limitations of the primary data, this hypothesis still requires testing in rigorous RCTs.

Spiritual Healing

Several CCTs have tested the effectiveness of therapeutic touch to reduce anxiety[77] or well-being[78] in cancer patients. Some of these studies have yielded positive results. However, due to weaknesses in study design, it remains unclear whether the observed effects were due to a specific therapeutic or a nonspecific (placebo) effect.

Other Therapies

Several other CAM treatments might improve the well-being of patients with cancer. Examples include mind-body programs for stress and well-being,[79] ginger for nausea, tai chi and other gentle exercise techniques for gaining strength, aromatherapy, massage, and relaxation techniques to reduce stress,[80] herbal medicines for depression, anxiety, indigestion, hot flushes in Tamoxifen patients,[81] pain[82] and other symptoms,[83] as well as acupuncture or homeopathy for pain.[83] The evidence in this area is, however, often anecdotal, inconsistent, and collectively unconvincing.[55,83,84]

These data suggest that CAM may have an important role in palliative/supportive cancer care. Unfortunately, the present evidence for most therapies is preliminary at best. This area clearly deserves more research; in particular, we need to know whether treatments are in any way superior to conventional methods of palliative/supportive cancer care.

To date, no CAM modality has been convincingly shown to reduce the tumor burden or prolong the life of cancer patients. Some of the therapies mentioned above may deserve further study in this respect. But until compelling evidence is available, cancer patients should be discouraged from using CAM as an alternative to conventional treatments. Some therapies, particularly those that are safe, can be tried as an adjunctive to conventional cancer therapy.

SAFETY ISSUES

Generally speaking, CAM safety issues are under-researched. Patients frequently perceive CAM as devoid of serious adverse events; 89% of New Zealand cancer patients, for instance, believe that CAM modalities are safe.[6] However, we know that this is not necessarily true.

TABLE 1. Toxicity Associated with Some Herbal and Other Dietary Supplements used by Cancer Patients

Name of ingredient	Toxicity/Interactions
Essiac	Contact dermatitis, gastrointestinal pain, hypokalemia, increased effect of antidiabetic drugs, decreased intestinal absorption of other drugs
Mistletoe	Allergic reactions including anaphylaxis, angina, bradycardia, cardiac arrest, diarrhea, fever, gastritis, gingivitis, headache, hepatitis, interactions with MAO inhibitors possible
Sho-saiko-to	Pneumonitis, pulmonary edema, thrombocytopenic purprea
St. John's wort	Enhances liver enzyme system (cytochrome P450) and P-glycoprotein transporter system, this can result in lowering of blood levels of a wide range of drugs
Hydrazine sulfate	Interaction with co-enzyme Q10 possible
Laetrile	Hepatotoxicity, nephrotoxicity
Melatonin	Increase in serum thyroxine, increased effect of barbiturates and morphine, safety of long-term use not established
714-X	None reported
Shark cartilage	Hepatitis, diarrhea
Thymus extract	Contamination with slow viruses

Many herbal or other dietary supplements are associated with a degree of toxicity. Table 1 summarizes adverse effects and potential interactions associated with some of the treatments discussed above.[83,85,86] In addition to direct toxicity, other indirect safety issues deserve a mention.

In the United States, Canada, and the United Kingdom, herbal medicinal products (HMPs) are, by and large, marketed as food supplements. As such, no rigorous regulation comparable to the pharmaceutical sector applies. In particular, the necessity for a manufacturer to demonstrate safety and quality of the marketed product is far less. Thus, contamination of HMPs has been reported on a regular basis. In particular, contamination with heavy metals is a problem that has been repeatedly associated with Asian HMPs.[87]

Adulteration with non-declared herbs or conventional drugs is a further problem with such HMPs of dubious quality.[88] For instance, when 2 609 Chinese herbal medicines were collected and analyzed in Taiwan, 24% of them were shown to be adulterated with synthetic drugs like acetaminophen, hydrochlorothiazide, indomethacin phenobarbital, theophylline, and corticosteroids.[89]

Underdosing is a further problem with HMPs. For example, whenever herbal food supplements from the US market are analyzed by independent experts, the findings reveal that in a substantial proportion of them, the active ingredient content differs marginally from label claims.[90]

In most countries, CAM providers are predominantly non-medically qualified practitioners. Most of these, one would hope, are probably adequately trained to do what they do. However, in the absence of adequate regulations, it is probable that some providers do not adhere to adequate standards of clinical practice. For example, we regularly hear of cases where CAM providers have delayed or hindered access to potentially life-saving conventional oncological treatment.[91,92] Changing prescribed treatments is a similar problem. There is preliminary evidence from areas other than oncology to suggest that a significant proportion of CAM providers would do this.[93]

Another problem can be the use of diagnostic techniques, which are invalid for diagnosing cancer or "precancerous" states. An example is the use of iridology, which would lead to false negative or false positive diagnosis.[94]

The attitude of the consumer toward CAM may constitute a further risk. For instance, about one quarter of CAM users would consult their doctor for a serious adverse effect of conventional medication while less than 1% would do the same in relation to a herbal remedy.[95] The plethora of lay books on CAM now available in every high street bookstore may also constitute a risk to patients. Preliminary evidence[96] suggests that this lay literature has the potential to put the health of the reader at risk if the advice from these books is being adhered to by seriously ill individuals. When we extracted the recommendations of 7 such books regarding cancer, we found no less than 133 different CAM modalities being advocated.[83] Even health food shops can present a risk to cancer patients. Researchers from Honolulu have shown that store personnel readily provide information that has the potential to harm cancer patients.[97]

A significant proportion of the UK daily press reports about CAM in a much more favorable tone than about mainstream medicine.[98] Unfortunately, this could lead to distrust in the latter and unjustified trust in the former which also might constitute a risk to cancer patients.

WHERE DO WE GO FROM HERE?

CAM has become a big issue for cancer patients, an issue that is unlikely to go away. Certain CAM modalities may turn out to be effective cancer cures but to date no such therapy has been identified. Several CAM approaches may be useful in palliative and supportive care. Other CAM modalities may play a role in cancer prevention,[83] a subject excluded from the above discussions. We should aim at dealing with CAM in the best possible way, so that the benefits of CAM are maximized and its risks minimized. This would require a multifactorial strategy.

1. Conventional health care professionals need to specifically ask their patients about CAM use. They also need to learn enough about the modalities involved to advise their patients responsibly.
2. Providers of CAM need to view their treatments realistically. In particular, they must be aware what these therapies can and cannot achieve for cancer patients.
3. Cancer patients also need to be equally realistic. They should bear one general rule in mind: if it sounds too good to be true, it probably is.
4. The media, when dealing with CAM, should abstain from misleading patients and raising false hopes—cheap sensationalism is a disservice to all.
5. Researchers should pick up the leads from promising preliminary results described above. There can be no shortcut to rigorous scientific investigation, and CAM is no exception to this rule.[99]
6. Finally, funding bodies should seriously reconsider their attitude toward CAM. One may love or hate CAM but in view of its increasing popularity, we need to know the essentials about its efficacy and safety. Without adequate funding, however, even these elementary questions will remain unanswered.

REFERENCES

1. Ernst E, Resch KL, Mills S, et al. Complementary medicine—a definition. *Br J Gen Pract.* 1995;45:506.
2. Ernst E, Cassileth BR. The prevalence of complementary/alternative medicine in cancer: a systematic review. *Cancer.* 1998;83:777-782.
3. Jones HA, Metz JM, Devine P. Rates of unconventional medical therapy use in patients with prostate cancer: standard history versus direct questioning. *Urology.* 2002;59:272-276.
4. Tough SC, Johnston DW, Verhoef MJ. Complementary and alternative medicine use among colorectal cancer patients in Alberta Canada. *Altern Ther Health Med.* 2002;8:54-64.
5. Ashikaga T, Bosompra K, O'Brien P, Nelson L. Use of complimentary and alternative medicine by breast cancer patients: prevalence, patterns and communication with physicians. *Supportive Care Cancer.* 2002;10:542-547.
6. Chrystal K, Allan S, Forgeson G, Isaacs R. The use of complementary/alternative medicine by cancer patients in a New Zealand regional cancer treatment centre. *N Z Med J.* 2003;116:1-8.
7. Kumar NB, Hopkins K, Allen K. Use of complementary/integrative nutritional therapies during cancer treatment: implications in clinical practice. *Cancer.* 2002;9:236-243.
8. Shen J, Andersen R, Albert PS, et al. Use of complementary/alternative therapies by women with advanced-stage breast cancer. *BMC Compl. Altern Med.* 2002;2:8-15.

9. Swisher EM, Cohn DE, Goff BA, et al. Use of complementary and alternative medicine among women with gynecologic cancers. *Gynecol Oncol.* 2002;84:363-367.

10. Standish LJ, Greene K, Greenlee H, Kim JG, Grosshans C. Complementary and alternative medical treatment of breast cancer: a survey of licensed North American naturopathic physicians. *Altern Ther.* 2002;8:74-81.

11. Long L, Huntley A, Ernst E. Which complementary and alternative therapies benefit which conditions? A survey of the opinions of 223 professional organisations. *Compl. Ther Med.* 2001;9:178-185.

12. Eisenberg D, David RB, Ettner SL, et al. Trends in alternative medicine use in the United States; 1990-1997. *JAMA.* 1998;280:1569-1575.

13. Kranz R, Rosenmund A. Über die Motivation zur Verwendung komplementärmedizinischer Heilmethoden. *Schweiz Med Wochenschr.* 1998;128:616-622.

14. Druss BG, Rosenheck RA. Association between use of unconventional therapies and conventional medical services. *JAMA.* 1999;282:651-656.

15. Furnham A. Why do people choose and use complementary therapies? In: Ernst E, ed. *Complementary Medicine: An Objective Appraisal.* Oxford: Butterworth Heinemann; 1996.

16. Astin JA. Why Patients Use Alternative Medicine: Results of a National Study. *JAMA.* 1998;279:1548-1553.

17. Ray PH. The emerging culture. American Demographics. *www.demographics.com* 1997.

18. Kaptchuk TJ, Eisenberg DM. The Persuasive Appeal of Alternative Medicine. *Ann Intern Med.* 1998;129:1061-1065.

19. Davidson J, Rampes H, Eisen M, Fisher P, Smith R, Malik M. Psychiatric disorders in primary care patients receiving complementary medicine. *Compr Psychiatr.* 1998;39:16-20.

20. Furnham A, Smith C. Choosing alternative medicine: a comparison of the beliefs of patients visiting a general practitioner and a homoeopath. *Soc Sci Med.* 1988;26:685-689.

21. Burstein HJ, Gelber S, Guadagnoli E, Weeks JC. Use of alternative medicine by women with early-stage breast cancer. *N Engl J Med.* 1999;340:1733-1739.

22. Wagner PJ, Jester D, LeClair B, Taylor AT, Woodward L, Lambert J. Taking the edge off why patients choose St John's wort. *J Fam Pract.* 1999;48:615-619.

23. Shumay DM, Maskarinec G, Gotay CC, Heiby EM, Kakai H. Determinants of the degree of complementary and alternative medicine use among patients with cancer. *J Altern Compl. Med.* 2002;8:661-671.

24. Wilkinson S, Gomella LG, Smith JA, et al. Attitudes and use of complementary medicine in men with prostate cancer. *J Urol.* 2002;168:2505-2509.

25. Ernst E, Willoughby M, Weihmayr TH. Nine possible reasons for choosing complementary medicine. *Perfusion.* 1995;11:356-359.

26. Finnegan MD. The Centre for the Study of Complementary Medicine: an attempt to understand its popularity through psychological, demographic and operational criteria. *Compl Med Res.* 1991;5:83-88.

27. Resch K, Hill S, Ernst E. Use of complementary therapies by individuals with "arthritis." *Clin Rheumatol.* 1997;16:391-395.

28. Garcia-Campayo J, Sanz-Carrillo C. The use of alternative medicines by somatoform disorder patients in Spain. *Br J Gen Pract.* 2000;50:487-488.

29. Jacobs J, Chapman EH, Crothers D. Patient characteristics and practice patterns of physicians using homeopathy. *Arch Fam Med.* 1998;7:537-540.

30. Chapman EH, Angelica J, Spitalny G, Strauss M. Results of a study of the homeopathic treatment of PMS. *J Am Inst Homeopath.* 1994;87:14-21.

31. Ernst E. Alternative views on alternative medicine. Letter to the editor. *Ann Intern Med.* 1999;131:229-230.

32. Sharma UM. Alternative choices of healing in North Staffordshire. *Compl Med Res.* 1989;3:1-4.

33. Dimmock S, Troughton PR, Bird HA. Factors predisposing to the resort of complementary therapies in patients with fibromyalgia. *Clin Rheumatol.* 1996;15:478-482.

34. Boon H, Brown JB, Gavin A, Kennard MA, Stewart M. Breast cancer survivors' perceptions of complementary/alternative medicine (CAM): making the decision to use or not to use. *Qual Health Res.* 1999;9:639-653.

35. Boon H, Stewart M, Kennard M, et al. Use of complementary/alternative medicine by breast cancer survivors in Ontario: prevalence and perceptions. *J Clin Oncol.* 2000;18: 2515-2521.

36. Risberg T, Vickers A, Bremnes RM, Wist EA, Kaasa S, Cassileth BR. Does use of alternative medicine predict survival from cancer? *Eur J Cancer.* 2003;39:372-377.

37. Italian Study Group for the Di Bella Multitherapy Trials. Evaluation of an unconventional cancer treatment (the Di Bella multitherapy): results of phase II trials in Italy. *BMJ.* 1999;318:224-228.

38. Buiatti A, Arniani S, Verdecchia A, Tomatis L. Results from a historical survey of the survival of cancer patients given Di Bella multitherapy. *Cancer.* 1999;86:2143-2149.

39. Ernst E, Cassileth BR. Cancer diets: fads and facts. *Cancer Prevent Int.* 1996;2:181-187.

40. Hildenbrand G. Five-year survival rates of melanoma patients treated by diet therapy after the manner of Gerson. A retrospective review. *Altern Ther Health Med.* 1995;4:29-37.

41. Downer SM, Cody MM, McCluskey P, et al. Pursuit and practice of complementary therapies by cancer patients receiving conventional treatment. *BMJ.* 1994;309:86-89.

42. Lissoni P, Giana L, Zerbini S, Trabattoni P, Rovelli F. Biotherapy with the pineal immunomodulating hormone melatonin versus melatonin plus aloe vera in untreatable advanced solid neoplasms. *Nat Immun.* 1998;16:27-33.

43. Xu GZ, Cai WM, Qin DX, et al. Chinese herb "destagnation" series I: combination of radiation with destagnation in the treatment of nasopharyngeal carcinoma (NPC): a prospective randomized trial on 188 cases. *Int J Rad Oncol Biol Phys.* 1989;16:297-300.

44. Kaegi E. Unconventional therapies for cancer: 1 Essiac. *CMAJ.* 1998;158:897-902.

45. Mansky PJ. Mistletoe and cancer: controversies and perspectives. *Semin Oncol.* 2002;29:589-594.

46. Kaegi E. Unconventional therapies for cancer: 3 Iscador. *CMAJ.* 1998;158:1157-1159.

47. Kleijnen J, Knipschild P. Mistletoe treatment for cancer: review of controlled trials in humans. *Phytomedicine.* 1994;1:255-260.

48. Pandha HS, Kirby RS. PC-SPES phytotherapy for prostate cancer. *Lancet.* 2002;359: 2213-2215.

49. DiPaola RS, Zhang H, Lambert GH, et al. Clinical and biologic activity of an estrogenic herbal combination (PC-SPEC) in prostate cancer. *N Engl J Med.* 1998;339:785-791.

50. Taille Adl, Kayek OR, Buttyan R, Bagiella E, Burchardt M, Katz AE. Effects of a phytotherapeutic agent; PC-SPES; on prostate cancer: a preliminary investigation on human cell lines and patients. *BJU Int.* 1999;84:845-850.

51. Oka H, Yamamoto S, Kuroki T, et al. Prospective study of chemoprevention of hepatocellular carcinoma with Sho-saiko-to (TJ-9). *Cancer.* 1995;76:743-749.

52. Alecu M, Ursaciuc C, Halalau F, et al. Photodynamic treatment of basal cell carcinoma and squamous cell carcinoma with hypericin. *Anticancer Res.* 1998;18:4651-4654.

53. Kaegi E. Unconventional therapies for cancer: 4 Hydrazine sulfate. *CMAJ.* 1998;158: 897-902.

54. Moertel CG, Fleming TR, Rubin J. A clinical trial of amygdalin (Laetrile) in the treatment of human cancer. *N Engl J Med.* 1982;306:201-216.

55. Jacobson JS, Workman SB, Kronenberg F. Research on complementary/alternative medicine for patients with breast cancer: a review of the biomedical literature. *J Clin Oncol.* 2000;18:668-683.

56. Lissoni P, Barni S, Ardizzoa A. A randomized study with pineal hormone melatonin versus supportive care alone in patients with brain metastases due to solid neoplasms. *Cancer.* 1994;73:699-701.

57. Kaegi E. Unconventional therapies for cancer: 6 714-X. *CMAJ.* 1998;158:1621-1624.

58. DeVere White RW, Hackman RM, Soares SE, Beckett LA, Sun B. Effects of a mushroom mycelium extract on the treatment of prostate cancer. *Urology.* 2002;60:640-644.

59. Ernst E. Antiangiogenic shark cartilage as a treatment for cancer? *Perfusion.* 1998;11:49.

60. Miller DR, Anderson GT, Stark JJ, Granick JL, Richardson D. Phase I/II trial of the safety and efficacy of shark cartilage in the treatment of advanced cancer. *J Clin Oncol.* 1998;16:3649-3655.

61. Ernst E. Thymus therapy for cancer? A criteria-based, systematic review. *Eur J Cancer.* 1997;33:531-534.

62. Spiegel D, Bloom JR, Kraemer HC. Effect of psychosocial treatment on survival of patients with metastatic breast cancer. *Lancet.* 1989;ii:888-891.

63. Spiegel D. Effects of psychotherapy on cancer survival. *Nature Rev Cancer.* 2002;2:338-389.

64. Li JH. A study on treatment of lung cancer by combined therapy of traditional Chinese medicine and chemotherapy. *Chung-Kuo Hsi I Chieh Ho Tsa Chih.* 1996;16:136-138.

65. Bagenal FS, Easton DF, Harris E, Chilvers CED, McElwain TJ. Survival of patients with breast cancer attending Bristol Cancer Help Centre. *Lancet.* 1990;336:606-610.

66. Cassileth BR, Lusk EJ, Guerry Dea. Survival and quality of life among patients receiving unproven as compared with conventional cancer therapy. *N Engl J Med.* 1991;324:1180-1185.

67. Gonzalez NJ, Isaacs NL. Evaluation of pancreatic proteolytic enzyme treatment of adeno-carcinoma of the pancreas, with nutrition and detoxification support. *Nutr Cancer.* 1999;33:115-116.

68. Vickers AJ. Can acupuncture have specific effects on health? A systematic review of acupuncture anti-emesis trials. *J Roy Soc Med.* 1996;89:303-311.

69. Spiegel D, Bloom JR. Group therapy and hypnosis reduce metastatic breast carcinoma pain. *Psychosom Med.* 1983;45:333-339.

70. Syrjala KL, Cummings C, Donaldson GW. Hypnosis or cognitive behavioral training for the reduction of pain and nausea during cancer treatment: a controlled clinical trial. *Pain.* 1992;48:137-146.

71. Hawkins PJ, Liossi C, Ewart BW, Hatira P, Kosmidis VH, Varvutsi M. Hypnotherapy for control of anticipatory nausea and vomiting in children with cancer: preliminary findings. *Psycho-Oncology.* 1995;4:101-106.

72. Zeltzer LK, Dolgin MJ, LeBaron S, LeBaron C. A randomized, controlled study of behavioral intention for chemotherapy distress in children with cancer. *Pediatrics.* 1991;88:34-42.

73. Sloman R, Brown P, Aldana E, Chee E. The use of relaxation for the promotion of comfort and pain relief in persons with advanced cancer. *Contemporary Nurse.* 1994;3:6-12.

74. Walker LG, Walker MB, Ogston K, et al. Psychological, clinical and pathological effects of relaxation training and guided imagery during primary chemotherapy. *Br J Cancer.* 1999;80:262-268.

75. Hauser SP. Alzoon—anticancer remedy or herbal concoction? *Schweiz Rundsch Med Prax.* 1997;86:1113-1115.

76. Leipner J, Saller R. Systematic enzyme therapy in oncology. *Forsch Komplementarmed.* 2000;7:45.

77. Samarel N, Fawcett J, Davis MM, Ryan FM. Effects of dialogue and therapeutic touch on preoperative and postoperative experiences of breast cancer surgery: an exploratory study. *Oncol Nurs Forum.* 1998;25:1369-1376.

78. Giasson M, Bouchard L. Effect of therapeutic touch on the well-being of persons with terminal cancer. *J Holistic Nurs.* 1998;16:383-398.

79. Targ EF, Levine EG. The efficacy of a mind-body-spirit group for women with breast cancer: a randomized controlled trial. *Gen Hosp Psychiatry.* 2002;24:238-248.

80. Petersen RW, Quinlivan JA. Preventing anxiety and depression in gynaecological cancer: a randomised controlled trial. *Br J Obstet Gynaecol.* 2002;109:386-394.

81. Munoz GH, Pluchino S. Cimifuga racemosa for the treatment of hot flushes in women surviving breast cancer. *Maturitas.* 2003;44(suppl 1):S59-S65.

82. Ware MA, Doyle CR, Woods R, Lynch ME, Clark AJ. Cannabis use for chronic non-cancer pain: results of a prospective survey. *Pain.* 2003;102:211-216.

83. Ernst E, Pittler MH, Stevinson C, White AR. *The Desktop Guide to Complementary and Alternative Medicine.* Edinburgh: Mosby; 2001.

84. Pan CX, Morrison RS, Ness J, Fugh-Berman A, Leipzig RM. Complementary and alternative medicine in the management of pain, dyspnea, and nausea and vomiting near end of life: a systematic review. *J Pain Symptom Manage.* 2000;20:374-387.

85. Bratman S, Girman AM. Handbook of herbs and supplements and their therapeutic uses. St Louis, MA: Mosby; 2003.

86. Herr SM, Ernst E, Young VSL. *Herb-Drug Interaction Handbook.* Nassua, NY: Church Street Books; 2002.

87. Ernst E. Toxic heavy metals and undeclared drugs in Asian herbal medicines. *Trends Pharmacol Sci.* 2002;23:136-139.

88. Ernst E. Adulteration of Chinese herbal medicines with synthetic drugs: a systematic review. *J Intern Med.* 2002;252:107-113.

89. Huang WF, Wen KC, Hsiao ML. Adulteration by synthetic therapeutic substances of traditional chinese medicines in Taiwan. *J Clin Pharmacol.* 1997;37:334-350.

90. Gurley BJ, Gardner SF, Hubbard MA. Content versus label claims in ephedra-containing dietary supplements. *Am J Health-Syst Pharm.* 2000;57:963-969.

91. Coppes MJ, Anderson RA, Egeler RM, Wolff JEA. Alternative therapies for the treatment of childhood cancer. *N Engl J Med.* 1998;339:846-847.

92. Oneschuk D, Bruera E. The potential dangers of complementary therapy use in a patient with cancer. *J Palliat Care.* 1999;15:49-52.

93. Moody GA, Eaden JA, Bhakta P, Sher K, Mayberry JF. The role of complementary medicine in European and Asian patients with inflammatory bowel disease. *Public Health.* 1998;112:269-271.

94. Ernst E. Iridology—not useful and potentially harmful. *Arch Ophthalmol.* 2000;118:120-121.

95. Barnes J, Mills SY, Abbot NC, Willoughby M, Ernst E. Different standards for reporting ADRs to herbal remedies and conventional OTC medicines face-to-face interviews with 515 users of herbal remedies. *Br J Clin Pharmacol.* 1998;45:496-500.

96. Ernst E, Armstrong NC. Lay books on complementary/alternative medicine: a risk factor for good health. *Int J Risk Safety Med.* 1998;11:209-215.

97. Gotay CC, Dumitriu D. Health food store recommendations for breast cancer patients. *Arch Fam Med.* 2000;9:692-698.

98. Ernst E, Weihmayr T. UK and German media differ over complementary medicine. *BMJ.* 2000;321:707.

99. White JD. Complementary and alternative medicine research: a national cancer institute perspective. *Semin Oncol.* 2002;29:546-551.

Dying and Death in Different Cultures

Chapter 11

Bereavement across Cultures

Richard T. Penson

INTRODUCTION

Bereavement is an inevitable part of life and an all too common part of cancer care. Death is a universal human experience about which science has taught us nothing. It is a taboo subject that draws morbid fascination or counter-phobic indifference. We have the unsubstantiated theories of science and psychology, religious superstitions and logical inconsistencies, and the pretensions of art and poetry. If there is nothing we can do about death, perhaps we should echo the collective unconscious and treat it as if it does not exist, high priests of the illusion that we can live forever? Confronted with the limits of treatment and subsequent death, support of the bereaved is one of the hardest tasks for the caregiver, and one of the most neglected.

Yet, there remains a responsibility to provide support for those grieving, care that goes beyond the death. A compassionate response helps both those who suffer and those who care. This chapter reviews the literature on culture and bereavement. Grief reactions, complicated and uncomplicated bereavement, counseling, cultural influences, and religious interpretations of bereavement are reviewed. The goals of this chapter are to enhance readers' understanding of cultural differences in grief, and promote culturally competent bereavement care. In what follows, the subject and important definitions are introduced. The theories of bereavement,

241

coping, and counseling are discussed, with a focus on perspectives on cancer, bereavement, and culture. As religious aspects of culture and bereavement have such a large influence on the experience, a separate section is devoted to religion. Insights throughout are supported with illustrations from the world literature and clinical practice.

Although the attempt is to present a global worldview, many of the insights have been formulated from a US perspective.

DEFINITIONS

Bereavement
The situation of anyone who has lost a person to whom they are attached.
Grief
The psychological and emotional reactions to bereavement.
Mourning
The ceremonies and practices of bereavement.

BEREAVEMENT

Grief is the psychological, behavioral, social, and physical reaction to the loss of someone or something that is closely tied to a person's identity. Grief is a universal, natural, but intensely individual aspect of human experience. Mourning represents the process by which people adapt to loss. Bereavement is the period after a loss during which grief is experienced and mourning occurs.[1-4]

The death of a loved one is widely acknowledged to be one of the most traumatic of life events.[5] Conjugal bereavement, sudden or traumatic death, and the death of a child are generally regarded the most severe types of loss.[6,7] Human beings need to belong, to feel valued, to achieve and find meaning. Death challenges all of these and the constant torture that there is now no value to life without the deceased whom you have lost, the biggest threat in life. C.S. Lewis eloquently observed that inherent in loving much, was that, at some point, much would be lost.[8] Grief is a sign of love, and love a virtue. Mourning is clearly a way of esteeming both the mourner and the dead. Within a social contract, it is clearly a time of profound pain, reflection, and adjustment. While in postmodern US culture, which honors the autonomous individual, and with our social connection challenged,[9] bereavement is very much seen as the unique response of an individual within the cultural context, destabilizing and isolating. Yet, in other cultures bereavement is far more certain and structured.[10]

While there are no pan-human categories for understanding death, there are core elements than can provide insight into the processes involved in bereavement. Rosenblatt, Walsh, and Jackson compared anthropologists' evaluations in 78 societies, representative of 186 world cultures, concluding that crying, fear, and anger were commonly and consistently experienced across all cultures and that most cultures provide social sanction for their expression.[11] There is some evidence that expressing grief more fully, translates into less lasting depression.[10] However, the grief response varies so much in character, duration, and magnitude with psychological, cognitive, and interpersonal disruptions that such a norm is hard to define. Furthermore, the interface with psychiatry is blurred. Up to 50% of widows may have transient but vivid hypnogogic hallucinations of the dead person, who is often felt to be near at hand.[6,7] Triggers and anniversaries can often prompt distress years later. Moreover, the psychosocial transition is usually unwelcome and ruminations resisted.

Bereavement is associated with declines in health, inappropriate health service use, elevated risk of depression, sleep disruption, increased consumption of tobacco, alcohol, and tranquillizers, increased depression and suicide, and excess mortality.[12,13] Yet, many individuals receive little or no support from clinicians for their grief during the bereavement period. Although much care may be marshaled, there is a universal guilt that more should be done.[14] For instance, a telephone interview study of 53 English-speaking relatives or close companions of adults who had died in the proceeding year at Massachusetts General Hospital (MGH) reported high satisfaction. However, there were complaints about the lack of privacy, dignity, and comfort, poor communication, excessive waiting for care, little attention to advanced directives, and little bereavement support. Over one third of relatives reported no contact with hospital health professionals after the death and of the 19% who sought professional help, none had been referred by their own, or the deceased's, physician.[15] Larger studies corroborate these findings.[16] Moreover, even in areas well served by palliative care, such as the United Kingdom, family's needs for additional information and emotional support continue to be great.[17]

There are a number of constructs that attempt to explain how individuals cope with grief. The task-based approach is the model most commonly used.[18] Kubler-Ross' seminal model describing loss, with the stages of denial, anger, bargaining, depression, and acceptance, has been criticized as inflexible.[19] Grief contains three essential elements: distress and missing the lost person, an urge to avoid or repress crying and searching and an urge to review and revise internal models.[6] While all these behaviors are common in bereavement, not all individuals experience all stages, some skip stages, while others regress through stages or experience different reactions concurrently. Increasingly, the phases of grief are seen in relation to the conceptual framework of attachment theory. Attachment theory informs much of the anthropologic view of social and structural factors that influence behavior. Attachment theory describes the bonds that are formed early in life with parental figures and derived from the need to feel secure and human information processing, the filtering of unwanted information. These concepts help divide the bereavement process into four phases: (1) shock: survivors have difficulty processing the loss and are stunned and numb; (2) yearning and searching: Pining with emotional turmoil, anger, self-reproach, bewilderment, or anxiety. Intense separation anxiety and denial of the reality of the loss; (3) disorganization and despair, depression and distraction lead to difficulty in planning future activities, and (4) reorganization and recovery: positive readjustment.[20] Though sorrow is intensely painful and psychologically draining, grief is a normal emotional response to the whole experience of loss.[21,22] Grief can be: (1) anticipatory, or (2) acute with pathologic variance of grief being: (1) chronic; (2) absent; (3) inhibited; (4) delayed; (5) unanticipated; or (6) abbreviated.

Classic Commentaries

Three studies have significantly framed research in the field of bereavement. In a seminal study of survivors post-disaster, Lindemann first called attention to issues related to loss, grief, and bereavement.[23] Three elements to bereavement were identified: (1) grief follows loss; (2) symptoms of grief vary among individuals; and (3) the outcome of grieving may be adaptive or nonadaptive. Subsequently, Parkes reported his observation of bereavement in a longitudinal study of London widows over 13 months.[24] More recently, Clayton studied 171 White men and women, and reported that increased use of alcohol, tranquilizers, hypnotics, and cigarettes, was associated with increased mortality in men under the age of 75 years during the first year of bereavement. In that particular study, however, poor physical or mental health before the loss proved to be a better predictor of negative outcomes.[25]

Optimal End-of-Life Care: Anticipating Bereavement

The quality of care at the end of a patient's life is very important to the family of the patient and can directly affect the way the family deals with the death of their loved one. In order to truly be effective in end-of-life care, the clinician needs to be certain that he or she addresses the pressing issues of the impending grief of the patient as well as that of the family and the caregivers.[22]

Good Death: Toward a Definition

The wish to plan and control major life events, including death is an important feature of self-identity in late modern societies.[26] Patients and family members define a "good" death based on physical comfort, the quality of personal relationships, finding meaning in their life and death, feeling some sense of control in the situation, and active preparations for death.[16] Whenever possible, the family should have the opportunity to be present at the actual time of death.[27] Yet individual wishes, particularly in the Western context, may conflict with the desires of the family. Nonetheless, at the time of death there are three cardinal rules: (1) we should take our cue from the family or partner and enable them to do things their way; (2) although talk is awkward it is right in the right place but there is rarely something that you can say that will make it better. If somebody wants to talk let them talk and if they are silent let them be silent; and (3) there are practical things to be done and these you should do. Immediately after the death, the bereaved need compassionate attention and validation of their loss, with time and permission to grieve.

In many non-Western societies, or with patients from non-Western contexts who increasingly live in the West, death rituals are more elaborate and protracted than those common in Western society. These exist in contrast with a largely rapid burial, discomfort at wakes, and the delay of a week between death and funeral in Western Christian burial.[10] This will be addressed in the sections "Cancer, Bereavement, Culture" and "Religious Aspects of Culture and Bereavement."

Complicated Grief

In 1944, Lindemann described "morbid grief reactions,"[23] Complicated or pathological grief occurs when normal bereavement, associated with psychiatric sequelae, overlaps with an adjustment disorder, major depression, substance abuse, or posttraumatic stress disorder. There is no clear definition and the cultural context has a profound influence on the interpretation of the intensity of loss and disruption caused by "excessive" grief. Nevertheless, there is greater consensus about absent, inhibited, delayed, conflicted, or chronic grief.[1,28] How long grief must persist to be considered pathologic remains a contentious matter of debate. Horowitz reported pathologic grief occurring within the first year of bereavement.[29] Jacobs reported highest levels of grief during the first 4 months of bereavement.[30] Parkes and Brown reported the level of depression and autonomic symptoms that differentiated one-year bereaved survivors from non-bereaved individuals in a long-term follow up study with some evidence that the symptoms persisted for up to 3 years after the death of a loved one.[6]

Parkes describes three typical types of abnormal grief: (1) traumatic loss; (2) conflicted grief; and (3) chronic grief.[31] Identifying compounding grief from earlier losses, unfinished business, and secondary gain may be necessary to enable the grief to be working through. While some argue for early intervention for major depressive disorders irrespective of bereavement status,[32] others advocate treatment be instituted only if symptoms persist beyond 1 year after the loss,[33,34] yet other diagnostic algorithms for diagnosing complicated grief mandate significant "separation distress," "traumatic distress," and disrupted functioning extending beyond 6 months.[35] Obviously suicidal ideation should always prompt urgent assessment.

Traumatic loss involves acute anxiety or even panic and reactions similar to posttraumatic stress disorder with an exaggeration of the period of shock and the withdrawal from society more pronounced. Conflicted grief follows an ambivalent attachment between spouse or partner with the immediate reaction often one of relief. There is often considerable unfinished business to be attended to and people often find themselves haunted by memories of the lost person and unsure or guilty about their reaction. Stormy relationships may to a degree be similar though more commonly characterized by conflicts with their family of the dead person. Chronic grief often arises from a relationship, which contained a considerable dependent element. Classically when the weak one in a mutually supportive system dies, it is the strong partner who collapses.

Gender and Age

There are significant gender differences in the experience of bereavement, though contradictory data exist.[36,37] Reactions appear to be more pronounced in mothers than fathers, and more widows seeking help for emotional problems.[36] On the other hand, widows' levels of anxiety and depression during the first year of bereavement have been reported to return to normal more quickly than those of widowers and the increased risk of a cardiovascular death appears to be greater in men than women.[37] Age, gender, and culture are also significant factors that influence emotional expression and processing during the course of grief. For instance, in old age, bereavement is less often unexpected and untimely and often, though not always, associated with less intense emotional disturbance.[38]

Predictors of Poor Outcome

Several factors have emerged that are clear predictors of poor outcome after bereavement. Many of these are codependent variables.[39] Clearly, the cultural context of the death is significant with sudden unexpected deaths being more difficult to process, though some studies have not found this to be so, perhaps again depending on the subject's age.[39-42] And though anticipated loss may mitigate the distress, the expectations and roles of the survivors more powerfully influence the outcome.

Past history of psychiatric illness is a major risk for maladaption after bereavement. More subtle morbidity has also been linked with a worse outcome. For example, lack of confidence, both in themselves and in others predicts a poor outcome,[43] as does certain aspects of the relationship between the bereaved and the lost, with clinging or ambivalent relationships being particularly important. The existence of a caring family who provide support appears to significantly influence outcome though it has been hard to measure and it is often the providers' perception of the family that is important rather than the numbers of available shoulders or active goodwill.

Other risk factors for abnormal grief reactions include: (1) poor social support; (2) being under 45 when the spouse dies suddenly or over 65 when the spouse has illness of 65 months or more; (3) ambivalent marital relationships; and (4) minimal funeral ceremony associated with a denial of the impact of death.[36,44]

Burnout

Of all work in oncology, it is arguable that bereavement care not only takes the greatest toll but benefits from the least resources and burnout is considerable. However, isolated physicians such as radiologists may be more at risk than palliative care physicians who work in a well-structured team.[45] Interestingly, the original reports about burnout from Freudenberg contain an essential element of grief. The term "burnout" was first used in the medical arena by Herbert Freudenberger in 1974.[46] Burnout comprises three key components: emotional exhaustion, depersonalization (treating people in an unfeeling, impersonal way), and low personal accomplishment.[45,47] Freudenberger, a distinguished psychologist who died in 2001, formulated this concept having worked alongside volunteers in the free clinic movement that served Vietnam veterans. He observed that the most dedicated and committed caregivers seemed especially at risk from burnout and that the condition was compounded by a sense of loss of idealism. He concluded: "If your idealism, the very motivation that led you to come into an institution... has been lost, then burnout has also within it the dynamics of mourning."[46]

Research

Much of the available information about the social and psychological consequences of death appears in retrospective studies. Still few studies have benefited from acceptable controls or random allocation of intervention. Nevertheless, studies in large numbers of patient,[24] have clearly and convincingly shown an association between bereavement and clinical depression and suicide. However, such a complicated multifaceted issue is clearly difficult to disentangle. It is clear that there is huge variation between and within subjects and over time. As an example, differences in quality of life as measured on the 100-point EORTC QTC-Q30 scale between well patients on adjuvant chemotherapy and unwell patients on palliative chemotherapy are approximately 10 points, while the variation within any individual from a good day to a bad day is approximately 20 points.[48]

COPING AND COUNSELING

Central to coping for the bereaved are getting information, opening options, and having personal support.[49] Ritual social support is an important way of reassuring people that they are not alone by offering relief of responsibilities during the early stage of grief, structured social calendar, and pastoral care. It is clear that the funeral is as much for the bereaved as the dead.[50] The funeral and memorial service incontrovertibly articulate the finality of the death. However, there are many cultures where a second ceremony marks final resting of the earth bound spirits of the dead which remain closed during the early period of mourning.[11] Formal ceremony may help mourners move out of their particular status and re-enter society while honoring the enduring memory of the lost. Rando identified the organized ritual of traditional religion as a helpful structure, while encouraging a closer calibration between ritual experts and psychological experts.[1] A consideration of age, gender, social role in the family, in the asking about feelings, function, goals, dreams, and responsibilities will improve an appreciation of how attitude and choices are informed. A very helpful way to evaluate the various influences within a family following bereavement is by a "relational network," mapping out on the family tree, the social and emotional connections between people and asking how each is coping. Such a "genogram" can identify both people at risk and ways to respond. Preparing or helping someone through bereavement by facing the reality of the situation, however, painful this may be, is sometimes profoundly affective and crystallized in Ira Byock's five questions/statements: (1) I love you; (2) Thank you; (3) I am sorry for ...; (4) I forgive you for ...; and (5) Good bye.[51] Responsibilities as well as hopes and dreams should be addressed.

Self-Help and Good Advice

Listed below are a few key points to coping or essential good advice taken from a chapter the author wrote for the UK Oncology text book: *Treatment of Cancer*, Bob Buckman's book *I don't know what to say* and Colin Murray Parkes' work.[10,52,53]

1. Grief, with its many ups and downs, lasts far longer than most people expect. Be patient with yourself.
2. Each person's grief is individual. You and your family will experience it and cope with it in your own way. You may feel there is nothing to live for. Be assured that many bereaved persons feel this way, but that a sense of purpose and meaning does return. The pain does lessen. There is nothing wrong with crying. It is a healthy expression of grief. Apathy, guilt, and anger are normal part of grief and sharing how you feel will help.
3. Avoid the use of illicit drugs and alcohol. Medication should be taken only under the supervision of your physician.
4. Friends and relatives may sometimes be uncomfortable around you. They want to ease your pain, but do not know how. Take the initiative if you can, and let them know how they can be supportive to you. Talk about your loved one so that they will feel freer to be able to do the same.
5. Consider putting off major decisions for at least a year. Avoid making hasty decisions about your loved one's belongings. Do not allow others to take over or to rush you. You can do it little by little whenever you feel ready.

Counseling

Proactively providing indicated counseling around the time of death appears to help shorten the period of distress after bereavement.[54] Psychological research suggests that the denial or avoidance of distressing thoughts may enable people to get through periods of crisis and is an appropriate defense.[55] Although cognitive behavioral therapy remains the backbone of psychological interventions, other components of care include training in self-management skills, problem-solving skills, self-discovery, group or relaxation therapy.[56] Nonetheless, denial is an unstable defense that cannot always be maintained and given appropriate support most people choose to express grief and process the emotion. Tears and fears abate with a period of adjustment and increasing ability to talk about distressing aspects. It is clear that colluding with initial denial can slow the process of adjustment. It remains a sad paradox that when a family is most aware of their need, they are least likely to be supported by the medical profession.[12] For instance, although at least 90% of National Cancer Institute Comprehensive Cancer Centers offer programs, worryingly, much of the response to the bereaved focuses more on the effort to continue services rather than on efforts to resolve grief.[57,58] Quality of life is not only worse for the primary caretaker of cancer survivors, but the period of bereavement clearly contains the most anguish for a family. Generally, counseling for bereaved people has been generic or directed to high-risk group.[59] Grief counseling guides uncomplicated "normal" grief to healthy completion with insight and adjustment. The positive impact of counseling the bereaved was pioneered by Colin Murray Parkes with a study of the effects of a comprehensive bereavement program. Twenty close relatives of patients who had died in a palliative care unit were compared with a matched group of twenty relatives of patients who had died of cancer in other wards of the same hospital.[60] Interviewed by telephone 2 weeks and 1 year after bereavement, relatives of the palliative care unit patients reported significantly fewer psychological symptoms and less lasting grief and anger. Factors thought to have contributed to the better outcomes were successful relief of pain, awareness of the coming death of the patient, and support given to relatives after bereavement. A larger study also reported better outcomes for the bereaved of those who died in hospice.[61] However, other studies have reported few or no significant differences.[62] Notably Kane's study used a longitudinal design and randomized participants to either hospice or traditional care.[62]

In another randomized clinical trial conducted to assess the effects of homecare management for terminally ill patients on spousal psychological distress during bereavement, 42 patients' spouses were randomly assigned to either an Oncology Homecare Group that received care from advanced practice nurse, a standard homecare group that received care from nurses with standard training, or an office care group that received standard care.[63,64] Psychologic stress was significantly less among spouses of patients in the Oncology Homecare Group compared to the other two groups suggesting that psychological distress can be positively influenced by nursing interventions. Yalom and Lieberman reported that spouses who examined the death rather than look away from it were better able to deal with their situation.[65] Caplan stressed the importance of helping people confront a crisis in manageable doses.[66] No one is strong enough to look at the whole horror of death without respite.

Over the first month, expression of grief should be encouraged and the person reassured that it is a normal human reaction. Assessment of the social support and coping strategies should identify practical or financial problems. Beyond a month, a clinician should screen for depression, consider referral for counseling, or should consider pharmacologic intervention. A recent review helpfully summarized the assessment, recommendations for interventions, and indications for referral.[4] These data suggest that a variety of interventions, including individualized counseling by a trained volunteer, professional counseling, or group therapy may offer benefit.[60,67] Clinician competence in end-of-life care requires skill and relationship building. The carer needs to be prepared to establish what is known, negotiate how information should be handled, share bad news clearly and compassionately, respond to emotions, set goals, and agree to a plan.[22] A comprehensive assessment should include a screen of the psychosocial domains, with a view to optimizing control of symptoms, maintaining psychological integrity, and finding meaning in the chaos.[21] What did the illness mean to them?[68] What are their coping styles?[69-71] What is the extent of the social network?[72] What are the strengths and weaknesses of major relationships with the medical team?[73] What are the major stressors?[74,75] What spiritual resources are available?[76] Are there psychiatric vulnerabilities (depression, anxiety, or drug dependence?)[36,70] Are there financial issues?[77]

While not all sadness can be treated with antidepressants, it is clear that grief work, though hard, is crucial and the failure to grieve or suppression of it may increase both mental and physical illness.[78] The use of medications may be helpful in treating the bereaved but their use should be adjunctive, symptomatic, and limited in time. It should be goal oriented with explicit parameters.[79]

Emergency Response

There is a general consensus that the best time to start more formal bereavement counseling is between 3 and 8 weeks after the event. Before this time the bereaved are often too wrapped up in their families whereas 2 months after the event there is often a reluctance to again open the trauma. Yet there are times when an emergency response is necessary. Emergency care is typically delivered by hospital or emergency medical social workers and chaplains. It is clear that during the September 11 tragedies, much of the support came through both emergency medical services and local pastoral care within New York.[80] In the emergency setting, brief education and support interventions are now designed to avoid a detailed exploration of traumatic experiences, help workers and victims recognize and understand reactions to the event and, as appropriate, to normalize those reactions.

Organized Bereavement Care

The British Organization, Cruse affiliated with many hospices, with over 200 branches in the United Kingdom provides an excellent example of organized bereavement care.[36] The name "Cruse" comes from the widow's cruse or jar or oil, which was blessed by the prophet Elijah with a promise that it would not run out until famine was gone from the land (1 Kings, chapter 8, versus 8-16). Trainee counselors spend a minimum of 20 hr in seminar discussion groups and 12 hr in experiential learning before 60 supervised sessions that are required for accreditation. Compassionate friend is a similar mutual help organization run for parents who have lost a child.[81] Much of the support by group counseling or through individuals is by "befriending" and the encouragement of mutual self-help clearly go a long way in providing psychological support. The clinician must remember that clearly negotiated decisions about withdrawal of support are crucial, as it is important to be proactive about the length of the intervention.

Psychiatric Referral

Social workers, psychologists, and psychiatrists have an important role though typically the interface between psychological and spiritual care is hazy. Many symptoms can be differently interpreted with grief tinged with projection (psychological), paranoia (psychiatric), alienation (social), or guilt (theological). It is clear that the appreciation of the experience is richest when all the different perspectives inform the situation. Referral to a psychiatrist is as dependent on personal wishes and prevailing dogma, as much as the issue at hand. Much of the difficulty with the process of care comes from the temptation to find simple solutions to complex problems. The best practice appears to be reflected by active integration between all available services with hospice volunteer, national organizations, ethnic, and religious services all being made available. A physician should refer to a psychiatrist if the patient has suicidal thoughts and psychotic symptoms, or after a failure of a trial of antidepressants. Immediate threat of danger to the patient, public, or staff requires immediate action. The decision to refer a patient with complicated bereavement is more controversial and should be considered when it has persisted for longer than 4 months, but, rather than constrained by criteria should be negotiated with patient and psychiatrist.

Grieving Children

The National Cancer Institute estimates that 24% of adults with cancer are parenting children under 18 years.[82] See also Chapter 5, this volume. Developmental milestones in children significantly affect response to loss, and this can be complicated by failure to communicate. Inversion of parenting may occur with older children finding themselves expected to care for a grief stricken parent. Children are helped by a simple and age appropriate explanation of death. Questions should be addressed honestly and directly. Euphemisms that are open to misinterpretation should be avoided. Children benefit from being involved in the planning of and participation in mourning rituals. Common concerns of bereaved children are: was it my fault, is it going to happen to me, and who is going to take care of me? These should be explicitly addressed. If the remaining parent is too distressed to be a support, other support should be mobilized.[83] Perhaps what children, and adults, most need is that we be "real" with them, as outlined in the *Velveteen Rabbit* by Marjorie Williams in which the new toy learns the rocking horse's wisdom, earned in his dedication to love.[84]

Parents should be encouraged to learn as much as possible about the child's perception of events. Learn about the children and how they feel, maximize their support system, talk about death and bereavement, and address common questions and concerns like, "should I make my child talk about things?" Find creative and age appropriate ways to celebrate the great things about the one who has died and say goodbye, role-play ahead of time what should be said and tell the truth, but perhaps not the whole truth.[85,86] General principles include: (1) let the child ask questions, but actively read between the lines and ask questions; (2) make sure the child understands that he or she is not to blame and that cancer is not contagious; (3) be realistic and optimistic; (4) respect the child's reaction; (5) take account of the child's personality and the experience that he or she has had, or has not had, to date; (6) inform the child's teacher or guidance counselor about the bereavement.

The wounds of bereavement to a mother after her child dies from cancer are life long. For example, one in-depth study examined bereaved Japanese mothers.[87] Japanese mothers clearly obsessed over the child's remains, belongings, and memories from specific sad memories to recollections from child's life as a whole, and allowing Japanese mothers to handle the remains and belongings appeared to be an important catalyst for adjustment. Respect is required in anticipating when sad memories may decrease and mothers may start recalling better memories as well. Clearly much of the loss related to loss of what the child symbolized or might have become. Mothers could articulate that they are angry with God that he would not save the life of the child. The same mother after a year and 10 months could finally articulate that she realized that nothing could bring her back to life as it used to be.[87]

Condolences

Medical training offers little guidance in the provision of bereavement care. As a consequence, clinicians are often uncertain of how to distinguish between normal and pathological grief reactions, and how to manage the bereaved's health care.[12] For instance, physicians rarely write letters of condolence.[88] Yet the contact between the physician and the bereaved can be extremely helpful although there is little consensus about appropriate action. Caregivers fear making mistakes, feel they have too little training and rarely address their own sense of loss.[12] It is true. In the managed care environments, clinicians are often too busy. In addition, they may feel that they did not know the patient well enough to write a genuine letter of condolence. The responsibility for writing the letter may not be clearly assigned to one member of the team, or there may be no mechanism to collate information about recent deaths. Still, writing condolence letters requires that the clinician overcomes his own often profound sense of loss, his sense of failure, as it is hard to know what to say when someone dies.

A flurry of very positive correspondence followed a recent *New England Journal of Medicine* sounding board article "The doctor's letter of condolence."[89] A number of institutions have successfully instituted "task forces" or "bereavement coordinators" who coordinate letters, bereavement counseling, and have information about community resources, support groups, and the services of the hospital chaplains.[90] However, a personal letter from the clinician to the patient's family or partner communicates compassionate care. The article helpfully listed suggested elements to a letter of condolence: (1) A direct expression of sorrow. This should not revisit clinical issues in order to avoid issues of legal liability; (2) Detail of the extent and depth of the relationship between clinician and patient; (3) A specific personal memory; (4) Reference to the patient's work, courage, or character, and (5) A statement that it was a privilege to have taken part in the patient's care.[89] Superficial attempts to assuage grief, such as, "It was meant to be," or "I know how you feel," should be avoided. Moreover, premature reassurance about adjustment is at best useless and worst, destructive.

Suggestions for Clinical Practice

The following bulleted list is taken from two resources. A chapter the author wrote for the UK Oncology text book: *Treatment of Cancer* and Walter Baile's and Bob Buckman's formulation of breaking bad news: CONES.[52,91] C.O.N.E.S., being an eponym for *C*ontext, getting the setting right, then starting with an *O*pening shot, before a clear *N*arrative of the issues that allows clarification of understanding. *E*motions have to be addressed, with an empathic response being one that: (1) identifies the emotion and (2) the source of that emotion and (3) demonstrates you have made the connection in a nonjudgmental fashion. Finally, it is essential to establish a plan and *S*ummarize. You should always negotiate an invitation to explore such sensitive issues.

- Be prepared: Anticipate needs
- Address your own sense of loss
- Be aware: make time for and give priority to important things
- If you feel unable, get trained, or staff your weaknesses
- Be informed: if you do not know ask
- If you make a mistake, assume too much, or are insensitive, apologize. People are amazingly forgiving
- Provide a direct expression of sorrow, with eye contact and touch
- Recall a specific personal memory. Refer to the patient's work, courage, character, or state that it was a privilege to have taken part in the patient's care
- Avoid premature reassurance about adjustment
- Address dreams and responsibilities. Ask about unfulfilled life goals
- Provide information about resources, support groups, and local services
- Broaden the team of people involved in support by involving hospital chaplains and social workers
- Proved psychotropic sedatives with clear goals in a set time frame
- Refer to a psychiatrist for (1) suicidal thoughts and psychotic symptoms, (2) failure of a trial of antidepressants, and (3) complicated bereavement that lasts longer than 4 months.

CANCER, BEREAVEMENT, CULTURE: SOME PERSPECTIVES

Cancer remains a leading cause of death and is predicted to overtake heart disease as the leading cause of death in the United States in the near future. Approximately 80% of American life ends in hospital.[92] Life and death have been "medicalized" to be sanitized. Although much of the rhetoric is changing from "war on cancer" to "living with" or surviving cancer, bereavement remains a testament to the failure of modern medical treatments and cancer and anticancer campaigns have replaced war and warfare as the modern crusade. Many elements of grief and mourning are strongly influenced by cultural aspects, but they are not immutable and evolve over time.[93] Briefly, culture in this instance is defined as a unified set of values, traditions, ideas, beliefs, standards of behavior, and possessions that are shared by an identifiable group of people.[94] In the broadest sense, cultural identity represents an integral aspect of a distinct group that is recognized by race, geography, age, education, gender, income, sexual orientation, taste, or character. It is also typically associated with judgment and separation; "One tends to apply the term 'culture or culturally different' to others and not to oneself."[95] For these reasons, cultural differences in oncology care remain fraught with sensitivities, justified by past abuses and the considerable potential for future abuse, and further compacted by suspicion and vulnerability. How do we cross and respect cultural boundaries in these contexts? The considerable variation between different religious and ethnic background is also to a large degree colored by national origin. Cultural groups tend to deliberately emphasize differences, particularly differences in major lifestyle events around birth, marriage, death and identifiable distinctions of diet, dress, and social interaction. Nevertheless, few people, no matter how tightly rigorous or orthodox, fully adhere to all that the textbook holds to be true, and there is considerable personal variation in an increasingly eclectic world made all the more a mixture by travel and technology. For instance, even Jehovah's Witness may break ranks over blood products.[96] The one absolute rule is that there are no absolutely hard and fast rules. However, there has to be a balance even within the Western cultural context. To seek balance and to enhance care, we must develop cultural competence. If we want to know what individuals think, we have to ask them and seek to understand their experiences accrued within a distinct cultural and historical framework.

Culture, Concepts, and Care

In 1944, Lindemann proposed that bereaved people need to separate from the memories of the deceased, readjust to the environment in which the deceased is missing and form new relationships.[23] Uncomplicated bereavement is not a mental disorder. Under normal circumstances, a grief reaction is not pathological and is an essential period of adaptation.[97] One wonderful commentary by Dickens perfectly describes both complicated and uncomplicated bereavement [98]. Here the jilted Miss Havisham barely lives with a broken heart, arrested in time and shrouded in her withered bridal dress, like "grave-clothes." Miss Havisham engages Pip to be a companion but her dark motivation is to use Estella, her ward, to wreak havoc on men's souls. The book turns beautifully to end with an interpretation of uncomplicated bereavement where Estella, suffering the lesson of loss, bent and broken, but better for the experience.[98] While an active attempt to make sense of the experience of loss and add significance of traumatic aspects of loss is clearly positive,[99] this view of bereavement may be too narrow and needs to be expanded. The 20th and 21st century models of the grief process emphasize the necessity for the survivor "to let go" in order to establish new relationships, yet for many people a healthy resolution of grief enables them to maintain a continuing bond with the deceased in their lives and communities.[100] The old model is based more on the cultural values of "Western" modernity and will be significantly molded by our ever-increasing multicultural and pluralistic society. Can we learn from each other? Can we integrate and can we, in medicine, acknowledge differences and treat patients equally across cultural divides? The death of any culture, threatens civilization.

In the past, disease- and system-based learning have dominated medical education. However, in cross-cultural interactions, the inductive, or patient-centered, approach is often invaluable. In this model, the patient, rather than the theory, is the starting point. This requires that the clinician and medical team become skilled observers of patient behavior in clinical settings. A sensitive exploration of a patient's culturally proscribed understandings of health, illness, and disease engenders a more complete sense of the values, assumptions, and expectations patients hold and effectively affirms the patients and their family's dignity and intrinsic worth.[101,102] Decisions are then based primarily on the patient and family, secondarily on the patient's immediate social and community context and their wider ethnic identity. Stereotyping "culture" as "the rare, quaint practices of unsophisticated peoples,"[103] and using outdated and inaccurate generalizations while attempting to be culturally sensitive are likely to reinforce negative biases which can lead to other adverse outcomes such as noncompliance.[104] Likewise, attributing correlates of social class and education to culture may also reinforce negative ethnic bias. Indeed, in studies of ethnic differences that controlled socioeconomic status, many group differences previously explained by culture disappeared.[105]

Cultural competence

Cultural competence is characterized by an individual or collective respect and response to the values and believes of specific people groups.[106] Cultural competence also improves satisfaction with care, compliance, and can aid in the clinician's interpretation of how the patients', their relatives' and significant others' understandings of the ways health, illness, and disease are shaped and expressed.[107] It is, for instance, important to understand the relevance of the conflict between "American" cultural values of individualism and self-determination, which mark freedom as individual autonomy,[108,109] which stands in marked contrast to "European" freedom, framed much more in a community context, and in the importance of the group over the individual, and reinforced in the face of national adversity.[110] Much of the Anglo American and British commitment to hospice and palliative care is still alien to other cultures where there is greater fatalism, and stronger respect for the traditional authority of the medical profession. Such paternalism remains perhaps strongest in Italy, France, Greece, and Japan.[108,111-113] Moreover, this is also changing perhaps most rapidly in Eastern Europe with the rapid change in political and economic climate.[111,114] Fundamental philosophical differences exist between "Western" thought about helping people cope with their eventual death, and terminally ill patients who are African American, American Indian or Native American, Asian Pacific Islander or Hispanic Latino, or first generation Caribbean Londoner, who may wish at all cost to prolong life and might rather pray for a miracle than accept hospice care.[115,116] Studies in United States indicate that patients often accept hospice care while everyone around them was still hoping for a miracle, and reported the common belief that God determined whether they lived or died rather than medical treatment or lack of it.[115] In such settings, open discussion and communication of goals remain a challenge. Thus, there remains a tension that exists within the diverse character of North America with the legitimacy of affirmative action being questioned. For example, while there has been a 17% drop in minority applications to Medical schools in California, Texas, Louisiana, and Mississippi (states that have been successful in reversing affirmative action policy),[117] minority patients are still five times more likely than their white counterparts to receive, or desire to receive, medical care from a minority physician.[118,119] Other research on African American and Hispanic patients in the context of AIDS were less likely to communicate their end of life issues to physicians and reluctant to use hospice for a variety of reasons, including economics, lack of knowledge, and mistrust of the system.[120] And still other studies indicate that non-Hispanic Whites were more likely to be race concordant with their physician compared to African American, Hispanic, and Asian American respondents. Among each race/ethnic group, respondents who were race concordant reported greater satisfaction with their physician compared with respondents who were not race concordant.[118] These findings are not only true in the North American context. For example, a study of the assessment and management of cancer symptoms in first-generation Caribbean Londoners, noted that respondents were also more likely to say that general practitioners, though not hospital doctors, could have tried harder to manage.[116] In other instances, while in North American "medical culture," informing patients of diagnosis and prognosis, both good and bad, is considered both respectful and obligatory,[121] in Native American culture "magical thinking," is used as a tool for healing the rift between mind and body that is caused by cancer and related treatments. As a consequence, it is often considered disrespectful and potentially harmful to predict a bad outcome.[122] Similar to studies on cancer in Tanzania and Ethiopia, in the Navajo philosophy of *nozho*, disclosing a bad diagnosis or prognosis is dangerous and disrespectful because "thoughts are things, thus one's thought and the language one chooses to use has the power to shape reality, and to control the outcome of events."[122-124] Yet another important means of gaining cultural competence is the inclusion of the perspectives of clinicians from culturally, linguistically diverse backgrounds. While a lack of minority clinicians (or clinicians who come from the same cultural groups) input could potentially compromise care since patients may either feel less comfortable or unable to fully communicate their needs to nonminority clinicians. In other instances, the patient may also choose to communicate such needs in his or her own language. Discussions about death, grief, and loss among a patient, a care giver, and the family of the same religious, socioeconomic and cultural background remain highly challenging, and even more so when they are from very different backgrounds.[125] Thus, communicating with a clinician from the same or similar cultural background can be profoundly comforting. These cultural differences are implicated in the patterns of communication between clinician and patient, the expectations of care, in patient satisfaction, and in the care that is actually received by both the patient and the family. For these reasons, the inclusion of culturally diverse insights from the multidisciplinary team can create a win-win situation since it can potentially assist in the effective communication and transmission of care to patients from culturally diverse backgrounds.[125]

We Die as We Live

Within the diversity of humankind, a given personality may be largely genetically determined. "Born miserable, die miserable," being scientifically defensible.[126-128] Thoughts reap actions; actions reap habits and habits destinies. We do die as we have lived. Respecting someone's coping style may resource them to again cope, to mobilize their coping strategies in the face of a greater threat like cancer or death. For example; many clinicians are potentially more vulnerable to burnout as they have a significant emphatic component to their personality.[129] Holland holds that specific personality types will flourish in a similar environment. The six categories being: (1) realistic: people who enjoy skills and tasks; (2) investigative: analytical and precise; (3) artistic: enjoying creativity and nonconfirmatory; (4) social: people who like to meet the physical and emotional needs of others; (5) enterprising: personality types who like persuading others to meet their own economic and organization goals; and (6) conventional; people who enjoy putting things in order.[129] From the patient point of view, Greer's Mental Adjustments to Cancer (MAC) scale has been the most accepted way of pigeon-holing patients response to a diagnosis of cancer: (1) Anxious preoccupation; (2) Helpless hopelessness; (3) Fighting spirit; and (4) Stoic denial.[130,131] Although this is a contentiously controversial area, and despite gross generalization, it may be helpful to identify an optimal environment in which each personality type is most likely to flourish.

Thus while one's own personal "culture" cannot be ignored, insight into our own biases remains essential for us to be informed about others. An appropriate understanding of cultural difference can contribute to the care, respect, and the dignity of the patients.[132] The golden rule, to treat others, as they would wish to be treated, is still the roughest of guides and requires that individuals, and in some contexts the family, be asked how they would wish to be treated. For example, the Christian, Muslim, Buddhist, Hindu, or Jewish patient will usually be honored to be asked by caring staff about the nature of his or her religious belief and cultural traditions. This is also an extraordinary opportunity for both sides to learn about others' traditions, cultural beliefs, interpretations, and acceptances. Indeed, while it may seem possible to manage an illness without regard to a patient's ethnic origin, a continued ignorance of the cultural needs of a dying patient and grieving family is simply unacceptable.

Collective Bereavement

Although the very reasonable emphasis is on the loss experienced by individuals, sometimes a group, through extraordinary or repeated trauma collectively experience bereavement, and this becomes an important part of their culture. Cultural bereavement was probably first described in Swiss mercenaries afflicted by *Heimweh*. A Swiss physician, Hoferus, described posttraumatic stress disorder following battle. Curiously this later became known as "nostalgia,"[133] reflecting the cumulative trauma of survivor guilt, anger, ambivalence, and violent separations, more than "shell shock." Although there is clear ethnic or cultural variation in posttraumatic stress reactions, it is poorly catalogued. Three examples will be used. Collective bereavement is perhaps most identified with the Jews following the Nazi Holocaust of World War II. Two more modern and evolving tragedies, the Middle East conflict over Palestine and displaced peoples, as illustrated by Cambodians refugees in the United States, will be reviewed.[134-136]

This atrocity of the Holocaust still significantly frames Jewish experience of emotional trauma, especially bereavement. A study of 41 women with cancer, who had sustained extreme trauma during the Holocaust, was compared with matched groups of cancer patients without Holocaust experience, a physically healthy group of female Holocaust survivors, and healthy women without a Holocaust past.[137] Psychological distress was far higher in Holocaust cancer patients than in either their non-Holocaust counterparts or in the group of healthy Holocaust survivors. An important finding by this group was that Holocaust survivors were unable to mobilize partial denial.[138] Even in successful psychotherapeutic treatment programs have found classical insight-oriented, interpretive counseling less than satisfactory.[139] Childhood exposure of subsequent generations to guilt-inducing and indirect communication, seem to relate significantly to negative outcomes.[140] Posttraumatic stress disorder is common in Holocaust survivors. Removing avoidance as a defense mechanism during psychotherapy may leave these survivors without an adequate way for coping with their trauma, subsequently increasing their vulnerability to psychopathology.[141]

The ongoing armed struggle in Israel and Palestine provides insight on culture and bereavement, with a clear link to national identity creating a "bereavement culture."[142] The commemoration of the fallen is an important part of Israel's recent civil religion. Ben-Gurion, Israel's first Prime Minister, said, "and death is not an ultimate nothingness but the life of each and every person interlaces not only with the life of his mother but is soaked into the life of his generation and generations to come." Yet, the rubble of death is cleared matter-of-factly behind TV reporters in contradistinction to the flowers and cordons that stand for a month or months as testimony to tragedy in times of peace. Secular Kibbutz require a code of mourning with minimal emotional expression marked by considerable restraint.[143] Silence being the hallmark of a Kibbutz funeral.[144] Younger generations are now more open to expressing emotions and talking about the deceased, curiously, more in line with historical and religious Jewish tradition.[145] Such differences may contribute to the conflict between ultra-orthodox *Hasidim* and progressive Jews, even within families, reflecting much of the complexity of a modern culture and compounded by the dispersal of the family, both within Israel and abroad. Much of modern Judaic culture strongly reflects the country of origin with considerable difference in funeral practices in the Jewish diaspora. There are considerable differences in the funeral practices between the Jews of Russia, Europe, North America, South America, Greece, Spain, Iran, Morocco (ie Sephardim), and Ethiopian Jewry. While in Russia, burying the dead and mourning are considered private issues with every family allowed to arrange this according to their own tradition and custom, other Jewish immigrant behaviors are more strongly dictated. For example, Ethiopian Jews require a middle man to first bring the bad news to the elders of the community who then tell the close relatives and there are strict rules about purity.[146] There is a mandated 7-day period of purification with ritual bathing receiving the *kase* (priest), formal dirges (*likso*), and the bereaved are comforted with coffee (*Buna*).

Among others, Eugene Brody, a critic of psychiatric "biologism" has highlighted how modern psychiatric interpretation values biology over culture.[147] And more recent studies have specifically highlighted cultural differences in patterns of bereavement. For example, Eisenbruch did seminal research immersing himself into the culture of Cambodian refugees and identifying cultural bereavement by mapping the experience of refugees and identifying how refugees gave meaning and structure to loss. Cambodians experienced culturally determined dreams and other perceptions during sleep that continued unabated in the wakened state and such dreams, craving, and nightmares were common. An annual ceremony (pcum-ben) to venerate the souls of the dead and incorporate the survivors into their community appeared to be particularly effective for those possessed by spirits or troubled by visitations of ghosts from the homeland. Bereaved Cambodia refugees commonly complain of shiikbaal (headache) as a psychosomatic illness. Eisenbruch concluded that even intrusive symptoms that were clearly quite distressing were not helped by psychiatric treatment and if anything, such amelioration appeared to prolong the trauma.[134] How the cultural experiences frame psychiatric disorders is fascinating. For instance, the cultural interpretation of the symptoms (somatization) thus allowing for a reformulation of classical posttraumatic stress disorder, and it is clear that there are concrete cultural pressures that proscribe how patients adjust and cope with distress and related symptoms.

RELIGIOUS ASPECTS OF CULTURE AND BEREAVEMENT

A religious dimension to life attempts, albeit tentatively, to make ultimate sense of experience. Existential crisis perhaps characterizes the 20th and 21st centuries in man's search for truth and for God.[148] Erikson remarked on his experiences in a concentration camp, "Man is not destroyed by suffering but by suffering without meaning".[149] Many of the transitions through difficult times have delegated, "official chaperones," often of religious background. An adequate understanding of the ways with which most of us cope psychologically with loss forms a crucial component of spiritual care and respect for religious language and assumption is as necessary as an appreciation of modern psychological theory. Religious backgrounds are probably most clearly distinguished by what one eats and how one disposes of the dead. However, labeling with cultural, ethnic, or religious titles can be deceptive and will rarely encompass all the aspects for an individual.

Each culture has a unique approach to dealing with loss and this should not be seen as a matter of taste but a vital connection to community and heritage. Yet, across the world and certainly in the Western context, processes of secularization, urbanization, and social mobility have resulted in a weakening of bonds with ritual, community, and family that previously served to buffer the experience of loss and buttress identity. A prominent postmodern theme has been the championing of individual rights against religious orthodoxy which reinforce adherence to collective and traditional interpretations. Sadly, wonderful aspects of reform, such as the emancipation of women, appear to lead to as much fragmentation as enrichment.

Spiritual and Existential Aspects of Bereavement

We live in an age when we are at risk of losing the respect for the sacred. Yet, everyone holds "spiritual" values about important relationships, and wrestles with issues of, "why?" The hospice movement is one way in which medicine has humanized itself, and increasingly is comfortable with opening space for the spiritual. There has been much commentary about existential or spiritual pain, with God *in absentia.* This has been helpfully developed in "total pain," formulated to include physical, psychological, social, emotional, and spiritual elements by Dame Cicely Saunders, the founder of the hospice movement in the United Kindgom.[150] One subsequent and very helpful reformulation is the concept of "biographical" pain, which can aid the clinician, the patient, and the family in their exploration of the unresolved distress that occurs in terms of losses and illness gains, and the consequences on identity in the context of unfulfilled life goals.[151,152]

The subsequent review of religious aspects of bereavement is not exhaustive, but intended to introduce major themes that relate religious interpretation to bereavement. The reader is referred to excellent commentary by Rabbi Julia Neuberger.[153]

Christianity

Although Christianity often reflects the diverse denominations and geographical idiosyncrasies of the faith, there is a central belief in a Savior, the Son of God who laid down his life for mankind. Starting as a Jewish sect, Christianity was adopted by Emperor Constantine in AD 313. The core sacraments of the Roman Catholic faith are: the Mass, Baptism, Confession, Anointing the Sick (previously called extreme unction), the Act of

Contrition (confession), and Requiem Masses (services held for the bereaved). Reformed with the protestant ethic of salvation by faith that Christ died for ones sins, the Bible is taken as the inspired word of God. The traditional strong belief in an after life, heaven or hell, means that attitudes to death include fear and hope more than anger and acceptance, and Christianity has the strongest concept of hell fire and damnation of any religious group. Although theologically meant to engender a sense of egalitarian liberty in the light of God's mercy, in the popular mind, the doctrine of original sin has often supported a guilt-ridden pessimism about the fate of one's soul. Greek orthodox faith often still sees the illness of cancer as a punishment.[154] Last rites are only performed in Roman Catholic and Orthodox traditions, not in Protestant faiths. Baptism can be a big issue around end of life care, understood by most Christians as the *sine qua non* of salvation. Non-baptized Christians, therefore, often seek baptism before death. If a loved one dies without receiving this sacrament, the bereaved may have great anxiety about whether or not their loved one's soul has been welcomed by God into heaven, and consequently, whether the two of them will ever be rejoined in the heavenly reunion and this can complicate bereavement. Providing pastoral care at the end of life, so that the family is reassured that their loved one has been returned to good standing with God, can reduce religious complications in bereavement.

Late 18th and early 19th century European "sentimentalization" of death brought in ornate funerals and the seeking of bedside reconciliation and confession to promote a "good death." Christ's birth and death are celebrated as Christmas (December 25) and Easter (Sunday following the Paschal Full Moon, as defined by Pope Gregory the 13th in 1583 AD Orthodox churches celebrate their Easter by the older Julian calendar), but are increasingly secular holidays. Dietary regulations and dress are not mandated. Last rites administered by a priest, involve a final confession. Some groups, notably influenced by Irish Catholics hold a wake, the ceremony of visiting the body prior to burial, sometimes displayed in an open casket. The funeral often takes a week to organize with procession, dark colors, and quietness marking the event, but with helpful personal commemoration and eulogy. Christian funerals are problematic for some because of they necessarily involving a public proclamation of faith. There is no fixed period of mourning.[153]

Islam

"Islam" means submission (to the will of God) and is divided into four main groups, *Sunni, Shi'a, Ismaili,* and *Ahmadiyya*. It is monotheistic, adheres to the *Qur'an* (Koran) as the holy teaching of the prophet Muhammad and has five main religious requirements: faith, prayer, giving alms, fasting, and the Hajj, the pilgrimage to Mecca. There is considerable concern about modesty in women, who in strict societies wear a veil (*chadur*), men cover themselves from waist to knee, older men cover their heads. At the extreme women are required by *purdah* to be kept from male society. Food should be *halal* (killed according to Islamic law) and no shellfish, except prawns, or alcohol is allowed. Ramadan is a month long fast, which moves around the year according to the Muslim lunar (360 day) calendar. It is common though not required for patients to refuse pain relief during this time and providing a glass of water and bowls for washing the mouth before prayers is an appropriate charity. Muslims may need the reassurance of an *Imam* that serious illness cancels the traditional proscriptions of the period of Ramadan. Reassurance that eating, drinking, and taking medication do not remove the dying person from Allah's favor can help ease bereavement. Muslims wash before prayers, which are offered at dawn, noon, mid-afternoon, just after sunset, and at night. Other festivals include "*Id al-Adha*," the feast of sacrifice, "*Id al-Fitr*," the breaking of the fast after Ramadan and it is appropriate to say happy "*Id*" (pronounced "eed") to make it clear that the festival is important.[153]

Devoted Muslims believe that death is part of Allah's plan and to struggle against it is wrong, and that God will judge according to the person's deeds, upon which the individual may be sent to heaven or to hell. A dying Muslim may typically want to sit or lie with his or her face turned toward Mecca. There are no official last rites, but a family will often stay by the bedside praying and whisper into the dying person's ear encouraging them to say, as there last words, "there is no God but Allah and Muhammad is his prophet" the call to pray. Non-Muslims are not permitted to touch the body and should wear rubber gloves, straighten the limbs, turn the head toward the right shoulder so the body may be buried with the face turned toward Mecca, eyes closed, the feet tied together with a thread around the toes and the face bandaged to keep the mouth closed, camphor is placed under the armpits and in orifices and the arms placed across the chest, and the unwashed body wrapped in a white cotton sheet. Muslims are buried and never cremated and it is an Islamic ideal to be buried in ones homeland. Some sects lament loudly and others practice serene stoicism. The period of mourning for bereaved family is 3 days after the funeral and the family visits the grave every Friday during the following 40 days.

Hinduism

Hindus believe a Supreme Being resides in each individual and the ultimate goal is the release of the individual soul from the cycle of birth, death, and rebirth to join the Supreme Being. There are various deities in the Hindu pantheon and many Hindus take comfort from figuring of *Vishnu,* the preserver and his incarnations as *Rama* or *Krishna* or *Brahma.* The *Vedas* or *Bhagavad Gita* are read aloud, and prayer, meditation, and physical exercise are often combined in *Hatha Yoga.* Hinduism has a strong requirement for modesty, patients typically unwilling to discuss problems in the genitourinary area, and requiring physical purity with daily bathing in running water. Traditional Hindu *Ayurvedic* medicine requires moderation in all things and reflects a strong link between virtue and health. Thus, if you live well, you will survive. Although there are no last rites, the *pandit* (Brahmin priest) is typically called and will perform the *puja* or act of worship. This often involves bringing Ganges water as a comfort to the dying person. Following the death, the ceremony known as Sreda, involving food brought by the Brahmins and rites for the dead are performed. Hindus are always cremated and the ashes are usually scattered on the river Ganges at Varanasi in India. This reflects a custom of floating burning *ghats* down the Ganges. Chief mourners often go into retirement, grief is expressed openly and communally, and the family is in mourning until the 13th day after the cremation with closure at the time of a special ceremony. Postmortems are not generally approved, but legally required postmortems are accepted provided the situation is explained. Crematoriums will usually be required to remove Christian symbols for the service and replace them with the symbol, *OM,* signifying the unity of and the presence of the Supreme Being in all living things.

Buddhism

There are two major Asian schools of Buddhism: *Mahayana* and *Teravada* Buddhism. Most Westerners who take on Buddhist practice identify with the Zen school. Buddhism centers around the disciplines of Siddhartha Gautama and his revelation of truth after which he was called Buddha. The four noble truths of Buddhism are: (1) Life is painful; (2) Pain originates from desire; (3) For pain to end, desire must end as well; and (4) The path to end this pain is righteous living. The *Bardö T'ödröl* (Tibetan Boof of the Dead) proposes that the art of living well and the art of dying well are one and the same. There is a doctrine of rebirth in Buddhism where one gradually approaches Nirvana, or perfection, where selfishness and separate identity are gone. For instance, despite the family emphasis on dependency, dying in Japan is thought to be a lonely task (*Sabishii*) and successful dying depends on strength and commitment to transcend the uncertainty and fear of death. The Japanese ideal is that death is "*ifagiyoku,*" without regret.[153] The religion is marked by rigorous discipline which recognizes that human existence and suffering are inextricably linked and demands a greater heightening of the awareness of this spirit in an attempt to reach a state of perfect freedom and peace. Given this, there was an understandable reluctance to blunt perception anyway. Many Buddhists are strict vegetarians or vegans and a considerable section of the Buddhist Community requires attention to modesty similar to the Hindu tradition. In Shinto Buddhism, purity is important and purification rituals such as salt throwing after a funeral or before a Sumo wrestling match or rinsing the mouth and hands with water before entering a shrine are important. Most Buddhists are cremated with the ceremony conducted by Bhikku (monks). Reverence of ancestors provides ritual ways of remaining connected with the deceased in socially accepted ways. As there is such considerable variation in patterns of dealing with terminal illness and bereavement in Buddhism, the individual and family involved must be consulted. Pastoral care of Buddhists can involve reading scriptures, chanting, meditating, or the sound of a bell. Clinicians should be cautious around calling in a Buddhist priest, however, because in some Asian Buddhist cultures, the priest only comes at the time of death.

Chinese attitudes and practices about death and dying are rooted in Asian cultural values such as filial piety, centrality of the family, and emphasis of hierarchy with strains of Confucianism, Buddhism, Taoism, and Local Folk Law.[155] Taoism is considered both a religion and philosophy emphasizing the independence of the individual and connection to natural forces of life. Important Chinese values are: (1) Collectivity rather than individuality with identity rooted in the group or family; (2) Hierarchical social structure with a centralized leadership rather than egalitarian democracy and paternal lineage; (3) Specific gender roles with the male being the head of the household; (4) Saving face with shameful behavior affecting the entire family lineage; (5) Harmony with conformity to rules; (6) An importance of filial piety with ancestor worship largely replaced by teaching children the importance of supporting parents; and (7) Restrained and indirect communication styles.

The Chinese are considerably more cautious often with a strong urge to return to their home country. While the fear of both medical personnel and technology may challenge a positive response, cautiously challenging behavior and personal connection from the clinician and the biomedical team are still important. This allows both respect and expression of feelings. However, for many Chinese families, talking about feelings or conflict is unacceptable and exploratory attempts at problem solving often are rebuffed with a request for concrete direction with respect to treatment or care.[154] Being culturally appropriate even though it requires considerable adjustment of one's own views may be the best way of expressing care.

Chinese American funerals are characterized by burning of incense or paper money or other symbolic possessions, hiring professional wailers or criers, white flowers in the hair, small gifts to guests who attend the funeral, large wreaths of flowers on the coffin, layering blankets on the deceased body before closing the casket, and elaborate funeral procession passing from the deceased's home to the cemetery. Subsequently, there is a large banquet and a picture of the deceased is hung in the family home (*Ching Ming*). There is a maximum time period for mourning of 49 days, entailing the practice of *Hung Sun* (walking the mountain or visiting the grave side). The Chinese are a good example of a geographic identity trumping religious affiliation.

Judaism

The two predominant denominations are the Ashkenazi originating in Europe and Sephardim originating in Spain, Portugal, or North Africa. Traditionally, Orthodox Jews believe in after life a world to come, although the precise nature of this is unclear, and the coming of a personal Messiah. However, many non-orthodox Jews (ie, Reform and Conservative) do not tend to believe in the physical after life and to what extent each believes in a personal God is also unclear.[153] The value of human life is infinite and beyond measure, a 100 years as important as a single second.[156] This life-affirming thread through Judaism is very strong particularly given the considerable periods of exile and prosecution. There also remains a strong desire not to give up hope and indeed all laws except three, the prohibition against murder, adultery, and incest, may be broken to save a human life even for few minutes (Talmud Yoma 85a). Highly Orthodox Jews are extremely modest, men keeping their heads covered or wearing (*yarmulkes*) and women wearing a wig (*sheitl*). Most Orthodox Jews abstain from eating pork or shellfish (ie, they avoid eating animals as specified in the Torah), and may require fully kosher or vegetarian food and no mixing of meat and milk.[153] Among the Orthodox, there is an absolute respect for Sabbath with the lighting of Sabbath candles on a Friday night at dusk and it is courteous to say *Shabbat shalom* meaning Sabbath peace. High holy days include the Jewish New Year commemorated 10 days after the Day of Atonement (*Yom Kippur*) and Passover celebrating the exodus from Egypt involves the *Seder* (passover meal) breast lamb and bitter herbs. There are no last rites in Judaism, but the dying Jew or family will often ask to see a Rabbi. When death is near, psalms are read and the dying person is encouraged to say the first line of the *Shema* prayer (Hear O Israel the Lord is our God the Lord is one), or a confessional prayer (*Vidui*). When the patient is expected to die in 3 days, they are termed as *goses*, fatally unwell as opposed to *terefah* in which there was no time constraint set on somebody who is critically ill. However, this is balanced by a commitment to dignity in the final days of life, and the Jewish patient is not bound to accept treatment at any expense in his or her final days.[157] The Talmud forbids euthanasia (Greek—"good death"). Moreover, traditional Jewish law (*Halacha*) prohibited organ donation because it would keep the *goses* alive past the natural time, though this is significantly changing with many Rabbis now believing that organ donation is compatible with Judaism (www.transplantforlife.org/). Burial occurs, if possible, within 24 hr or at the most 48 hr of death. There is considerable resistance to postmortem examination. When the death occurs, people stay by the body for 8 min while a feather is placed over the nose and mouth to check if the breathing has completely stopped. As a person breathes his last breath, many Jews will open a window to let the spirit escape from the room. This may not always be possible in the hospital, but the door may be opened symbolically to achieve the same effect. Close relatives may tear their clothes. The oldest son or nearest relative closes the eyes. Traditionally, the body is placed on the floor where the feet face toward the door, covered with a sheet and a candle placed beside it and is not left alone until burial. However, some of these practices mix religious prescription with ethnic folk customs. Many congregations have a *chevra kaddisha* (holy assembly) of men and women who wash and prepare the body for the funeral. Judaism's funeral and bereavement rituals are quite extensive and detailed. This is usually very helpful to the bereavement process: the bereaved have socially sanctioned ways of mourning within the context of family and community. In Israel, Jews are buried in shrouds not coffins. During the funeral service, the Rabbi may perform a traditional cutting of the shirt near the heart. In Judaism, there is also a prescribed 7 days of official mourning after the death, a period called *Shiva*, when a family sits in mourning and recites an Aramaic prayer called *kaddish* three times a day. There is a *Shloshin* ceremony 30 days after burial with prayers and *Kaddish* recited at the grave. Twelve months after the burial, a memorial service, *Yizkor*, is held at the grave.

Sikhism

Sikhism has its origins in Hinduism and Islam following the founder, Guru Nanak of the 16th century with a community approach much like a military fellowship centered around the *Gurdwara* or "center of learning" and the book of Sikhism, the *Guru Granth Sahib*, which is read aloud to dying Sikhs. There are five essential symbols of Sikhism, the *Kesh* or uncut hair left long and worn in a bun by both men and women covered by a turban in men and older women. The *Kangha is* a cone, which keeps the bun in place. The *Kara,* the steel bangle that all Sikhs wear, the *Kirpan* or ceremonial daggera, and the *Kaccha* or underpants/shorts worn by all Sikhs at all times. Dietary prohibitions include never eating *halal* meat and tobacco is expressly forbidden. Sikhs are vegetarian. Sikhs believe in a series of reincarnation, with the ultimate objective being for the soul to reach perfection and be reunited with God, and *Karma* being the influence of the previous life. Unlike Hindus, the cycle can be altered by exceptionally virtuous action. Last rites are a family affair. A nurse is typically asked to close the eyes and the family will straighten the limbs and wrap the body in plain sheets. Sikhs are cremated wearing their five symbols with men wrapped in a white cotton shroud and women wrapped in red. Cremation occurs within 24 hr of death, if possible, and while there remains a desire for the oldest son to light the funeral pyre, this is often achieved by a family member pushing the button, which starts the process at the crematorium. The ashes are collected and scattered on water ideally in the river Sutlej at Anandpur in the Punjab where Sikhism was founded. The family is in mourning for about 10 days, although this varies. The end of mourning is marked by a celebration (*Bhaug*) held at the family home.

Internet

The Internet has attracted considerable attention as a means to improve health and health care delivery.[158,159] While there are certain ethical and medical problems with the use of the Internet for diagnosis and treatment of medical problems, the use of the Internet may facilitate connection of the well resourced and mitigate distress and isolation. Individuals from culturally and linguistically diverse backgrounds may feel more comfortable initially disclosing concerns with anonymity than with their clinician.[159,160] Given the increasing importance of the Internet as a tool for health care, a list of web resources and readings is included.

Internet: Resources

1. National Cancer Institute: http://www.cancer.gov/cancer_information
2. Massachusetts General Hospital Cancer Renter Resource Room http://www.cancer.mgh.harvard.edu/resources
3. Massachusetts commission on end-of-life care. Listing end-of-life and bereavement resources in Massachusetts http://www.end-oflifecommission.org/
4. THEOS (They Help Each Other Spiritually) telephone: 1-412-471-7779

5. American Association of Retired Persons: http://www.aarp.org/griefandloss
6. CRUSE in the UK: http://www.crusebereavementcare.org.uk (telephone: 0870 1671677)
7. Counseling for Loss: http://www.counselingforloss.com
8. Aging With Dignity http://www.agingwithdignity.org (1-888-5-WISHES (594-7437)
9. America's Voices for the Dying: 1-800-989-9455
10. American Hospice Foundation: http://www.americanhospice.org 1-202-223-0204
11. Children's Hospice International http://www.chionline.org (1-800-242-4453)
12. Compassion in Dying: http://www.compassionindying.org (1-503-221-9556)
13. GriefNet: http://www.griefnet.org
14. Hospice Foundation of America (HFA) http://www.hospicefoundation.org (1-800-854-3402)
15. Hospice Net: http://www.hospicenet.org
16. National Center for Grieving Children and Their Families: http://www.grievingchild.org (1-503-775-5683)
17. National Hospice & Palliative Care Organization (NHPCO): http://www.nhpco.org (1-800-658-8898)
18. US National Hospice Foundation http://www.hospiceinfo.org 1-800-338-8619. Bereaved Families Online offers support for people who have lost an immediate family member: http://www.inforamp.net/~bfo/
19. Cancer Care, Inc. provides a special section on end of life and bereavement as well as online bereavement groups facilitated by certified social workers: http://www.cancercare.org/campaigns/end_life1.htm
20. Grief and Loss in the Workplace provides guidelines and resources for co-workers, managers, and supervisors: http://www.umich.edu/~hraa/griefandloss/reactions.html
21. GriefNet offers numerous discussion and support groups for bereaved persons (in email listserv format) and a variety of resources related to death and major losses: http://griefnet.org/
22. Grief Recovery Online features message boards, chat groups, and resource listings. Spanish language groups are available: http://www.groww.org/
23. Growth House offers extensive grief and bereavement sections, including a chat room and information about general and family bereavement, pregnancy loss, and infant death, and helping

children with grief and illness: http://www.growthhouse.org/
death.html

24. HospiceNet offers extensive information about grief and bereavement including issues regarding children and adolescents:
http://www.hospicenet.org/html/bereavement.html

25. KidsAid is an online support group for children dealing with any
kind of loss. It includes artwork, stories, and poems: http://kid-
said.com/

26. WidowNet is an information and support group resource for, and
by, men and women of all ages, religious backgrounds and sexual
orientations who have suffered the death of a spouse or life partner: http://www.fortnet.org/WidowNet/

27. American Counseling Association offers ethical standards for the
practice of online counseling: http://www.counseling.org/gc/
cybertx.htm

28. The International Society for Mental Health Online suggests principles for the online provision of mental health services:
http://www.ismho.org/suggestions.html

29. National Board for Certified Counselors: http://www.nbcc.org/ethics/
wcstandards.htm

CONCLUSION

"Never does one feel oneself so utterly helpless as in trying to speak
comfort for great bereavement." Jane Welsh Carlyle

In this chapter, the relationship between cultural difference and bereavement is discussed in a primarily Western context. Talking about death,
dying, and the process of coping with loss still remain taboo subjects.
Bereavement is an inevitable part of everyone's life. People cope, or fail to
cope, in culturally diverse ways. Bereavement may be one of the hardest
tasks for health care professionals confronted with the limitations of our
endeavors. The clinician and the medical staff have a responsibility to provide grieving families with support and care, care that goes beyond the
death. A compassionate response helps both those who suffer and those
who care.

REFERENCES

1. Rando TA. *Treatment of Complicated Mourning*. Champaign IL:Research Press; 1993.
2. Switzer DK. *The Dynamics of Grief*. Nashville, TN and New York, NY:Abingdon Press; 1970.

3. Freud S. Mourning and melancholia, In: Strachey J, ed. *The Standard Edition of the Complete Psychological Works of Sigmund Freud*, London:Hogarth Press; 1917.

4. Casarett D, Kutner JS, Abrahm J. Life after death: a practical approach to grief and bereavement. *Ann Intern Med.* 2001;134(3):208-215.

5. Rabkin JG, Struening EL. Live events, stress, and illness. *Science.* 1976;194(4269):1013-1020.

6. Parkes CM, Brown RJ. Health after bereavement. A controlled study of young Boston widows and widowers. *Psychosom Med.* 1972;34(5):449-461.

7. Worden J. *Grief Counseling and Grief Therapy.* New York: Spring Publishing; 1991.

8. Lewis C. *Gried Observed.* San Francisco, CA: Harper; 2001.

9. Pappano L. *The Connection Gap: Why Americans Feel so Alone.* Piscataway, NJ: Rutgers University Press; 2001.

10. Parkes C, Laungani P, Young B. *Death and Bereavement Across Cultures.* London: Routledge; 1996.

11. Rosenblatt P, Walsh R, Jackson B. *Grief and Mourning in Crossed Cultural Perspective.* New York, NY: Hras Press;1976.

12. Prigerson HG, Jacobs SC. Perspectives on care at the close of life. Caring for bereaved patients: "all the doctors just suddenly go." *JAMA.* 2001;286(11):1369-1376.

13. Schaefer C, Quesenberry CP, Jr., Wi S. Mortality following conjugal bereavement and the effects of a shared environment. *Am J Epidemiol.* 1995;141(12):1142-1152.

14. Ferris TGG, et al. When the patient dies: a survey of medical housestaff about care after death. *J Palliat Med.* 1998;1(3):231-239.

15. Billings J, Kolton E. Family satisfaction and bereavement care following death in the hospital. *J Palliat Med.* 1999;2:33-49.

16. Hanson LC, Danis M, Garrett J. What is wrong with end-of-life care? Opinions of bereaved family members. *J Am Geriatr Soc.* 1997;45(11):1339-1344.

17. Higginson I, Wade A, McCarthy M. Palliative care: views of patients and their families. *BMJ.* 1990;301(6746):277-281.

18. Corr CA, Nabe CM, Corr DM. *Death and Dying, Life and Living.* 2nd ed. Pacific Grove, CA:Brooks/Cole Publishing Company; 1997.

19. Kubler-Ross E. *On Death and Dying.* New York, NY: Macmillan Publishing Company Inc; 1969.

20. Bowlby J. *Attachment and Loss.* Vol 3. New York, NY:Basic Books, Inc.; 1980.

21. Block SD. Perspectives on care at the close of life. Psychological considerations, growth, and transcendence at the end of life: the art of the possible. *JAMA.* 2001;285(22): 2898-2905.

22. von Gunten CF, Ferris FD, Emanuel LL. The patient–physician relationship. Ensuring competency in end-of-life care: communication and relational skills. *JAMA.* 2000;284(23):3051-3057.

23. Lindemann E. Symptomatology and management of acute grief. *Am J Psychiatry.* 1944;101:141-148.

24. Parkes CM. The first year of bereavement. A longitudinal study of the reaction of London widows to the death of their husbands. *Psychiatry.* 1970;33(4):444-467.

25. Clayton PJ. Bereavement and depression. *J Clin Psychiatry.* 1990;51(suppl):34-38; discussion 39-40.

26. Giddens A. *Modernity and Self-identity: Self and Society in the Late Modern Age.* Cambridge: UK Polity Press; 1991.

27. Green M. Roles of health professionals in institutions. In: S.F.a.G.M. Osterweiss M, ed. *Bereavement: Reactions, Consequences and Care.* Washington DC: National Academy Press; 1984.

28. Raphael B. *The Anatomy of Bereavement.* New York, NY: Basic Books, Inc., 1983.

29. Horowitz M, et al. Pathological grief: an intensive case study. *Psychiatry.* 1993;56(4): 356-374.

30. Jacobs S, et al. The measurement of grief: age and sex variation. *Br J Med Psychol.* 1986;59(Pt 4):305-310.

31. Parkes C, Weiss R. *Recovery from Bereavement.* New York, NY: Basic Books; 1983.

32. Zisook S, Downs NS. Diagnosis and treatment of depression in late life. *J Clin Psychiatr.* 1998;59(suppl 4):80-91.

33. Horowitz MJ, Bonanno GA, Holen A. Pathological grief: diagnosis and explanation. *Psychosom Med.* 1993;55(3):260-273.

34. Horowitz MJ, et al. Diagnostic criteria for complicated grief disorder. *Am J Psychiatry.* 1997;154(7):904-910.

35. Prigerson HG, et al. Consensus criteria for traumatic grief. A preliminary empirical test. *Br J Psychiatry.* 1999;174:67-73.

36. Parkes C. *Bereavement Studies of Grief in Adult Life.* 3rd ed. London: Routledge; 1996.

37. Osterweiss M, Solomon F, Green M. *Bereavement: Reactions, Consequences and Care.* Washington DC: National Academy Press; 1984.

38. Cumming E, Henry W. *Growing Old.* New York: Basic Books; 1961.

39. Parkes C. Risk Factors in Bereavement: Implications for the prevention and treatment of pathologic grief. *Psychiatric Ann.* 1990;20:308-313.

40. Lundin T. Morbidity following sudden and unexpected bereavement. *Br J Psychiatry.* 1984;144:84-88.

41. Helsing KJ, Szklo M. Mortality after bereavement. *Am J Epidemiol.* 1981;114(1):41-52.

42. Helsing KJ, Szklo M, Comstock GW. Factors associated with mortality after widowhood. *Am J Public Health.* 1981;71(8):802-809.

43. Parkes C. Attachment, bonding and psychiatric problems after bereavement in adulthood. In: Parkes C, Stevenson-Hinde J, Marris P. ed. *Attachment Across the Life Cycle.* London: Routledge; 1991.

44. Vachon ML. Grief and bereavement following the death of a spouse. *Can Psychiatr Assoc J.* 1976;21(1):35-44.

45. Ramirez AJ, et al. Mental health of hospital consultants: the effects of stress and satisfaction at work. *Lancet.* 1996;347(9003):724-728.

46. Freudenberger H. Staff burnout. *J Social Issues.* 1974;30:159-165.

47. Maslach C, Leiter M. *The Truth About Burnout: How Organizations Cause Personal Stress and What to Do About It.* Palo Alto, CA: Jossey-Bass; 1997.

48. Cohen SR, Mount BM. Living with cancer: "good" days and "bad" days—what produces them? Can the McGill quality of life questionnaire distinguish between them? *Cancer.* 2000;89(8):1854-1865.

49. Kfir N, Slevin M. *Challenging Cancer: From Chaos to Control.* London: Routledge; 1999.

50. Walter T. *Funerals and How to Improve Them.* London: Hodder and Stoughton; 1990.

51. Byock IR. Growth: the essence of hospice. From a physician's point of view. *Am J Hosp Care.* 1986;3(6):16-21.

52. Penson R, Slevin M. Communication with the cancer patient. In: Price P, Sikora K. ed. *Treatment of Cancer,* New York, NY:Arnold; 2002: 1187-1198.

53. Buckman R. *I Don't Know What to Say: How to Help and Support Someone Who Is Dying.* New York, NY: Vintage Books; 1992.

54. Schulz R, et al. Involvement in caregiving and adjustment to death of a spouse: findings from the caregiver health effects study. *JAMA.* 2001;285(24):3123-3129.

55. Suls J, Fletcher B. The relative efficacy of avoidant and nonavoidant strategies: a meta-analysis. *Health Psychol.* 1985; 4: 249–288.

56. Houldin AD, McCorkle R, Lowery BJ. Relaxation training and psychoimmunological status of bereaved spouses. A pilot study. *Cancer Nurs.* 1993;16(1):47-52.

57. Coluzzi PH, et al. Survey of the provision of supportive care services at National Cancer Institute-designated cancer centers. *J Clin Oncol.* 1995;13(3):756-764.

58. Bromberg MH, Higginson I. Bereavement follow-up: what do palliative support teams actually do? *J Palliat Care.* 1996;12(1):12-17.

59. Raphael B. Preventive interventions with the recent bereaved. *Arch J Psychiatry.* 1977;34:1454.

60. Cameron J, Parkes CM. Terminal care: evaluation of effects on surviving family of care before and after bereavement. *Postgrad Med J.* 1983;59:73-78.

61. Ransford HE, Smith ML. Grief resolution among the bereaved in hospice and hospital wards. *Soc Sci Med.* 1991;32(3):295-304.

62. Kane RL, et al. The role of hospice in reducing the impact of bereavement. *J Chronic Dis.* 1986;39(9):735-742.

63. Kissane DW. Family-based grief counselling. *Aust Fam Physician.* 1994;23(4):678-680.

64. Kissane DW, Bloch S. Family grief. *Br J Psychiatr.* 1994;164(6):728-740.

65. Yalom ID, Lieberman MA. Bereavement and heightened existential awareness. *Psychiatry.* 1991;54(4):334-345.

66. Caplan G. *Principles of Preventive Psychiatry.* New York, NY: Basic Books; 1964.

67. Vachon ML, et al. A controlled study of self-help intervention for widows. *Am J Psychiatry.* 1980;137(11):1380-1384.

68. Barkwell DP. Ascribed meaning: a critical factor in coping and pain attenuation in patients with cancer-related pain. *J Palliat Care.* 1991;7(3):5-14.

69. Derogatis LR, Abeloff MD, Melisaratos N. Psychological coping mechanisms and survival time in metastatic breast cancer. *JAMA.* 1979;242(14):1504-1508.

70. Weisman AD. *On Death and Denying.* New York, NY: Behavioral Publications; 1972.

71. Miller SM. Monitoring versus blunting styles of coping with cancer influence the information patients want and need about their disease. Implications for cancer screening and management. *Cancer.* 1995;76(2):167-177.

72. Goodwin JS, et al. The effect of marital status on stage, treatment, and survival of cancer patients. *JAMA.* 1987;258(21):3125-3130.

73. Cassem EH. Care and management of the patient at end of life. In: Chochinov HM, ed. Breibart W. Handbook of psychiatry in palliative medicine, Oxford:Oxford University Press; 2000: 13-24.

74. Temoshok LR. Psychological response and survival in breast cancer. *Lancet.* 2000;355(9201):404-405; discussion 405.

75. Temoshok L. Personality, coping style, emotion and cancer: towards an integrative model. *Cancer Surv.* 1987;6(3):545-567.

76. Smith ED. Addressing the psychospiritual distress of death as reality: a transpersonal approach. *Soc Work.* 1995;40(3):402-413.

77. Cella DF, et al. Socioeconomic status and cancer survival. *J Clin Oncol.* 1991;9(8):1500-1509.

78. Morgan DM. Not all sadness can be treated with antidepressants. *W V Med J.* 1980;76(6):136-137.

79. Hollister L. Psychotherapy, drugs in the dying and bereaved. *J Thanatol.* 1972;2:623-629.

80. Ruzek JI. Providing "Brief Education and Support" for emergency response workers: an alternative to debriefing. *Mil Med.* 2002;167(9 suppl):73-75.

81. Stephens S. *Death Comes Home.* London:Mullberry; 1972.

82. Survey NHI. *National Cancer Institute, Division of Cancer Control and Population Sciences, Office of Cancer Survivorship.* 1992.

83. Worden JW. *Children and Grief: When a Parent Dies.* New York, NY: The Guilford Press; 1996.

84. Williams M. *Velveteen Rabbit.* Garden City: Doubleday; 1922.

85. Sahler OJ. The child and death. *Pediatr Rev.* 2000;21:350-353.

86. Rauch PK, Muriel AC, Cassem NH. Parents with cancer: who's looking after the children? *J Clin Oncol.* 2002;20(21):4399-4402.

87. Saiki-Craighil S. The grieving posters of the Japanese mothers who have lost a child to cancer, part II; establishment of new relationship from the memories. *J Pediatr Oncol Nurs.* 2001;18:268-275.

88. Tolle SW, Elliot DL, Hickam DH. Physician attitudes and practices at the time of patient death. *Arch Intern Med.* 1984;144(12):2389-2391.

89. Bedell SE, Cadenhead K, Graboys TB. The doctor's letter of condolence. *N Engl J Med.* 2001;344(15):1161-1164.

90. Grall T. Bereavement program helps to meet families' needs. *Oncol Nurs Forum.* 1998;25(5):828.

91. Baile W, et al. SPIKES-A six-step protocol for delivering bad news: application to the patient with cancer. *Oncologist.* 2000;5:302-311.

92. Nuland S. *How We Die: Reflections On Life's Final Chapter.* New York, NY: Random House; 1994.

93. Rubin SS, Schechter N. Exploring the social construction of bereavement: perceptions of adjustment and recovery in bereaved men. *Am J Orthopsychiatry.* 1997;67(2):279-289.

94. Saleeby D. Culture, theory and narrative: the intersection of meanings in practice. *Soc Work.* 1994;139:352-361.

95. Groce NE, Zola IK. Multiculturalism, chronic illness, and disability. *Pediatrics.* 1993;91 (5 Pt 2):1048-1055.

96. Jensen R. *Letter to Watch Tower Bible and Tract Society, dated March 1, 2000: page 1 of main text and page 4 of enclosure.* 2000.

97. Skodol A, Spitzer R. ICD-9 and DFM-3: A comparison. In: Spitzer R, Williams J, Skodol A, eds. *International Perspective on DFM-3.* Washington DC: American Psychiatric Association Press; 1983.

98. Dickens C. *Great Expectations.* New York, NY:Penguin; 2003.

99. Stroebem A, van dem Bout J, Schuth O. Misconception about bereavement: the opening of a debate. *J Death Dying.* 1994;29:1987-2003.

100. Klass D, Silverman P, Nickman S. *Continuing Bonds: New Understandings Of Grief.* New York, NY: Taylor & Francis; 1996.

101. Brody H. *Stories of Sickness.* New Haven, CT: Yale University Press; 1987.

102. Detzner DF. Life histories: conflict in southeast Asian refugee families. In: Gilgun J, et al., eds. *Qualitative methods in family research.* Newbury Park: Sage Publications; 1992; 85-102.

103. Marcus L, Marcus A. From soma to psyche: the crucial connection. (Perspectives on behavioral and cross cultural medicine addressed to first-year residents). Part 1. It ain't what you do—its the way how you do it: style as substance. *Fam Med.* 1988;20(5):368-373.

104. Lopez S, Grover K, Holland D. Development of culturally sensitive psychotherapists. *Prof Psychol Res Practice.* 1989;20:269-276.

105. Stein RE, Jessop DJ. Measuring health variables among Hispanic and non-Hispanic children with chronic conditions. *Public Health Rep.* 1989;104(4):377-384.

106. Leninger M. *Culture Care Diversity and Universality: A Theory of Nursing.* Vol publication 15-2401. New York, NY: National League for Nursing press; 1992.

107. Dyck I. The immigrant client: issues in developing culturally sensitive practice. *Can J Occup Ther.* 1989;56(5):248-255.

108. Delvecchio Good M, et al. American oncology and the discourse on hope. *Cult Med Psychiatry.* 1990;14:59-79.
109. Fielo SB, Degazon CE. When cultures collide: decision making in a multicultural environment. *Nurs Health Care Perspect.* 1997;18(5):238-243.
110. Surbone A. The quandary of cultural diversity. *J Palliat Care.* 2003;19(1):7-8.
111. Kakai H. A double standard in bioethical reasoning for disclosure of advanced cancer diagnoses in Japan. *Health Commun.* 2002;14:361-376.
112. Seale C. Changing patterns of death and dying. *Soc Sci Med.* 2000;51(6):917-930.
113. Eisinger F, et al. Cultural basis for differences between US and French clinical recommendations for women at increased risk of breast and ovarian cancer. *Lancet.* 1999;353:919-920.
114. Luczak J. Palliative care in eastern Europe. In: Clark D, Hockley J, Ahmedzai S. eds. *New Themes in Palliative Care.* Buckingham: Open University: 1997;170-194.
115. Reese DJ, et al. Hospice access and use by African Americans: addressing cultural and institutional barriers through participatory action research. *Soc Work.* 1999;44(6): 549-559.
116. Koffman J, Higginson I, Donaldson N. Symptom severity in advanced cancer, assessed in two ethnic groups by interviews with bereaved family members and friends. *J R Soc Med.* 2003;96:10-16.
117. Hawkins B. Hostile environment: reducing applications to medical school nationwide. *Black Issues in Higher Education.* 1997;14:18-20.
118. Laveist T, Nuru-Jeter A. Is doctor–patient race concordance associated with greater satisfaction with care? *J Health Soc Behav.* 2002;43:296-306.
119. Gray B, Stoddard JJ. Patient–physician pairing: does racial and ethnic congruity influence selection of a regular physician? *J Community Health.* 1997;22(4):247-259.
120. Curtis JR, et al. The quality of patient–doctor communication about end-of-life care: a study of patients with advanced AIDS and their primary care clinicians. *Aids.* 1999;13(9):1123-1131.
121. Annas G. *The Rights of Patients.* Carbondale, IL: Southern Illinois University Press; 1989.
122. Carrese JA, Rhodes LA. Western bioethics on the Navajo reservation. Benefit or harm? *JAMA.* 1995;274(10):826-829.
123. Beyene Y. Medical disclosure and refugees. Telling bad news to Ethiopian patients. *West J Med.* 1992;157:328-332.
124. Harris J, Shao J, Sugarman J. Disclosure of cancer diagnosis and prognosis in Northern Tanzania. *Soc Sci Med.* 2003;56:905-913.
125. Butow PN, Tattersall MH, Goldstein D. Communication with cancer patients in culturally diverse societies. *Ann N Y Acad Sci.* 1997;809:317-329.
126. Bouchard TJ, Jr., McGue M. Genetic and environmental influences on human psychological differences. *J Neurobiol.* 2003;54(1):4-45.
127. Markon KE, et al. Normal and abnormal personality traits: evidence for genetic and environmental relationships in the Minnesota Study of Twins Reared Apart. *J Pers.* 2002;70(5):661-693.
128. Reif A, Lesch KP. Toward a molecular architecture of personality. *Behav Brain Res.* 2003;139(1-2):1-20.
129. Holland J. *Making Vocational Choices: A Theory of Vocational Personalities and Work Environment.* Odessa, FL: Psychological assessment results; 1985.
130. Greer S, Moorey S. Adjuvant psychological therapy for patients with cancer. *Eur J Surg Oncol.* 1987;13(6):511-516.
131. Greer S, Watson M. Mental adjustment to cancer: its measurement and prognostic importance. *Cancer Surv.* 1987;6(3):439-453.

132. Chochinov HM, et al. Dignity in the terminally ill: a cross-sectional, cohort study. *Lancet.* 2002;360(9350):2026-2030.

133. Zwingmann C. The nostalgic phenomenon and it's exploitation. In: Zwingmann C, Psister-Ammende M. eds. *Obliterating and After.* New York, NY: Verlag; 1973.

134. Eisenbruch M. From post-traumatic stress disorder to cultural bereavement: diagnosis of southeast Asian refugees. *Soc Sci Med.* 1991;33(6):673-680.

135. Parson E. Ethnicity and traumatic stress: the intersecting point in psychotherapy. In: F. CR, ed. *trauma and its weight; study and treatment of posttraumatic stress disorder,* Brunner/Mazel, EO; 1985.

136. Kleinman A. *Rethinking Psychiatry: From Cultural Category to Personal Experience.* New York, NY:Free press; 1991.

137. Peretz T, et al. Psychological distress in female cancer patients with Holocaust experience. *Gen Hosp Psychiatr.* 1994;16(6):413-418.

138. Baider L, Peretz T, Kaplan De-Nour A. Effect of the holocaust on coping with cancer. *Soc Sci Med.* 1992;34(1):11-15.

139. Fonagy P. The transgenerational transmission of holocaust trauma. Lessons learned from the analysis of an adolescent with obsessive-compulsive disorder. *Attach Hum Dev.* 1999;1(1):92-114.

140. Lichtman H. Parental communication of Holocaust experiences and personality characteristics among second-generation survivors. *J Clin Psychol.* 1984;40(4):914-924.

141. Trappler B, et al. Holocaust survivors in a primary care setting: fifty years later. *Psychol Rep.* 2002;91(2):545-552.

142. Witzutum E, Malkinson R, Rubin S. Death, bereavement and traumatic loss in Israel: a historical and cultural perspective. *Israeli J Psychiatr Related Sci.* 2001;38:157-170.

143. Rubin N. *Unofficial Memorial Rites in an Army Unit.* Social forces service studies. 1985.

144. Kalekin F, Fishman D, Klingman A. Bereavement and mourning in non-religious Kibbutz. *Death Stud.* 1988;12:253-272.

145. Lamm N. *Jewish Way in Death and Mourning.* New York, NY: Jonathan David; 1969.

146. Budowskid D, Baruchafl J. Ethiopian Jews in cultural transition: family and life cycle. Jerusalem: Betachin; 1994.

147. Brody EB. The new biological determinism in socio-cultural context. *Aust N Z J Psychiatry.* 1990;24(4):464-469.

148. Hewitt H. *Searching for God in America.* Orange, CA: Word. 515;1996.

149. Hoare C. *Erikson on Development in Adulthood: New Insights from Unpublished Papers.* Oxford: Oxford University Press; 2002.

150. Clark D. 'Total pain', disciplinary power and the body in the work of Cicely Saunders, 1958-1967. *Soc Sci Med.* 1999;49(6):727-736.

151. Bury M. Chronic illness as biographical disruption. In: Gabe J, Bury M. eds. *The Sociology of Health and Illness: A Reader.* London:Routledge: 2003;167-182.

152. McGrath P. Spiritual pain: a comparison of findings from survivors and hospice patients. *Am J Hosp Palliat Care.* 2003;20(1):23-33.

153. Neuberger J. *Caring for Dying People of Different Faiths.* London: Austen Cornish Publishers; 1987.

154. Boston P. Understanding cultural differences through family assessment. *J Cancer Educ.* 1992;7(3):261-266.

155. Yick AG, Gupta R. Chinese cultural dimensions of death, dying, and bereavement: focus group findings. *J Cult Divers.* 2002;9(2):32-42.

156. Jakobovits I. *Jewish Medical Ethics: A Comparative and Historical Study of the Jewish Religious Attitude to Medicine and Its Practice.* New York, NY: Philosophical Library; 1959.

157. Goldman A. *Judaism: Contemporary Issues.* New York, NY: Shengold Publishers Inc.; 1978.
158. Penson RT, et al. Virtual connections: internet health care. *Oncologist.* 2002;7(6):555-568.
159. Baker L, et al. Use of the Internet and e-mail for health care information: results from a national survey. *JAMA.* 2003;289(18):2400-2406.
160. Rillstoneand S. Hutchinson, Managing the reemergence of anguish: pregnancy after a loss due to anomalies. *J Obstet Gynecol Neonatal Nurs.* 2001;30:291-298.

CHAPTER 12

The Unmet Need

Addressing Spirituality and Meaning through Culturally Sensitive Communication and Intervention

Christopher A. Gibson, Hayley Pessin, Colleen S. McLain,
Ami D. Shah, and William Breitbart

INTRODUCTION

As humans, we all experience various stressors throughout our lives. Serious illnesses, such as cancer, often engender severe stress and tax an individual's ability to function at all levels. An important question is how are humans able to incorporate such stressful situations into their lives without allowing them to interrupt or destroy their ability to function? Research has begun pointing to the value and importance of spiritual and religious mechanisms in individuals facing serious illness, especially as to how they give meaning to the situation presenting itself to the individual (Breitbart et al., 2000). As with all psychological phenomena, cross-cultural factors play a major role in shaping how the individual creates and utilizes such mechanisms. Each culture has its own, unique, set of beliefs about the meaning of illness and culturally appropriate responses to it.[1] However, Kinzie,[2] has noted that Western clinicians "are dominated by value systems of clinical humanistic psychology which promote self-aggrandizement and self-satisfaction, autonomy and rejection of authority, relativity in values, situational ethics, apology (rather than restitution), and avoidance of long-term relationships and responsibility" (p. 47). These values often differ from the values of other cultures, and can pose treatment and communication obstacles. Clinicians who are insensitive to patient's cultural and ethnic values and beliefs are often viewed as being rude, ignorant or uncaring.[3] This chapter will give the clinician guidelines on communicating with culturally and ethnically diverse patients about spirituality. It will also describe the current interventions aimed at enhancing the role of spirituality and meaning in patient's lives in the face of their illnesses.

SPIRITUALITY AND MEANING

Puchalski and Romer[4] have defined spirituality as that which allows a person to experience *transcendent meaning* in life. Spirituality is a construct that involves concepts of "Faith" and/or "Meaning," according to Karasu[5] and Brady et al.[6] Faith is a belief in a higher transcendent power, not needed to be identified as God, and not necessarily achieved through rituals or beliefs of an organized religion.

It should be noted that, the terms "spirituality" and "religion" are often used interchangeably, but are coming to be viewed as distinct elements, with religion often being viewed as an *external* set of specific beliefs and practices, and spirituality as more of a self-created and motivated set of *internal* beliefs and practices.[7] However, in reviewing the literature on cross-cultural differences in spirituality, such a distinction becomes murky. Zinnbauer[8] notes that individuals define spirituality and religiousness quite differently, and that for some ethnic groups (especially those with strong religious ties), such distinctions are difficult to make. They strongly suggest that future research should take into account the ambiguity of the terms at the popular level as well as variations in meanings according to demographic and ethnic groups. Musick[64] stresses that when one separates religion from spirituality, it often becomes a concept that is difficult to utilize or measure effectively. In our own studies, we have often witnessed patients who, upon being asked to rate how "spirituality" and "religious" they are, respond with some confusion. Considering such factors, we will therefore present some findings on religion and religiosity, in addition to spirituality, in this chapter.

One important outlet of individual spiritual beliefs is by attaining a sense of meaning in one's life. As humans, we strive to incorporate and synthesize a vast inner and outer world in order to make "meaning" out of our past and current experiences. For example, researchers theorize that religious beliefs may play a role in assisting patients in the construction of meaning out of experiences of suffering, that are often an inherent part of an illness which may in turn facilitate acceptance of their situation.[9] Importantly, recent studies have found that religion and spirituality generally play a positive role in patients' coping with illnesses such as cancer or HIV.[6,10,11] Spiritual well-being in general, and a sense of meaning and peace of mind, in particular, appear to have a substantial benefit on psychological distress at the end of life. Brady and colleagues[6] found that cancer patients who reported a high degree of meaning in their lives were better able to tolerate severe physical symptoms more than patients who reported lower scores on meaning/peace. For instance, patients with a high sense of meaning reported high satisfaction with their quality of life despite pain and fatigue to a greater degree than patients with a low sense of meaning.

Park and Folkman[12] reviewed the concepts of "meaning" in the context of stress and coping, and described conceptual models for meaning in relation to traumatic events and coping. They describe meaning as a general life orientation, as personal significance, as causality, as a coping mechanism and as an outcome. Thus, positive psychological changes and an improved sense of meaning in life have been associated with cancer illness for instance.[13] Cancer professionals have also witnessed many examples of positive life change and positive reappraisals of the value and meaning of life in their work with patients.[14-16]

CROSS-CULTURAL DIFFERENCES IN SPIRITUALITY, MEANING, AND COPING WITH LIFE-THREATENING ILLNESS

In exploring how people cope with the *threatened psychological state* that results from living with a serious, possibly fatal, illness such as cancer, a person's ethnicity determines, at least partially, the way they will employ spirituality and meaning in this endeavor. For all cultures, spiritual and religious practices play an important role in how the individual copes with a serious illness, such as cancer.[17] However, the evidence is mixed in regard to whether people of different ethnicities use similar or different coping strategies in the face of serious disease. On a very general level, it appears that individuals from traditional, Western cultures use different coping strategies than individuals from non-Western cultures.[18] These differences likely exist because of variation in basic values and cultural norms between these broad cultural groupings, such as reliance on the family and others for social support, and the value of individual vs group effort.

A common distinction that is often made in the coping literature is between active and avoidant coping strategies.[19] Active coping strategies are behavioral and psychological responses intended to change the nature of the stressor itself and how the individual conceptualizes it. Avoidant coping strategies lead people into activities and mental states that keep them from directly addressing stressful events. This distinction is important to keep in mind when examining the ways that some cultures and ethnicities utilize spirituality and religion in coping with illness.

Once someone, regardless of culture, is diagnosed with such an illness, images of suffering, pain, loss, loneliness, and possible death may arise. For example, in relation to cancer, Johnson and Spilka[65] wrote, "Potential terminality becomes a salient issue, along with expectations of pain, anguish, and suffering. Physical problems are compounded with a host of psychological difficulties, not the least of which are feelings of isolation, separation, dependency, and helplessness" (p. 21). Therefore, it is likely that in all such instances, coping strategies, whether conscious or not, are put into action. Further, coping with a physical illness such as cancer is quite complex and brings with it a great deal of uncertainty. Therefore, active coping mechanisms that are adaptive in most situations may be less so with regard to coping with terminal illness.[20] It is therefore important for Western clinicians to not view their own, ethno-centric conceptions of "proper" coping techniques in the face of illness as the model for their non-Western patients to strive for.

An exhaustive review of the literature on cultural and ethnic differences in spirituality, religiosity, and meaning in the face of illness is beyond the scope of this chapter. However, we would like to briefly summarize relevant findings for three ethnic and cultural groups Western clinicians are more likely to encounter in their practices (African Americans, Hispanics, and Asians Pacific Islanders), as well as one less common, but growing cultural grouping (sub-Saharan Africans).

African Americans

Hunt[21] examined the coping styles of a group of women with stage II and recurrent breast cancer and found that African American women were more likely to use a repressive coping style, while White females were more likely to use an active coping style, regardless of education level. Hunt examined whether or not religiosity accounted for the relationship between repressive coping style and race implying that higher levels of religiosity lead to more repressive coping. However, this hypothesis was not supported, leaving the question of how exactly religiosity impacts the coping styles of African Americans unanswered.

It may well be that African Americans turn to religion more often than non-Hispanic Whites because the relation between religion and well-being is stronger among that group. Others suggest that because African

Americans face more discrimination and barriers, both in general and in relation to healthcare, "they must find alternate avenues to success and well-being" (p. S220).[22] Therefore, they often turn to God and the Church as sources of support and assistance. For instance, Jordan and colleagues,[23] found that among a group of people with rheumatoid arthritis, African Americans used hoping/praying more than non-Hispanic Whites, whereas non-Hispanic Whites ignored their pain more than African Americans. Musick et al.[22] investigated the relationship between religious activity and depression among a group of elderly African American and non-Hispanic Whites, all of whom had a serious physical illness. Results demonstrated that the relationship between religious attendance and positive affect and depressive symptoms was stronger among African Americans than Whites. Several other analyses have shown that, overall, African Americans endorse participation in religious activities more so than Whites.[24]

With such findings in mind, clinicians should endeavor to support the desired spiritual and religious involvement of patients from this culture. The spiritually sensitive approach of the "Witness Project" cancer education program for African American women is an excellent example of such advice being put into practical application.[25] This is a culturally competent and sensitive community based cancer education program that realized that one way effective way to reach and educate African American women was through the voices of church leaders. The Witness Project partners with local churches in an attempt to better educate African American women about cancer, screening methods, and available treatments.

Hispanics

Ell and Nishimoto[66] identified a number of important differences in coping between non-Hispanic Whites and Hispanic (Puerto Rican) cancer patients. They found that individuals of Hispanic descent and individuals of low socioeconomic status tended to have more difficulty accepting a cancer diagnosis. Importantly, Hispanics were more likely to rely on religion as a means of coping than Whites. Such findings highlight the relative importance of spirituality and religion as a tool for coping among individuals from Hispanic backgrounds. For many Hispanics, spirituality and religion are closely intertwined concepts. Spirituality is often expressed through organized religion, particularly Roman Catholicism. The family is an important conduit of expression of spiritual and religious activity, and can be seen in the impact that numerous Catholic rituals have throughout the life cycle: baptism, confirmation, First Holy Communion, marriage, and death. These religious events are occasions to strengthen family relationships, as well as to extend family boundaries by including close friends, which in circumstances of medical illness, often begins to include the relevant health care providers. Hispanics also often express their spirituality through folk healers, such as Curanderas (Mexican Americans), Spiritualists (Puerto Ricans), and Santeras (Cuban Americans). These healers represent a belief system with roots in American Indian, African, and Catholic faiths[26] and should be viewed as important components of overall treatment for patients who utilize them.

Asian Pacific Islanders

As with most ethnic classifications, Asian Pacific Islanders are not a homogeneous group. Over 30 distinct ethnic groups exist within this category. Clinicians should always be aware of such diversity within an ethnic group and must avoid clustering individuals into simple, and thus artificial, classifications. With this caveat in mind, we will focus this section on findings for four such groups: Fillipinos, Japanese, Korean, and Chinese.

Chinese

Traditional Chinese Medicine employs a holistic approach to address illness in which body, mind, and spirit are considered indivisible entities that cannot be easily separated into individual components. Health, in this paradigm, is considered a state of equilibrium among body, mind, and spirit, while illness is characterized as an imbalance in the interplay between these entities. Unlike conventional Western medicine, which seeks to *combat or wage war on* disease (for instance, by killing bacteria or removing diseased tissue), Chinese philosophy "regards disease as symptomatic of the patient's bodily dysfunction and inner disharmony."[27] As such, traditional Chinese Medicine addresses illness by both treating the physical body *and* the patient's sense of "inner balance." Practitioners of Chinese Medicine employ treatments that involve acupressure, *qigong*, and massage therapies as these modalities address both mind and body, and serve as important spiritual outlets for many Chinese patients. Western clinicians need to be aware of these alternative modalities and encourage their use as needed to ease the mental burden of physical illness.

Another factor that highly influences the Chinese approach to illness is religion. Although there are many religions practiced by individuals of Chinese descent, the most common is Buddhism. In discussing meaning, one important difference between Western and Buddhist approaches to physical illness is in the role of acceptance. For many Westerners, meaning-making centers around finding a *purpose* and/or rational *cause* for the illness and its effects on one's life. For many Buddhists, purpose and cause are viewed as artificial human impositions, whereas *acceptance* of the illness and its effects is the more accepted goal of meaning-making. This difference is apparent in the differentiation between pain and suffering.[28] For many Westerners, such terms are interchangeable. However, in the Buddhist tradition, pain and suffering are quite distinct, in that pain is accepted as a natural part of illness, while suffering is composed of our attempts to try and make some rational justification for the existence and cause of the pain. The ultimate goal, in the Buddhist tradition, would be to strive for *acceptance* of the pain. Western clinicians may have a natural inclination to view such acceptance as the patient giving up hope or resigning his or herself to fate rather than fighting. Clinicians should endeavor to better understand the motivations of such acceptance as possibly being culturally appropriate and "healthy," and not inevitably a sign of hopelessness and despair. This recommendation is equally relevant in the context of research on hopelessness in this group, in that our current measures of hopelessness may contain items which do not adequately allow for such acceptance. For example, in the Beck Hopelessness Inventory[61] items such as "I can look forward to more good times than bad times" and "When I look ahead to the future I expect that I will be happier than I am now" may elicit negative responses if answered from a standpoint of acceptance, and thus serve as artificial indicators of our Western conception of hopelessness and despair.

Filipino

Within the Filipino community, health care decisions and methods of coping with serious illness are significantly influenced by both family bonds and a sense of fatalism. Nishimoto and Foley noted that when an individual of Filipino descent falls ill, his or her family often assumes a prominent role, in which they "pamper the patient, not allowing him to do self care."[29] While the high level of care offered by family members does provide the patient with much needed support during his or her time of illness, it may also allow the patient to assume a passive role in the face of illness. This tendency toward passivity is also noted in their religious beliefs, as Filipinos "often see illness as the will of God, and although they will pray devoutly for God's will to occur, they believe 'it is best to leave things in the hands of God.'"[29] By assuming such a passive role, patients may become less amenable to clinician recommendations for activities such as physical therapy and daily exercise. Clinicians should realize that much of a patient's resistance to such recommendations may emanate from traditional family values and religious beliefs that complicate his or her ability to comply. As such, it may be extremely beneficial for clinicians to enlist the support of family members when making such recommendations.

Japanese

Japanese individuals, like Filipinos, tend to be extremely family-oriented. They are reluctant about accepting outside help when caring for family members and, as such, clinicians should be attuned to signs of over-exhaustion and exertion on the part of their patient's family. When such signs do arise, clinicians ought to actively refer those families to services, such as home-nursing care programs, that may help alleviate the burden. Many Japanese are also practicing Buddhists and as such are prone to assuming an attitude of acceptance, as described above, in relation to their illness.

Koreans

Within the Korean community, as with the Chinese, Filipino, and Japanese communities, family-dynamics factor significantly into approaches to healthcare. All major decisions, including those pertaining to healthcare, are often left to the discretion of the eldest male family member. In a study conducted by Kimlin Tan Ashing and colleagues, the dominance of this patriarchal family model was found to be a source of strain for Korean women coping with breast cancer. One woman noted that "My family expects me to work and function the same as before the surgery [for breast cancer]. It saddens me."[30] These stoical family expectations appear to have a demoralizing effect on the patient's spirit. However, Ashing also notes that many of these women "became more religious as a result of their diagnosis" and "felt that their faith helped them cope with their breast cancer."[30]

Sub-Saharan Africans

Ngu[31] has noted that traditional Africans tend to focus on spiritual and moral issues as illness progresses, and lessen their focus on material concerns. Such concerns tend to focus on familial relationships. This focus becomes a major tool for coping among people from this culture, and is often their way of attempting to create meaning for their suffering. One major difference between Western culture and sub-Saharan African culture is in their approach to illness and death. In Western cultures, illness and death are private affairs, meant to be dealt with by the individual and their close relations. In sub-Saharan African culture, death and illness are often more social events.[32] Western clinicians should be aware of this difference when treating individuals from this culture, and be careful to not impose their cultural view of these events on the patient. For example, such patients may be dismayed at Western hospitals restrictions on visiting hours and the number of visitors they may receive.

WHY MIGHT SUCH DIFFERENCES EXIST?

With regard to differential outcomes of certain types of coping with respect to culture, it is possible that religious coping is more effective for individuals from many cultures. Although there is little, if any, empirical literature available that explains *why* spirituality and religion play such a prominent role in regard to coping with illness among many cultures, we do know that is *does*. Relying on God and religion enables patients from many cultures to remain more psychologically adjusted when faced with dire circumstances. Although it does not specifically address it, the Musick et al.[22] study mentioned above indirectly supports this proposition, in that the relationship between religious activity and psychological well-being was stronger among African Americans than Whites. This illuminates the important differences in the way different cultures utilize spirituality in coping with serious illness such as cancer. Consequently, clinicians should be aware of the ways their patients utilize and construct spirituality and religiosity in their lives. More importantly, learning *how* to communicate about such issues is an essential skill for health care clinicians in today's ethnically diverse climate.

GUIDELINES FOR EFFECTIVE COMMUNICATION ABOUT SPIRITUALITY

To alleviate sources of spiritual pain, a careful assessment and active intervention is often required by the clinician. Communicating about spirituality with patients effectively requires comfort in several domains. This includes: a basic knowledge of common spiritual concerns and sources of spiritual pain, as well as the principles and beliefs of the major world religions; good communication skills, such as active and empathetic listening and the ability to identify and highlight spiritually relevant issues; an awareness and acknowledgment that there are many mysteries and unanswerable questions associated with human existence; and the ability to remain open, empathic, and available to the patient's struggle with spiritual issues and their search for meaning.[33] Therefore, it is recommended that clinicians assess their own skill sets, knowledge, and time limitations before entering into discussions of spiritual matters. In addition, clinicians working with severely medically ill populations should seek specialized training to deal better with complicated spiritual issues. Of course, discussions of spirituality should not be limited to clinicians. It is also important to effectively utilize an interdisciplinary team such as members of pastoral and palliative care services. Referrals to chaplains should be approached as if they are as important as referrals to any other specialist and an essential part of comprehensive care.[34] Patients should be made aware as early as possible in treatment that pastoral care is available and clinicians should endeavor to make more active referrals as it becomes clear that spiritual issues are salient.

In terms of addressing multicultural issue, clinicians discussing spiritual matters should have a basic understanding of the principles of the major world religions (Buddhism, Christianity, Islam, and Judaism) as the patient's religious beliefs and practices may be intertwined with their spiritual beliefs.[33] Therefore, clinicians should always inquire directly from the patient how their own culture may impact such beliefs. The following general guidelines are intended to provide the clinician with tools that should enable the clinician to engage in discussions with patients that are sensitive to cultural belief regardless of their specific cultural identity, acknowledging that the need for meaning and a sense of purpose is universal.

The American Academy of Hospice and Palliative Medicine offers the following guidelines for clinicians when communicating about spiritual issues.[33,35,36] First, it is important to recognize that every patient is an individual and has a unique belief system that should be honored and respected. A patient's spiritual views may or may not incorporate religious beliefs, as spirituality is considered the more inclusive category. Therefore, initial discussions should focus on broad spiritual issues and then, when appropriate, on more specific religious beliefs. Clinicians should maintain appropriate boundaries and avoid discussions of their own religious beliefs, as it is usually not relevant. However, in some cultures where there is a significant overlap between spiritual/religious figures and "healers," such as Chinese, Native American, or some African tribal cultures[28,32,37] sharing personal beliefs may be more appropriate, if it is intended to serve the needs of the patient. In the end, the patient is the best arbitrator of what should be considered most relevant to their treatment needs. Ultimately, the goal of any exploration of spiritual and religious beliefs, is to foster hope and integrate meaning into a patient's life, as this is a more important aspect of providing spiritual healing than any adherence to a particular belief system or religious affiliation.

TAKING A SPIRITUAL HISTORY

A spiritual history should be taken as early in the treatment as possible, as it provides an opportunity to give more comprehensive care and serves in building a relationship with a patient. Several general communication strategies should help to illicit patient concerns around spiritual concerns. These include the use of open-ended questions, asking patients to say more about a subject as a follow-up question, acknowledging and normalizing patient concerns, the use of empathetic comments in response to patient concerns, and inquiring about patient's emotions around these issues.[38] There are several methods to taking a spiritual history. Puchalski[39] recommends the acronym FICA to structure a spiritual history, which stands for Faith and Belief, Importance, Community, and Address. A good assessment should include the following questions[4,39,40]: (1) Do you consider yourself a spiritual or religious person? (2) What gives your life meaning? (3) Do the religious or spiritual beliefs provide comfort and support or cause stress? (4) What importance do these beliefs have in your life? (5) Could these beliefs influence your medical decisions? (6) Do you have beliefs that might conflict with your medical care? (7) Are you part of a spiritual or religious community? Are they important to you or a source of support? (8) What are your spiritual needs that someone should address? How would you like these needs to be addressed as part of your healthcare? In addition to these more open-ended questions, there also exist several formal assessment tools.[41,42] Most importantly, it should be noted that although a detailed spiritual assessment can be very helpful in eliciting the beliefs that are relevant to good patient care, this should not be looked upon as a one time discussion but rather the beginning of a dialogue that should continue throughout a patient's care. This type of assessment should serve to let the patient know that the clinician is open to these discussions should they wish at any time as concerns arise and give the message that they will be met in a supportive and respectful manner.[43]

DIFFICULTIES ASSESSING SPIRITUALITY

Spirituality is often quite difficult to assess as it is personal as well as social. As such there are several pitfalls to avoid in these discussions, which include[38]: (1) trying to solve unsolvable problems, as "spiritual suffering" cannot be fixed in the way many medical problems can be addressed, (2) attempting to answer unanswerable questions such as what happens after death, (3) going beyond one's professional role or area of expertise, (4) imposing personal religious beliefs on the patient, (5) providing premature reassurance, as it may come across as simplistic or cut patients off from expressing more troublesome feelings. Instead, simply being present, actively listening, offering empathetic responses, and trying to understand the patient's point of view will foster a productive dialogue and offer great comfort to the patient.

If a patient does not have an existing religious or spiritual belief system, it is not recommended to imply or recommend that they become more religious or spiritual, as it is disrespectful and may be more alienating to a patient.[43] Furthermore, some patients may not feel comfortable discussing religious beliefs with their caregivers, as one study demonstrated that a third of patients asked stated they were uncomfortable discussing their religious beliefs with their physicians.[44] In these cases, the patient's wishes should be respected and the discussion should be redirected to topics that assist the patient in coping with their illness or maintaining a sense of meaning or hope.[39] However, this initial discussion will convey the message that spiritual concerns may be discussed in the future if it becomes needed.

BARRIERS TO COMMUNICATION

There may be several factors that inhibit effective communication with patients about spirituality.[43,45-48] First, other areas of concern such as physical, emotional, and social problems may take precedence in a patient's mind and may cause him or her to delay addressing spiritual issues.[35] Spiritual pain may manifest itself as physical symptoms which patients may find easier to express.[49] Spiritual pain may overlap with symptoms of psychological distress such as feelings of guilt, hopelessness, meaningless, a sense of fear or dread about the future.[33] Several additional factors have been cited as contributing to the avoidance of these discussions, including a lack of time on the part of the clinician, a lack of training in this area, fear of projecting one's own beliefs onto the patient, and concerns about patient autonomy.[47] Finally, clinicians may feel that these discussions are inappropriate, as they are outside of their area of expertise or intrusive to the patient's privacy, and may experience some discomfort around pursuing these topics.[43,46-48] Nevertheless, the majority of studies have demonstrated that in fact the opposite is true, as patients welcome these discussions.[41,44,50] This was particularly true in the context of major medical events such as surgery, major illness, terminal illness, or death[51] and remained true for the majority of patients even if they reported that they were not religious.[63] Such discussions should be not be avoided, but may just require more consideration on the part of the clinician to overcome barriers to these discussions.

INTERVENTIONS FOR SPIRITUAL SUFFERING

Psychotherapeutic interventions aimed at specifically addressing spiritual suffering among cancer patients generally differ in their focus on spiritual/religious issues more existential issues of meaning. Although the broad goal of any of the interventions is similar, this difference is important from a cross-cultural perspective in that patients from cultures that have more of a focus on spiritual/religious means of coping may benefit more from interventions. Similarly, patients from cultures that focus more on active, individualistic coping may reject the spiritual/religious focus of these therapies and therefore gain more from those therapies focused on issues of meaning. The argument could be made that issues of meaning in dealing with cancer are more "broad based" and less driven by belief systems than issues of spirituality or religiosity. Therefore, they may cut across cultural boundaries more effectively and thus be more easily digested by a wider range of cultures and ethnicities. It should be noted that such an argument is purely speculative and is not backed by any direct empirical knowledge that the authors are aware of. A general recommendation to clinicians endeavoring to begin a therapeutic program to address issues of spirituality and meaning would be to consider their patient population's cultural make-up very closely and choose an intervention type that most closely matches it. If the patient population is quite diverse, then interventions focused on meaning may be the more easily and broadly acceptable. Future research should endeavor to determine if such differences exist and to what degree interventions with these different focuses are accepted by patients from varying cultures.

NONTRADITIONAL INTERVENTIONS

In discussing available, spiritually oriented interventions, it should be noted that several complimentary and/or alternative interventions (ie, yoga, massage, meditation, acupuncture, etc.) are now coming into use by a wide variety of patients (see Chapter 10 by Ernst, this volume), which may also be utilized as potential sources of spiritual strength by such populations.[52] Such nontraditional, complementary and alternative therapies, may be quite appealing to some ethically diverse cancer patients (see chapter 10 this volume).[53]

Certain individual in non-Hispanic populations (ie, African American, African, Chinese) may not fully believe that they will receive adequate medical treatment by mainstream medical professionals. Such beliefs may lead to a general distrust of the traditional medical system as a whole.[54] It is also possible that individuals from culturally diverse groups may be more likely to view a diagnosis of cancer as uncontrollable or terminal than non-Hispanic Whites, particularly those who are upper middle class.[67] Therefore, it would be logical that they would be more likely to engage in avoidant, passive strategies because they may view active, approach-strategies as a waste of time and effort. In other words, it may be that they do not feel that their efforts will pay off from engaging in mainstream interventions. They may believe that there is no investment from clinicians in their health, not only because they believe their illnesses are uncontrollable, but because they simply believe their voices will go unheard in such systems. This difference in evaluation may be related to the higher mortality rates of minorities for some diseases.[54] In this vein, such patients may not be "giving up" on mainstream medical care and interventions, but instead may be turning to something that they can count on, that is, God and/or their own, innate sense of spirituality. For these reasons, clinicians should always be aware of such mediating factors when dealing with ethnically diverse populations. Such awareness, in and of itself, often allows the clinician to intervene more effectively and circumvent many potential miscommunications. Future research should also endeavor to explore cross-cultural differences in the utilization and effectiveness of such interventions with culturally diverse patients.

SPIRITUAL/RELIGIOUS FOCUSED INTERVENTIONS

Cole and Pargament[55] have developed a group intervention with a focus on spiritual/religious issues for people with cancer. This group is based on the assumption that struggles over the issues of control, identity, relationships with others, and meaning often arise among cancer patients, and that spirituality can often provide answers to these conflicts. Therefore, the intervention is designed to address control, identity, relationships, and meaning. It should be noted that this intervention is of the type that directly addresses spirituality, religiosity, and God. Therefore, this intervention may be more appropriate for people who hold spiritual and/or religious beliefs before beginning the therapy and/or come from cultural backgrounds that are more open to such issues.

Similarly, Rousseau[56] has also outlined an approach for the treatment of spiritual suffering that is composed of the following steps: (1) controlling physical symptoms; (2) providing a supportive presence; (3) Encouraging life review to assist in recognizing purpose value and meaning; (4) exploring guilt, remorse, forgiveness, reconciliation; (5) facilitating religious expression; (6) reframing goals; (7) encourage meditative practices, focus on healing rather than cure. Rousseau has presented an interesting approach to spiritual suffering, but, considering the aforementioned cultural factors, it may not be applicable to all patients nor is it an intervention that many clinicians may feel comfortable providing considering its heavy emphasis on religion.

MEANING-BASED INTERVENTIONS

In contrast to interventions with a distinct spiritual/religious focus, Greenstein and Breitbart[57] have designed an intervention to directly address issues of meaning in advanced stage cancer patients. This intervention, based upon the writings of Victor Frankl, and Irvin Yalom, is called "Meaning Centered Group Psychotherapy (MCGP)," and is the first use of these principals specifically targeting the needs of severely medically ill. This therapy is designed to alleviate depression and anxiety by assisting group members to find meaning in their lives in spite of their illnesses. An advantage of this therapy is that it does not focus directly on spirituality and God, but rather approaches the crises that cancer patients face by addressing the "crises" of meaning that such an illness engenders in patients. We have conducted a preliminary analysis of the efficacy of these groups. Our analyses revealed substantially significant effects for spiritual well-being and end-of-life despair (hopelessness and desire for hastened death). We also analyzed responses to a specific item from the Schedule of Attitudes Toward Hastened Death,[58] focusing on a sense of meaning. Responses to the item "Despite my illness, my life has meaning and purpose" increased substantially (and significantly) following this intervention. At the beginning of treatment, roughly 40% of study participants indicated that they did not perceive a sense of meaning and purpose in their lives. *After* the intervention, none of the study participants perceived their life as meaningless. Importantly, an analysis of the data from the 2-month follow-up assessment demonstrated that the benefits of this intervention continued to grow after treatment had concluded. In addition, since group interventions are not always feasible due to logistic restraints and/or patient preference, we are developing an individual version of this intervention as well[59] for patients who cannot or do not prefer to be in a group.

For Frankl,[60] life has meaning and never ceases to have meaning. It is our intention that achieving such a sense of purpose and meaning can help to reduce the distress experienced by many cancer patients. However, it must be considered that what one may hold as meaningful may change over time. Frankl suggests that each individual has the freedom to choose their attitude toward suffering by finding a sense of meaning and purpose in the face of their anguish. For Frankl, this quest to find meaning within the contents of our lives and within our existence is a primary motivating force in humans, and thus cuts across cultural boundaries.

This essential mutability of meaning has been very apparent in our groups. For example, some common themes noted in the early sessions include feelings of helplessness, anger, betrayal, injustice, physical concerns, as well as interpersonal concerns such as isolation, dependency, envy, fear of death. As the groups progress, we have noted in later sessions that themes such as the afterlife, uncertainty about the future, loss of identity, meaninglessness, and previous experiences with illnesses, or the sudden death of other family members and or close friends come to the forefront.

This progression in focus on broader, more existential themes is in keeping with Frankl's conception of culturally independent human meaning-making. We feel that it is this metamorphosis of meaning that results in the positive outcomes we have noted in the groups so far and that, we hope, cuts across many of the cultural boundaries we have discussed in this chapter.

REFERENCES

1. Miller MA. Culture, spirituality, and women's health. *J Obstet Gynelcol Neonatal Nurs.* 1995;257-263.
2. Kinzie D. Cultural aspects of psychiatric treatment with Indochinese patients. *Am J Social Psychiatry.* 1985;1:47-53.
3. Klessig J. Cross-cultural medicine a decade later. *West J Med.* 1992;157:316-322.
4. Puchalski CM, Romer AL. Taking a spiritual history allows clinicians to understand patients more fully. *J Pall Med.* 2000;3:129-137.
5. Karasu BT. Spiritual psychotherapy. *Am J Psychotherapy.* 1999;53:143-162.
6. Brady M, Peterman A, Fitchett G, Mo M, Cella, D. A case for including spirituality in quality of life measurement in oncology. *Psycho-Oncology.* 1999;8:417-428.
7. Richards PS, Bergin AE. A spiritual strategy for counseling and psychotherapy. Washington, DC: American Psychological Association; 1997.
8. Zinnbauer BJ, Pargament KI, Cowell BJ, Rye M, Scott AB. Religion and spirituality: unfuzzing the fuzzy. *J Scientific Study Religion.* 1997;36(4):549-564.
9. Koenig HG, George LK, Peterson, BL. Religiosity and remission of depression in medically ill older patients. *Am J Psychiatry.* 1998;155(4):536-542.
10. Baider L, Russak SM, Perry S, et al. The role of religious and spiritual beliefs in coping with malignant melanoma: an Israeli sample. *Psycho-Oncology.* 1999;8:27-35.
11. Nelson C, Rosenfeld B, Breitbart W, Galietta M. Spirituality, depression and religion in the terminally ill. *Psychosomatics.* 2002;43:213-220.
12. Park C, Folkman S. Meaning in the context of Stress and Coping. *Rev Gen Psychol.* 1997;1:115-144.
13. Andrykowski MA, Brady MJ, Hunt JW. Positive psychosocial adjustment in potential bone marrow transplant recipients: cancer as a psychosocial transition, *Psycho-Oncology.* 1993;2:261-276.
14. Taylor SE. Adjustment to threatening events: a theory of cognitive adaptation. *Am Psychologist.* 1983;38:1161-1173.
15. Davis CG, Nolen-Hoeksma S, Larson J. Making sense of loss and benefiting from the experience: Two construals of meaning. *J Pers Soc Psychol.* 1998;75:561-574.
16. Lazarus RS, Folkman S. *Stress, Appraisal and Coping.* New York, NY: Springer; 1984.
17. Mazanec P, Tyler MK. Cultural considerations in wend-of-life care. *Am J Nurs.* 2003;103(3):50-58.
18. Barg FK, Gullatte MM. Cancer support groups: Meeting the needs of African Americans with cancer. *Semin Oncol Nurs.* 2001;17(3):171-178.
19. Holahan CJ, Moos RH. Risk, resistance, and psychological distress: A longitudinal analysis with adults and children. *J Abnorm Psychol.* 1987;96:3-13.
20. Hilton BA. The relationship of uncertainty, control, commitment, and threat of recurrence to coping strategies used by women diagnosed with breast cancer. *J Behav Med.* 1989;12:39-54.
21. Hunt ME. Exploring the repressive coping styles of Non-hispanic white and African-American women with newly diagnosed stage II and recurrent breast cancer: The impact

of religiosity and under-reporting of stressful life events. *Dissertation Abstracts International: Section B: The Sciences & Engineering.* 2001;62(3-B):1580.

22. Musick MA, Koenig HG, Hays JC, Cohen HJ. Religious activity and depression among community-dwelling elderly persons with cancer: The moderating effect of race. *J Gerontol Soc Sci.* 1998;53B:S218-S227.

23. Jordan MS, Lumley MA, Leisen JC. The relationships of cognitive coping and pain control beliefs to pain and adjustment among African-American and Caucasian women with rheumatoid arthritis. *Arthritis Care Res.* 1998;11(2):80-88.

24. Taylor RJ, Chatters LM, Jayakody R, Levin JS. Black and White differences in religious participation: a multisample comparison. *Scientific Study Religion.* 1996;35:403-410.

25. Erwin DO. Cancer education takes on a spiritual focus for the African-American faith community. *J Cancer Educ.* 2002;17:46-49.

26. Canive JM, Castillo D. Hispanic veterans diagnosed with PTSD: assessment and treatment issues. *NCPP Clin Quart.* 1997;7(1).

27. Chan C, Ho P, Chow E. A body-mind-spirit model in health: an Eastern approach. *Soc Work Health Mental Care.* 2001;34(3-4):261-282.

28. Gordon JS. Asian Spiritual Traditions and their usefulness to practitioners and patients facing life and death. *J Alternative Complimentary Medicine.* 2002;5:603-608.

29. Nishimoto P, Foley J. Cultural beliefs of Asian Americans associated with terminal illness and death. *Semin Oncol Nurs.* 2001;17(3):179-189.

30. Ashing T, Padilla G, Tejero J, Kagawa-Singer M. Understanding the breast cancer experience of Asian American women. *Psycho-Oncology.* 2003;12:38-58.

31. Ngu VA. Dying with dignity: Spiritual considerations are all important. *World Health Forum.* 1991;12:394-395.

32. Olweny CLM. Cultural issues in sub-saharan Africa. In: Doyle D, Hanks GW, MacDonald N, eds. *Oxford Textbook of Palliative Medicine.* New York, NY: Oxford Medical Publications; 1998:787-791.

33. Storey P, Knight, C. *UNIPAC Two: Alleviating Psychological and Spiritual Pain in the Terminally Ill, American Academy of Hospice and Palliative Medicine.* C, Larchmont, NY: Mary Ann Liebert, Inc; 2001.

34. Thiel MM, Robinson MR. Physicians' collaboration with chaplains: difficulties and benefits. *J Clin Ethics.* 1997;8:94-103.

35. Doyle D. Have we looked beyond the physical and psychosocial? *J Pain Symptom Manage.* 1992;7(5):302-311.

36. Hay MW. Developing guidelines for spiritual caregivers in hospice: Principles for spiritual assessment. Presented at: The National Hospice Organization Annual Symposium and Exposition; Nov 6-9, 1996; Chicago, IL.

37. Chan KS, Lam Z, Chun R, Dai D, Lung A. Chinese patients with terminal cancer. In: Doyle D, Hanks GW, MacDonald N, eds. *Oxford Textbook of Palliative Medicine.* New York, NY: Oxford Medical Publications; 1998;793-795.

38. Lo B, Ruston D, Kates LW, et al. Discussing religious and spiritual issues at the end of life: A practical guide for physicians. *JAMA.* 2002 Feb 13;287(6):749-754.

39. Puchalski CM. Spirituality and health: the art of compassionate medicine. *Hospital Physician.* Mar 2001;30-36.

40. Koenig HG. An 83-year-old woman with chronic illness and strong religious beliefs. *JAMA.* 2002 Jul 24-31;288(4):487-493.

41. Maugens TA. The Spiritual history. *Arch Fam Med.* 1996;5:11-16.

42. McBride JL, Arthur G, Brooks R, Pilkington L. The relationship between a patient's spirituality and health experiences. *Fam Med.* 1998;30:122-126.

43. Post SG, Puchalski CM, Larson DB. Physicians and patient spirituality: professional boundaries, competency, and ethics. *Ann Intern Med.* 2000 Apr 4;132(7):578-583.

44. King DE, Bushwick B. Beliefs and attitudes of hospital inpatients about faith healing and prayer. *J Fam Pract*. 1994;39:349-352.
45. Clayton CL. Barriers, boundaries, & blessings: Ethical issues in physicians' spiritual involvement with patients. *Med Humanities*. 2000;21:368–376.
46. Cohen CB, Wheeler SE, Scott DA. Walking a fine line: Physician inquiries into patients' religious and spiritual beliefs. *Hastings Cent Rep*. 2001;31(5):29-39.
47. Ellis M, Vinson D, Ewigman B. Addressing spiritual concerns of patients: Family physicians' attitudes and practices. *J Fam Pract*. 1999;48:105-109.
48. Sloan RP, Bagiella E, Powell T. Religion, spirituality, and medicine. *Lancet*. 1999;353: 664-667.
49. Kearney M. Spiritual care of the dying. In Chochinov HM, Breitbart W, editors, *Handbook of psychiatry in palliative medicine*. Oxford: Oxford University Press. 2000; 357–373.
50. Anderson JM, Anderson LJ, Felsenthal G. Pastoral needs for support within an inpatient rehabilitation unit. *Arch Phys Med Rehab*. 1993;74:574-578.
51. Maugans TA, Wadland WC. Religion and family medicine: A survey of physicians and patients. *J Fam Pract*. 1991;32:210-213.
52. Cassileth BR, Vicker AJ. Complementary and alternative therapies. *Urol Clin North Am*. 2003;30:369-376.
53. Chiu L. Spiritual resources of chinese immigrants with breast cancer in the USA. *Int J Nursing Stud*, 2001;38:175-184.
54. Die-Trill M. The Patient from a Different Culture. In: Holland JC, Ed. *Psycho-Oncology*. New York, NY: Oxford University Press; 1998:857-866.
55. Cole B, Pargament K. Recreating your life: A spiritual/psychotherapeutic intervention for people diagnosed with cancer. *Psycho-Oncology*. 1999;8:395-407.
56. Rousseau P. Spirituality and the dying patient. *J Clin Oncol*. 2000;18:2000–2002.
57. Greenstein M, Breitbart W. Cancer and the experience of meaning: A group psychotherapy program for people with cancer. *Am J Psychother*. 2000;54(4):486-501.
58. Rosenfeld B, Breitbart W, Galietta M, et al. Schedule of Attitudes toward Hastened Death: Measuring desire for death among terminally ill cancer patients. *Cancer*. 2000;88:868-875.
59. Gibson C, Breitbart W. The Search for Meaning: Meaning-Centered Psychotherapy for Advanced Cancer Patients Program Manual. Unpublished manuscript. 2003.
60. Frankl VF. *Man's Search for Meaning*. 4th edn Massachusetts: Beacon Press; 1959/1992.
61. Beck AT, Weissman A, Lester D, Trexler L. The measurement of pessimism: the Beck Hopelessness Scale. *J Consult Clin Psychol*. 1974;42:861-865.
62. Breitbart W, Rosenfeld B, Pessin H, et al. Depression, hopelessness, and desire for hastened death in terminally ill patients with cancer. *J Am Med Assoc*. 2000;284:2907-2911.
63. Ehman JW, Ott BB, Short TH, Ciampa RC, Hansen-Flaschen J. Do patients want physicians to inquire about their spiritual or religious beliefs if they become gravely ill? *Arch Intern Med*. 1999;159:1803-1806.
64. Musick MA, Koenig HG, Larson DB, Mathews D. Religion and spiritual beliefs. In: Holland JC, ed. *Psycho-Oncology* New York, NY: Oxford University Press; 1998:780-790.
65. Johnson, SC, Spilka, B. Coping with breast cancer: the roles of clergy and faith. *J. Relig and Health*. 1991; 30: 21–33.
66. Ell, K, Nishimoto. Coping resources in adaptation to cancer: an analysis of tyl socioeconomic and racial differences. *Soc Serv Rev*. 1989; 63: 443–446.
67. Gregg, J Curry, RH. Explanatory models for cancer among African-American women at two Atlanta neighborhood health centers: the implications for a cancer screening program. *Soc. Sci & Med*. 1994; 39: 519–526.

Index

Korean breast cancer patients, family
dynamics of, 288
Kübler-Ross, Elisabeth, 243

L

Lactose, 145
as heart disease risk factor, 148–149
Lactulose, as laxative, 208
Laetrile, 227
toxicity of, 231
La Lique Nationale Contre Le Cancer,
174
Language barriers
to health care access, 21
to physician-patient communication, 25,
26
to treatment adherence, 22
Latina women, 157, 158
Laxatives, 208
Lethargy, opioids-related, 208
Leukemia
acute, Down syndrome-related, 111
acute myeloid, in elderly patients,
94–95
lymphoblastic, pediatric, 110–111
pediatric, 109
stem cell transplantation treatment for,
113
Lewis, C. S., 242
Lidocaine, as neuropathic cancer pain
treatment, 211
Life expectancy
of elderly cancer patients, 92–93
ethnic factors in, 99
geographical factors in, 98–99
Life priorities, recording of, 161
Lifestyle
Lifestyle, as cancer risk factor, 137–138,
139–140, 146–148
Liver, *N*-hydroxylation in, 148
Liver cancer, aflatoxins-related, 140
Local anesthetics, as neuropathic cancer
pain treatment, 211
Loss
anticipated, 247
grief as response to, 244
stages of, 243
traumatic, 246
Low-density-lipoprotein cholesterol (LDL),
143–144
oxidation of, 145

Lung cancer
asbestos-related, 142
complementary and alternative treatment
for, 228
in elderly people, 97
as mortality cause, in women, 137
rates of, ethnic differences in, 145–146
smoking-related, 147
synergistic interaction with asbestos in,
142
tea-based prevention of, 150
Lymphoma
Burkitt's, 111
in elderly patients, 92–93
pediatric, 109
stem cell transplantation treatment for,
113

M

Macrobiotic diet, 225
Magnesium citrate, 208
Malnutrition, in elderly patients, 79, 82–83
radiation-induced esophagitis associated
with, 94
Mammography, 93
Managed care
effect on childhood cancer treatment, 115
effect on older patients' health care, 98
effect on physician-patient
communication, 115
institutional racism of, 195
Massachusetts General Hospital, 243
Massage therapy, 222, 230, 286
McGill Pain Questionnaire, 200
MDR-1, in elderly leukemia patients, 94–95
Meaning-based interventions, 295–296
Meat, fried
as genotoxic carcinogen source, 147
as saturated fat source, 148
Meclizine, as opioids-related nausea
treatment, 208–209
Medicaid coverage, for children, 114
Medical language
ambiguity of, 25
patients' misunderstanding of, 22
Medical power of attorney, 121
Medical practice, ethical principles of, 17
Medical profession, paternalism of, 257–258
Medicare coverage, regulations for, 189
Medicare Hospice Benefit, 117
Mediterranean diet, 144